Making Health Policy

Second edition

Understanding Public Health Series

Series editors: Ros Plowman and Nicki Thorogood, London School of Hygiene & Tropical Medicine.

Throughout the world, there is growing recognition of the importance of public health to sustainable, safe and healthy societies. The achievements of public health in nineteenth-century Europe were for much of the twentieth century overshadowed by advances in personal care, in particular in hospital care. Now, as we move into the new century, there is increasing understanding of the inevitable limits of individual health care and of the need to complement such services with effective public health strategies. Major improvements in people's health will come from controlling communicable diseases, eradicating environmental hazards, improving people's diets and enhancing the availability and quality of effective health care. To achieve this, every country needs a cadre of knowledgeable public health practitioners with social, political and organizational skills to lead and bring about changes at international, national and local levels.

This is one of a series of books that provides a foundation for those wishing to join in and contribute to the twenty-first-century regeneration of public health, helping to put the concerns and perspectives of public health at the heart of policy-making and service provision. While each book stands alone, together they provide a comprehensive account of the three main aims of public health: protecting the public from environmental hazards, improving the health of the public and ensuring high quality health services are available to all. Some of the books focus on methods, others on key topics. They have been written by staff at the London School of Hygiene & Tropical Medicine with considerable experience of teaching public health to students from low, middle and high income countries. Much of the material has been developed and tested with postgraduate students both in face-to-face teaching and through distance learning.

The books are designed for self-directed learning. Each chapter has explicit learning objectives, key terms are highlighted and the text contains many activities to enable the reader to test their own understanding of the ideas and material covered. Written in a clear and accessible style, the series is essential reading for students taking postgraduate courses in public health and will also be of interest to public health practitioners and policy-makers.

Titles in the series

Analytical models for decision making: Colin Sanderson and Reinhold Gruen
Controlling communicable disease: Norman Noah
Economic analysis for management and policy: Stephen Jan, Lilani Kumaranayake, Jenny Roberts, Kara Hanson and Kate Archibald
Economic evaluation: Julia Fox-Rushby and John Cairns (eds)
Environmental epidemiology: Paul Wilkinson (ed.)
Environmental health policy: Megan Landon and Tony Fletcher
Financial management in health services: Reinhold Gruen and Anne Howarth
Global change and health: Kelley Lee and Jeff Collin (eds)
Health care evaluation: Sarah Smith, Don Sinclair, Rosalind Raine and Barnaby Reeves
Health promotion practice: Maggie Davies, Wendy Macdowall and Chris Bonell (eds)
Health promotion theory: Maggie Davies and Wendy Macdowall (eds)
Introduction to epidemiology, Second Edition: Ilona Carneiro and Natasha Howard
Introduction to health economics, Second Edition: Lorna Guinness and Virginia Wiseman (eds)
Issues in public health, Second Edition: Fiona Sim and Martin McKee (eds)
Making health policy, Second Edition: Kent Buse, Nicholas Mays and Gill Walt
Managing health services: Nick Goodwin, Reinhold Gruen and Valerie Iles
Medical anthropology: Robert Pool and Wenzel Geissler
Principles of social research: Judith Green and John Browne (eds)
Public Health in History: Virginia Berridge, Martin Gorsky and Alex Mold
Understanding health services: Nick Black and Reinhold Gruen

Forthcoming titles

Sexual health: a public health perspective: Kaye Wellings, Kirstin Mitchell and Martine Collumbien
Conflict and health: Natasha Howard, Egbert Sondorp and Annemarie ter Veen (eds)
Environment, health and sustainable development, second edition: Sari Kovats and Emma Hutchinson (eds)

Making Health Policy

Second edition

Kent Buse, Nicholas Mays and
Gill Walt

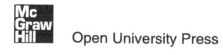
Open University Press

Open University Press
McGraw-Hill Education
McGraw-Hill House
Shoppenhangers Road
Maidenhead
Berkshire
England
SL6 2QL

email: enquiries@openup.co.uk
world wide web: www.openup.co.uk

and Two Penn Plaza, New York, NY 10121-2289, USA

First published 2005
Second edition published 2012

Copyright © London School of Hygiene & Tropical Medicine, 2012

A catalogue record of this book is available from the British Library

ISBN-13: 978-0-33-524634-2 (pb)
ISBN-10: 0-33-524634-6 (pb)
eISBN: 978-0-33-524635-9

Library of Congress Cataloging-in-Publication Data
CIP data applied for

Typesetting and e-book compilations by
RefineCatch Limited, Bungay, Suffolk
Printed in the UK by Bell & Bain Ltd, Glasgow

Fictitious names of companies, products, people, characters and/or data that may be used
herein (in case studies or in examples) are not intended to represent any real individual,
company, product or event.

The *McGraw·Hill* Companies

"Making Health Policy is a must-read for those studying and working in global health. It provides a unique introduction to core concepts in global health policy and brings politics to the core of public health. Why do some issues get more attention than others? Why is evidence-based policy making so difficult? How can we understand and study power in the health system? This book provides answers to these crucial questions."
Devi Sridhar, James Martin Lecturer in Global Health Politics, Oxford University, UK

"This is an excellent and accessible introduction to the politics of health policy making by three of the world's leading scholars on the subject. If anyone thinks that improving the health of a population is solely about getting the interventions and policy content right, this book will surely disavow them of that belief. Political dynamics matter, and the authors draw on the most up-to-date research to provide practitioners and students with clear, sensible, evidence-based guidance on how to manage these dynamics."
Jeremy Shiffman, Associate Professor of Public Administration and Policy, American University, USA

"Having used the earlier edition of this book, I would highly recommend it. The book provides an outstanding mix of policy theories, described in clear and accessible terms, with up-to-date and engaging examples from across the world that illustrate the application of those theories. Frequent activities throughout the book provide openings for greater student engagement in the subject matter. It's a great resource for teaching."
Sara Bennett, Associate Professor, Johns Hopkins School of Public Health, USA

"This book is excellent and unique in the way it addresses complexity within the field of global health and policies in a simplified and practical way. Each chapter is structured to include Activities and Feedback, which fosters reflection and adult learning. This approach makes the book ideal for teaching at all levels of university. I highly recommend it."
Göran Tomson, Professor of International Health Systems Research, Karolinska Institute, Sweden

"This book is an excellent teaching tool on policy making in the field of public health. It is very clearly structured and written, and provides a wealth of concrete examples to illustrate new concepts ... One of the key strengths is to highlight the political nature of health policy making, not presenting it as a technocratic process, but very much part of power dynamics at the local, national and global level."
Chantal Blouin, Associate Director, Centre for Trade Policy and Law, Carleton University/University of Ottawa, Canada

"A great introduction and reference for health policy students, offering clear and concise explication of key theories about policy making and applied to the health sector. This book unravels the complex world of health politics and decision-making, making it comprehensible for many who have difficulty understanding the system they work in, or aspire to enter the world of health policy to make a difference."
Professor Vivian Lin, School of Public Health, La Trobe University, Australia

Contents

Overview of the book   1

 1 The health policy framework   4
 2 Power and the policy process   20
 3 The state and the private sector in health policy   47
 4 Agenda setting   64
 5 Government and the policy process   84
 6 Interest groups and the policy process   105
 7 Policy implementation   128
 8 Globalizing the policy process   148
 9 Research, evaluation and policy   169
10 Doing policy analysis   191

Glossary   211
Acronyms   217
Index   219

Overview of the book

Introduction

This book provides a comprehensive introduction to the study of power and process in health policy. Much of what is currently available deals with the content of health policy – the 'what' of policy. This literature may use medicine, epidemiology, organizational theory or economics to provide evidence for, or evaluation of, health policy. Legions of doctors, epidemiologists, health economists and organizational theorists develop technically sound solutions to problems of public health importance. Yet, surprisingly little guidance is available to public health practitioners who wish to understand how issues make their way onto policy agendas (and how to frame these issues so that they are better received), how policy makers treat evidence (and how to form better relationships with decision makers), and why some policy initiatives are implemented while others languish. These political dimensions of the health policy process are rarely taught in schools of medicine or public health – but are profoundly important in determining public health outcomes.

Why study health policy?

The book integrates power and process into the study of health policy. It views these two themes as integral to understanding policy. Who makes and implements policy decisions (those with power) and how decisions are made (process) largely determine the content of health policy and, thereby, ultimately people's health. To illustrate this point, take the case of developing HIV policy in a low income country. Were health economists primarily involved in advising the health minister, it is likely that prevention would be emphasized (as preventive interventions tend to be more cost-effective than curative ones). If, however, the minister also consulted representatives of people living with HIV, as well as the pharmaceutical industry, it is likely that greater emphasis would be placed on treatment and care. In the unlikely event that powerful feminist organizations had the ear of the minister, they might lobby for interventions to empower women to protect themselves from unwanted and unprotected sex. The reconciliation of different views and the resulting policy depends on the power of various actors in the policy arena as well as the process of policy making (e.g. how widely groups are consulted and involved). Whether or not behavioural, curative or structural HIV interventions are given priority will impact on the trajectory of an HIV epidemic.

All activity is subject to politics. For example, research into public health problems requires funding. In many universities, bench scientists and social scientists compete with each other for funds to support their research. Politics will determine the allocation of public funds to different research areas and academic disciplines and private firms will invest in those researchers and endeavours that are most likely to lead to the highest rates of return. Politics does not end with funding, as politics is likely to govern access to study populations and even publication. Unfavourable findings can be blocked or distorted by project sponsors and they can be disputed or ignored by decision makers or others who find them inconvenient. Politics is omnipresent. For this reason, understanding the politics of the policy process is arguably as important as understanding how medicine improves health. Stated differently, while other academic disciplines may provide necessary evidence to improve health, in the absence of a robust understanding of the policy process, technical solutions will likely be insufficient to change practice in the real world.

This book is for those who wish to understand the policy process so that they are better equipped to influence it in their working lives. It is intended as a guide for students and professionals who wish to improve their skills in navigating and managing the health policy process – irrespective of the health issue or setting.

Structure of the book

Conceptually, the book is organized according to an analytical framework for health policy developed by Walt and Gilson (1994). The framework attempts to simplify what are in practice highly complex relationships by describing them in relation to a 'policy triangle'. The framework draws attention to the 'context' within which policy is formulated and executed, the 'actors' involved in policy making, and the 'processes' associated with developing and implementing policy – and the interactions between them. The framework is useful as it can be applied in any country, to any policy, and at any policy level. A diverse range of theories and disciplinary approaches, particularly from political science, international relations, economics, sociology, and organizational theory are drawn upon throughout the book to support this simple analytical framework and provide further explanations of policy process and power.

Ten chapters cover different stages of the policy process. Chapter 1 provides an introduction to the importance and meaning of policy, an explanation of the policy analysis framework, and demonstrates how it can be used to understand policy change. Chapter 2 describes a number of theories which help explain the relationship between power and policy making, including those which deal with how power is exercised by different groups, how political systems and governments transform power into policies, how power is distributed, and how power affects decision making processes.

Chapter 3 introduces the state and the private for-profit sector. It traces the changing roles of these two important sectors in health policy and, thereby, provides a contextual backdrop to understanding the content and processes of contemporary health policy making. Agenda setting is the focus of the fourth chapter. Chapter 5 returns to actors by focusing on the different institutions of government and the influence they wield. Chapter 6 looks at actors outside government. Different types of interest groups in the health sector are compared in terms of their resources, tactics and success in the policy process.

Chapter 7 returns to the policy process by exploring policy implementation. It contrasts and reconciles 'top-down' and 'bottom-up' approaches to explaining implementation (or more often lack thereof). Chapter 8 shifts the focus to the global level and examines the role of various global actors in health policy processes and the implications of increasing global interdependence on domestic policy making. Chapter 9 looks at policy evaluation and explores the linkages between research and policy. The final chapter is devoted to doing policy analysis. It introduces a political approach to policy analysis, provides tips on gathering information for analysis, and guidance for presenting analysis. The aim of the chapter is to help you to develop better political strategies to bring about health reform in your professional life.

Each chapter presents an overview, learning objectives, key terms, activities, feedback, and a brief summary and list of references. A number of the activities ask you to reflect on various aspects of a specific health policy which you select on the basis of having some familiarity with it. It would be helpful to begin to set aside documents related to your chosen policy for later use. These could be government documents, independent reports or articles from the popular press. You may also like to save Tweets and blogs related to the topic.

Acknowledgements

The first edition of this book built upon Gill Walt's *Health Policy: An Introduction to Process and Power* (1994). For this second edition we have updated the text, where possible, and revised parts of it in response to comments and suggestions from students and colleagues received since the first edition in 2005. We have made no significant structural changes. Rather, we have concentrated on incorporating additional theoretical perspectives and new and more recent examples and references.

We were very fortunate to have excellent research assistance from Stefanie Tan and Penny Robertson in updating statistics and in identifying and summarizing new material, especially relevant examples to illustrate general points. Stefanie also commented very helpfully on the draft chapters from the perspective of a recent student using this text.

References

Walt G (1994) *Health policy: an Introduction to Process and Power*. London: Zed Books.

Walt G and Gilson L (1994) Reforming the health sector in developing countries: the central role of policy analysis. *Health Policy and Planning* 9: 353–70.

The health policy framework

Overview

In this chapter you are introduced to why health policy is important and how to define policy. You will then go on to consider a simple analytical framework that incorporates the notions of context, process and actors, to demonstrate how they can help explain how and why policies do or do not change over time.

Learning objectives

After working through this chapter, you will be better able to:

- understand the framework for analysing health policy used in this book to define the following key concepts:
  - policy
  - context
  - actors
  - process
- describe how health policies are made through the inter-relationship of context, process and actors
- understand a related way of looking at policy making that sees it as occurring through the ongoing interaction among interests, ideas and institutions.

Key terms

Actor. Short-hand term used to denote any participant in the policy process that affects policy, including individuals, organizations, groups and even the government.

Content. Substance of a particular policy which details its constituent parts (e.g. its specific objectives).

Context. Systemic factors – political, economic, social or cultural, both national and international – which may have an effect on health policy.

Epistemic community. Policy community marked by shared political values, and a shared understanding of a problem and its causes.

Ideas. The values, evidence, anecdote and argument that shape policy, including the way a policy problem or solution is presented.

Interest. What an actor or group stands to gain or lose from a policy change.

Institutions. The 'rules of the game' determining how government and the wider state operate. Institutions can be formal structures and procedures, but also informal norms of behaviour that may not be written down.

Policy. Broad statement of goals, objectives and means that create the framework for activity. Often takes the form of explicit written documents, but may also be implicit or unwritten.

Policy elite. Specific group of policy makers who hold high positions in a policy system, and often have privileged access to other top members of the same, and other, organizations.

Policy makers. Those who make policies in organizations such as central or local government, multinational companies or local businesses, clinics, or hospitals.

Policy process. The way in which policies are initiated, formulated, developed, negotiated, communicated, implemented and evaluated.

Why is health policy important?

In many countries, the health sector is a major part of the economy. Some see it as a sponge – absorbing large amounts of national resources to pay for the many health workers employed. Others see it as a driver of the economy, through innovation and investment in bio-medical technologies or production and sales of pharmaceuticals, or through ensuring an economically productive population. Most citizens come into contact with the health sector as patients or clients, through using hospitals, clinics or pharmacies; or as health professionals, such as nurses, doctors, medical auxiliaries, pharmacists or managers. Because the nature of decision making in relation to health often involves matters of life and death, health is often accorded a special position in comparison to other social issues.

Health is affected by many decisions that go beyond the treatment provided by the health care system, for example, poverty, the physical environment and education all can have an impact on health status. Policies in these areas are therefore likely to affect people's health, for example, economic policies, such as taxes on cigarettes or alcohol may influence people's behaviour.

Understanding the relationship between health policy and health, and the impact that other policies have on health, is important because it may help to tackle some of the major health problems of our time – such as rising obesity. Health policy guides choices about which health technologies to develop and use, how to organize and finance health services, or which drugs will be freely available. To understand these relationships, it is necessary to better define what is meant by health policy.

What is health policy?

In this book you will often come across the terms policy, public policy and health policy. *Policy* is often thought of as decisions taken by those with responsibility for a given policy area – it may be in health or the environment, in education or in trade. The people who make policies are referred to as *policy makers*. Policy may be made at many levels – in central or local government, in a multinational company or local business, in a school or hospital. Policy makers are sometimes referred to as *policy elites* – a specific group of decision makers who have high positions in an organization, and often privileged access to other top members of the same, and other, organizations. For example, policy elites in government include the members of the prime minister's cabinet, all of whom would be able to contact and meet the top executives of a multinational company or of an international agency, such as the World Health Organization (WHO).

Policies are made in the private and the public sectors. In the private sector, multinational conglomerates may establish policies for all their companies around the world, but allow local companies to decide their own policies on conditions of service. For example, corporations such as Anglo-American and Heineken introduced antiretroviral therapy for their employees living with HIV in Africa in the early 2000s before many governments did so. However, private sector corporations have to ensure that their policies are made within the confines of public law, made by governments.

Public policy refers to government policy or the policies of government agencies. For example, Thomas Dye (2001) says that public policy is whatever governments choose to do or not to do. He argues that failure to decide or act on a particular issue also constitutes policy. For example, many countries have taken no legislative action requiring the use of child seats for young children in vehicles while others have regarded it as a priority for action.

When looking for examples of public policy, you should look first for statements or formal positions issued by a government, or a government department. These may be couched in terms that suggest the accomplishment of a particular purpose or goal (e.g. the introduction of needle exchange programmes to reduce harm among people who inject drugs) or to resolve a problem (e.g. charges on cars to reduce traffic congestion in urban areas).

Policies may refer to a government's health or economic policy, where policy is used as a field of activity, or to a specific proposal – 'From next year, it will be university policy to ensure students are represented on all governing bodies'. Sometimes policy is called a programme. The government's school health programme may include a number of different policies: precluding children from starting school before they are fully immunized, providing medical inspections, subsidized school meals and ensuring sex education in the school curriculum. The programme is thus the embodiment of policy for school children. In this example, it is clear that policies may not arise from a single decision but could consist of bundles of decisions that lead to a broad course of action over time. These decisions or actions may or may not be intended, defined or even recognized as policy in a formal document or statement.

As you can see, there are many ways of defining policy. Thomas Dye's simple definition of public policy being what governments do, or do not do, contrasts with the more formal assumption that all policy is made to achieve a particular goal or purpose.

Health policy may cover public and private policies about health. In this book, health policy is assumed to embrace courses of action (and inaction) that affect the set of institutions, organizations, services and funding arrangements of the health and health care system. It includes policy made in the public sector (by government) as well as policies in the private sector. But because health is influenced by many determinants outside the health system, health policy analysts are also interested in the actions and intended actions of organizations external to the health system which have an impact on health (for example, the Ministry of Transport or the food, tobacco or pharmaceutical industries).

Analysing health policy

Just as there are various definitions of what policy is, so there are many ideas about the analysis of health policy, and its focus: an economist may say health policy is primarily about the allocation of scarce resources for health; a planner may see it as a way to influence the determinants of health in order to improve public health; and for a doctor it may be all about health services to individuals (Walt 1994). Health policy is inextricably linked to politics and deals explicitly with who influences policy making, and how they exercise that influence under different conditions.

As you will see, this book places health policy within a framework that incorporates politics. Politics cannot be divorced from health policy. If you are applying epidemiology, economics, biology or any other professional or technical knowledge to everyday life, politics will affect you. No one is unaffected by the influence of politics. For example, scientists may have to focus their research on the issues funders are interested in, rather than the questions they want to explore; in prescribing drugs, health professionals may have to take into consideration potentially conflicting demands of hospital managers, government regulations and people's ability to pay. They may also be visited by drug company representatives who want to persuade them to prescribe particular drugs, and who may use incentives to encourage them to do so. Most activities that impact on health are subject to the ebb and flow of politics.

Devising a framework for incorporating politics into health policy needs to go beyond the point at which many health policy analysts stop: the *content* of policy. Much health policy focuses on a particular policy, describing what it purports to do, the strategy to achieve set goals, and whether or not it achieved them. For example, during the 1990s attention was on the financing of health services, with analysts asking questions such as:

- Which would be a better policy to raise funds for services – the introduction of user fees or a social insurance system?
- Which public health services should be contracted out to the private sector – cleaning services in hospitals or blood banks or others?
- Which policy instruments are needed to undertake major changes such as these – legislation, or regulation or incentives?

These are the 'what' or content questions of health policy. But they cannot be divorced from the 'who' and 'how' questions. Who makes the decisions? Who implements them? Under what conditions will they be introduced and executed, or ignored? In other words, the content is not separate from the politics of policy making. For example, in Uganda, when the president saw evidence that utilization of health services had fallen dramatically after the introduction of charges for health services, he overturned the earlier policy of his Ministry of Health. To understand how he made that decision, you need to know something about the political *context* (an election coming up and the desire to win votes); the power of the president to introduce change; and the role of evidence in influencing the decision, among other things.

You may have found it tricky to define these terms. This is because 'policy' is not a precise or self-evident term. For example, Anderson (1975) says policy is 'a purposive course of action followed by an *actor* or set of actors in dealing with a problem or matter of concern'. But this appears to make policy an 'intended' course of action, whereas many would argue that policies are sometimes the unintended result of many different decisions made over time, including decisions not to do anything. Policies may be expressed in a whole series of instruments: practices, statements, regulations and laws. They may be implicit or explicit, discretionary or statutory. Also, the word 'policy' does not always translate well: in English a distinction is often made between policy and politics, but in many European languages the word for policy is the same as the word for politics.

The 'health policy triangle'

The framework used in this book acknowledges the importance of looking at the *content* of policy, the *processes* of policy making and how power is used in a particular health policy context. This means exploring the role of the nation state, international organizations, the groups making up national and global civil society, as well as the private sector, to understand how they interact and influence health policy. It also means understanding the processes through which such influence is played out (e.g. in formulating policy) and the *context* in which these different actors and processes interact. The framework (Figure 1.1) focuses on content, context, process and actors. It is used in this book because it helps to explore systematically the somewhat neglected place of politics in health policy and it can be applied to high, middle and low income countries.

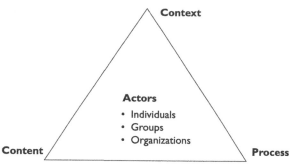

Figure 1.1 Policy analysis triangle

Source: Walt and Gilson (1994)

The health policy triangle is a highly simplified representation of a complex set of inter-relationships, and may give the impression that the four factors can be considered separately. This is not so! In reality, actors are influenced (as individuals or members of groups or organizations) by the context within which they live and work; context is affected by many factors such as political instability or ideology, by history and culture; and the process of policy making – how issues get on to policy agendas, and how they fare once there – is affected by actors, their position in power structures, their own values and expectations. And the content of policy reflects some or all of these factors. So, while the policy triangle is useful for helping to think systematically about all the different factors that might affect policy, it is like a map that shows the main roads but that has yet to have contours, rivers, forests, paths and dwellings added to it.

The actors who make or influence policy

As you can see from Figure 1.1, actors are at the centre of the health policy framework. Actor may be used to denote individuals (a particular statesman – Nelson Mandela, the ex-President of South Africa, for example), organizations such as the World Bank or multinational companies such as Shell, or the state or government. However, it is important to recognize that this is a simplification. Individuals cannot be separated from the organizations within which they work and any organization or group is made up of many different people, not all of whom speak with one voice and whose values and beliefs may differ.

In the chapters that follow, you will look at many different actors and ways of differentiating between them in order to analyse who has influence in the policy process. For example, there are many ways of describing groups that are outside the realm of the state. In international relations it has been customary to talk about non-state actors (actors outside government). Political scientists talk about interest or pressure groups. In the development literature, these groups are usually referred to as civil society organizations (organizations which fall between the state and the individual or household). What differentiates all these actors from government or state actors and political parties is that they do not seek formal political power for themselves, although they do want to influence those with formal political power.

Sometimes many different groups get together to demonstrate strong feelings about particular issues – these are called social movements or people's movements. For example, the 2000s were marked by a global social movement loosely united under the anti-globalization banner. It organized major protests at the annual meetings of the World Trade Organization, the International Monetary Fund and the Group of Eight (G8) among others, against what was perceived as the unfair, unregulated and greedy power of multinational corporations and banks.

Actors may try to influence the policy process at the local, national, regional or international level. Often they become parts of networks to consult and decide on policy at all of these levels. At the local level, for example, community health workers may interact with environmental health officers, teachers in local schools, or local businesses in the implementation of health policy. At the other end of the spectrum, actors may be linked with others across state borders. For example, they may be members of intergovernmental networks (i.e. government officials in one department of government in one country, learning lessons about policy alternatives with government officials from another country); or they may be part of policy or *epistemic communities* – networks of professionals who get together at scientific meetings or collaborate on research projects. Others may form issue networks – coming together to act on a particular issue. In Chapter 6 you will learn more about the differences between these groups and their roles in the policy process.

To understand how much actors influence the policy process means understanding the concept of power, and how it is exercised. Actors may seek to influence policy, but the extent to which they will be able to do so will depend, among other things, on their perceived or actual power. Power may be characterized by a mixture of individual wealth, personality, level of or access to knowledge, or authority, but it is strongly tied up with the organizations and structures (including networks) within which the individual actor works and lives as well as the position or office that the individual holds. Sociologists and political scientists talk about the interplay between 'agency' and 'structure'. 'Agency' refers to the power or capacity of actors to act independently and to make their own free choices. 'Structure', by contrast, denotes the arrangements which limit the choices and opportunities available to specific actors. In practice, the power of actors (agents) is intertwined with the structures (organizations) to which they belong. You will look more closely at the notion of power in Chapter 2 but in this book it is assumed that power is the result of the interaction between agency and structure.

Activity 1.2

Make a list of the different actors who might be involved in making policy on AIDS in your country. Place the actors into different groups.

Feedback

You might have grouped actors in different ways and in each country the list will differ and will change over time. The examples below may or may not apply to your country but they give an idea of the sorts of categories and actors you might have thought of. Where you do not know them, do not worry. There will be explanations in later chapters:

- government (e.g. ministries of health, education, the interior)
- international non-governmental organizations (e.g. Médecins Sans Frontières)

- national non-governmental organizations (e.g. of people living with HIV, faith-based organizations)
- pressure/interest groups (e.g. the Treatment Action Campaign)
- international organizations (e.g. WHO, UNAIDS, the World Bank)
- bilateral agencies (e.g. DFID, SIDA)
- funding organizations (e.g. the Global Fund, PEPFAR)
- private sector companies (e.g. Anglo-American, Heineken, Merck & Co)
- researchers (e.g. from universities, think tanks)

Contextual factors that affect policy

Context refers to systemic factors – political, economic and social, local, regional, national and international – which may have an effect on health policy. There are many ways of categorizing such factors, but one useful way is provided by Leichter (1979):

- *Situational factors* are more or less transient or idiosyncratic conditions which may influence policy (e.g. wars, droughts). These are sometimes called 'focusing events' (see Chapter 4). These may be a one-off occurrence, such as an earthquake which leads to changes in hospital building regulations, or much longer diffused public recognition of a problem. For example, the advent of the HIV epidemic (which took time to be acknowledged as an epidemic on a world scale) gradually produced new treatment and control policies on tuberculosis (TB) because of the inter-relationship of the two diseases – people living with HIV are more susceptible to diseases, and latent tuberculosis may be triggered by HIV.
- *Structural factors* are the relatively unchanging elements of the society. They may include the political system, and extent to which it is open or closed and the opportunities for civil society to participate in policy discussions and decisions; structural factors may also include the type of economy and the employment base. For example, where wages for nurses are low, or where workloads are unrealistically high, countries may suffer migration of these professionals to other societies where there is a shortage or better working conditions. Other structural factors that will affect a country's health policy will include demographic features or technological advance. For example, long-term care costs rise for countries with ageing populations, as their health care needs increase with age. Technological change has increased the number of women giving birth by caesarean section in many countries. Among the reasons given are increasing professional reliance on high technology that has led to reluctance among some doctors and midwives to take any risks, and a fear of litigation. And, of course, a country's national wealth will have a strong effect on which health services can be afforded.
- *Cultural factors* may also affect health policy. In societies where formal hierarchies are important, it may be difficult to question high officials or elder statesmen. The position of ethnic minorities or linguistic differences may lead to certain groups being poorly informed about their rights, or receiving services that do not meet their particular needs. In some countries where women cannot easily access health services (because they have to be accompanied by their husbands) or where there is considerable stigma about the disease (for example, tuberculosis or HIV), some authorities have developed systems of home visits or 'door-step' delivery. Religious factors can also strongly affect policy, as was seen by the insistence of

President George W. Bush in the early 2000s that sexual abstinence be promoted over the delivery of condoms in controlling sexually transmitted infections such as HIV. This affected policy in the US as well as many other countries, where NGO reproductive health services were heavily curtailed or their funds from the US were cut if they failed to comply with President Bush's cultural mores on sexual health.

- *International or exogenous factors* leading to greater inter-dependence between states, and influencing sovereignty and international cooperation in health may also affect health policy (see Chapter 8). Although many health problems are dealt with by national governments, some demand cooperation between national, regional or multilateral organizations. For example, the eradication of polio has taken place in many parts of the world through national and regional action, sometimes with the assistance from international organizations such as the WHO. However, even if one state manages to immunize all its children against polio and to sustain coverage, the polio virus can be imported by people who have not been immunized crossing the border from a neighbouring country.

All these contextual factors are complex, and unique in both time and setting. For example, in the nineteenth century, Britain sought to introduce public policies to control sexually transmitted disease in the countries of the British Empire. Dominant colonial assumptions, regarding how the categories of race and gender operated in societies under colonial rule, produced policies that reflected the prejudices and assumptions of the ruling imperial power, rather than policies sensitive to local culture. Levine (2003) describes how in India, female sex workers were required to register with the police as prostitutes, a policy prompted by the British belief that prostitution carried neither shame nor stigma in India. Colonial policies on prostitution frequently focused on brothels, requiring them to be registered with the local authorities. In Britain, however, brothels were illegal and policies concerning female sex workers focused exclusively on those who 'walked the streets'.

An illustrative example of how context affects policy is given by Shiffman and colleagues (2002). They compared reproductive rights in Serbia and Croatia, where governments advocated measures to encourage women to have more children. The authors argued that these pro-natalist policies were due to perceptions by elites in both countries that national survival was at stake. Elite perceptions were shaped by several factors: one was a shift from a socialist philosophy committed to female emancipation to a more nationalist ideology that held no such pretensions. Another was the comparison made by elites between low fertility rates among Serbs in Serbia and Croats in Croatia, and higher fertility rates in other ethnic groups in both countries.

To understand how health policies change, or do not, implies an ability to analyse the context in which they are made, and an attempt to assess how far any, or some, of these sorts of factors may influence policy outcomes.

Activity 1.3

Consider AIDS policy in your own country. Identify some contextual factors that might have influenced the way policy has (or has not) developed. Bear in mind the way context was divided into four different factors in the description above.

Feedback

Each setting is unique, but the sorts of contextual factors you may have identified are:

Situational

- a new prime minister/president coming to power and making AIDS policy a priority
- the death of a famous person acknowledged publicly to be due to AIDS
- new research findings on the prevalence of HIV in specific population groups

Structural

- the role of the media or NGOs in publicizing, or not, the AIDS epidemic – relating to the extent to which the political system is open or closed
- evidence of growing mortality from AIDS made public – perhaps among a particular group such as health workers

Cultural

- The actions of religious groups – both negative and positive – with regard to people living with HIV or towards sexual behaviour
- Prevailing norms concerning sex work, homosexuality, concurrent sexual partnerships, injecting drug use, and the position of women in society

International

- The role of international donors – the extra funds brought in by global initiatives such as the Global Fund to Fight AIDS, TB and Malaria
- Technical norms and standards promoted by international agencies, for example, WHO's guidelines for AIDS treatment initiation
- Drug donations or tiered pricing by pharmaceutical companies

The processes of policy making

Process refers to the way in which policies are initiated, developed or formulated, negotiated, communicated, implemented and evaluated. The most common approach to understanding policy processes is to use what is called the 'stages heuristic' (Sabatier and Jenkins-Smith 1993). This means breaking down the policy process into a series of steps, but acknowledging that this is a model, and does not necessarily represent exactly what happens in the real world. It is nevertheless helpful to think of policy making occurring in these different stages:

- *Problem identification and issue recognition*: explores how some issues get on to the policy agenda, while others do not even get discussed. In Chapter 4 you will go into this stage in more detail.

- *Policy formulation*: explores who is involved in formulating policy, how policies are arrived at, agreed upon, and how they are communicated. The role of policy making in government is covered in Chapter 5 and that of interest groups in Chapter 6.
- *Policy implementation*: this is often the most neglected phase of policy making and is sometimes seen as quite divorced from the first two stages. However, this is arguably the most important phase of policy making because if policies are not implemented, or are diverted or changed at implementation, then presumably something is going wrong from the point of view of the policy originator – and the policy outcomes may not be those which were sought. These issues are discussed in Chapter 7.
- *Policy evaluation*: identifies what happens once a policy is put into effect – how it is monitored, whether it achieves its objectives and whether it has unintended consequences. This may be the stage at which policies are changed or terminated and new policies introduced. Chapter 9 covers this stage.

There are caveats to using this useful but simple framework. First, it makes it look as if the policy process is linear – in other words, proceeding smoothly from one stage to another, from problem recognition to implementation and evaluation. However, it is seldom so clear or obvious a process. It may be at the stage of implementation that problem recognition occurs or policies may be formulated but never reach implementation. In other words, policy making is seldom a fully *rational* process – it is iterative and affected by interests – i.e. actors. Many people agree with Lindblom (1959) that the policy process is one which policy makers 'muddle through'. This is discussed in more detail in Chapter 2.

Nevertheless, the 'stages heuristic' has lasted for a long time and continues to be useful. It can be used for exploring national as well as international policies in order to try to understand how policies are transferred around the world.

While the policy triangle (see Figure 1.1) provides a useful framework for simplifying the extremely complex, dynamic, and inter-active nature of policy making, some feel it pays too little attention to other factors that explain why and how policies change. John (1998) and Howlett et al. (2009), for example, refer to the importance of the interaction of ideas, institutions and interests (or actors) in changing policy. The notion of *ideas* provides a useful lens for looking at how policies are framed and presented, because as ideas change, or issues are re-defined and re-packaged, so policy may be affected – making it more or less palatable to different interest groups. When you read the case study below on TB, you will learn how the framing and packaging of the policy response to TB through the 'DOTS' strategy radically changed prevailing ideas about TB control. Alcohol provides a different example, where the alcohol industry favours ideas that stress self-regulation and individual responsibility, and the public health community prefers ideas that promote taxation, and restrictions on sales and marketing. These ideas reflect competing values of individual versus collective responsibility – as well as underlying interests – profits made from selling alcohol versus a role to protect health.

Institutions can mean two things in the social sciences: an organization such as the World Health Organization, or the rules, authority and values of an organization, and the ways in which it makes decisions or acts (democratically or autocratically, centrally or devolved). This second meaning of institution is clearly important in analysing how policy processes are shaped and influenced. *Interests* refer to actors who may be individuals or groups, organized or informal and who want to see policy that furthers their goals or at least does not threaten their attainment.

Other analysts have stressed other concepts useful to understanding policy change. Shiffman and Smith (2007), for example, refer to 'issue characteristics' which may affect policy. By characteristics, they mean specific features of a particular issue (which could be a problem or a solution). For example, having credible indicators – clear measures that show the severity of the problem – may affect how far the issue is perceived as urgent or not. If evidence for a specific issue is contested, or uncertain, it may be more difficult to argue for change. Shiffman and Smith also stress the role of ideas (and how evidence is framed) as being important to understanding change in the policy process.

Shiffman and Smith's (2007) framework builds on the policy triangle's notions of actors and context (although they use the term environment for context), but gives greater space for consideration of ideas (the ways in which those involved with the issue understand and portray it) and issue characteristics. In their framework, institutions are perceived as part of actor power (and may neglect somewhat the sense of institutions as norms and rules).

In the case of John's or Howlett et al.'s 'ideas, institutions and interests' framework, and Shiffman and Smith's 'actor power, ideas, environment and issue characteristics' framework, there is significant overlap with the policy triangle of actors, context, process and content. The policy triangle reminds us more about processes – and how useful it is to understand the cycle of policy making from agenda setting to implementation and evaluation, but its broad approach can be enhanced by adding ideas and institutions (when thinking about actors and how they influence policy), in thinking about the rules and norms of organizations when considering policy processes, and in considering issue characteristics when considering the content of a particular problem and how actors are likely to respond to it.

Activity 1.4

The following case study on the rise and fall of policies on tuberculosis, largely extracted from Jessica Ogden and colleagues (2003), describes the different stages of the policy process, looking at context and actors as well as process.

As you read it, apply the health policy triangle:

1 Identify and write down who were the actors.
2 What processes can you identify?
3 What can you discern about the context?
4 What part did content play in determining policy?
5 Are there examples of interests, ideas, institutions or issue characteristics that enhance understanding of the policy process?

Case Study 1: getting TB on the policy agenda and formulating the DOTS policy

1970s: the era of neglect and complacency

Throughout the 1970s, TB control programmes were being implemented in many low and middle income countries, with only modest success. Only one international NGO, the International Union Against Tuberculosis and Lung Disease (the Union), explored ways of improving TB programmes, largely through the efforts of one of its public health physicians, Karel Styblo. Styblo and the Union developed a control strategy using a standardized short-course regimen (six months) that would be feasible and effective in developing countries. At the time, most TB programmes were using much longer drug regimens, and the public health community disagreed about best practice in TB treatment.

Yet, the international health policy context in the 1970s militated against support for the development of the Union's vertical approach to TB control. This was the period when the WHO, and in particular its then Director-General, Halfdan Mahler, espoused the goal of 'Health for All by the Year 2000'. This was to be achieved through concerted action to improve and integrate basic primary health care within the health care systems of poor countries, rather than promoting vertical (specialized) disease control programmes.

The late 1980s: resurgence and experimentation

Interest in and concern over TB re-emerged from the mid-1980s as increasing numbers of cases, and alarming rises in multi-drug-resistant disease, were seen in industrialized countries. It was increasingly evident that TB and HIV were linked, and many deaths from TB were linked to HIV.

Several international agencies initiated a process to get TB back on the international health policy agenda. The World Bank highlighted TB control as a highly cost-effective intervention. The *Ad Hoc* Commission on Health Research, made up of distinguished experts, also identified TB as a neglected disease. Members of the Commission met Styblo, and were impressed with his approach. The WHO expanded its TB Unit, and appointed Arata Kochi, an ex-UNICEF official, as its new head. One of his first appointments was an advocacy and communications expert.

The 1990s: advocacy opens up the window of opportunity

The WHO TB programme switched from a primarily technical focus to intensive advocacy in 1993. One of the first signs was a major media event in London in April 1993 declaring TB a 'Global Emergency'. The second was the branding of a new TB policy – DOTS – Directly Observed Therapy, Short-course. DOTS relied on five components: directly observed therapy (where health workers watched patients taking their drugs); sputum smear testing; dedicated patient recording systems; efficient drug supplies; and political commitment.

This branding process was initially hotly contested in the TB community. The political and operational experts wanted to push the new strategy (which downplayed the importance of new vaccine and drug developments for TB) while the technical and scientific experts (including many in the academic community) were concerned that the new WHO strategy not only oversimplified TB control measures, but indicated less funding to research and development.

From 2001: moving to consensus – the partnership years

By the 2000s, however, contestation had been transformed into consensus. By then, WHO had launched annual reports presenting credible global estimates of the scale of the TB epidemic, providing concrete data on which to base advocacy for greater investment in TB control. The TB community negotiated three ways forward; first, launching a Global Partnership to Stop TB in 2001. Second, it agreed a global strategy to stop TB, which included DOTS, but also research on diagnostics, drugs and vaccines. Third, it advocated the inclusion of TB among the diseases covered by the Global Fund, launched in 2002. This secured an exponential increase in funding for TB. The first global assessment of the DOTS/Stop TB Strategy (Glaziou et al. 2011) suggests that between 4.6 and 6.3 million lives were saved between 1995 and 2009.

Feedback

1 Actors
You may have named the following as actors:
1 Karel Styblo, Halfdan Mahler, Arata Kochi (and the organizations within which they worked, which provided the base for their influence: the Union, WHO, UNICEF)
2 an unnamed advocacy and communications expert
3 the World Bank; the *Ad Hoc* Commission on Health Research
4 networks: of public health advocates; TB specialists; technical and scientific experts interested in new drugs and vaccines research for TB
5 the Stop TB Partnership or the Global Fund to Fight AIDS, TB and Malaria.

2 Processes
The story is divided into decades that suggest a stage of neglect in the 1970s (with TB programmes being implemented in many countries but with no special attention to improving their impact); a stage when a problem was recognized in the 1980s as connections were made between the HIV epidemic and increasing TB cases through research and experience. Then came the agenda-setting 1990s when concerted action put TB back on the international policy agenda and the 2000s when the Stop TB strategy was implemented and an evaluation suggested it was effective in saving lives.

One of the important *ideas* that influenced the dissemination of the new TB strategy was the way it was promoted and marketed as DOTS. You might also mention that announcing TB as a Global Emergency was an idea that drew attention to the issue – supported by the launch of flagship epidemiological reports. And you could speculate that the Stop TB Partnership would have marked an *institutional* shift in the way TB policy was decided.

3 Context
Some of the points you might make under context would be: complacency in the industrialized world up to the end of the 1980s, because TB was thought to be conquered. This was not true in low income countries, partly because of the relationship between TB and poverty. You might mention that WHO was promoting its 'Health for All' policy, which subscribed to integrated health care, and rejected special, vertical programmes, which was how TB programmes had been designed. You could also say that resources for TB increased significantly from 2002.

4 Content
You may have noted references to the technical content of TB policy such as short-course drug regime, what DOTS stood for and different views on what TB policy should be. You might also have observed that the later Stop TB strategy was broader than DOTS. You might also have noted that it was only when there was sufficient evidence linking TB to HIV that the former really started getting global attention. These could all be described as issue characteristics.

Using the health policy triangle

You can use the health policy triangle to help analyse or understand a particular policy or you can apply it to plan a particular policy. The former can be referred to as analysis *of* policy, the latter as analysis *for* policy.

Analysis *of* policy is generally retrospective and explanatory – it looks back to explore the determination of policy (how policies got on to the agenda, were initiated and formulated) and what the policy consisted of (content). It also includes evaluating and monitoring the policy – did it achieve its goals? Was it seen as successful?

Analysis for policy is usually prospective – it looks forward and tries to anticipate what will happen if a particular policy is introduced. It feeds into strategic thinking about how to modify policy and may lead to policy advocacy or lobbying. For example, following a multi-disciplinary study to inform HIV prevention policy among high risk groups in Pakistan, the government commissioned a prospective analysis of the major policy recommendations made by the researchers. This involved a survey of relevant policy elites who were asked to express their level of agreement with 15 statements concerning each recommendation where each question related to a variable associated with presumed policy success. This survey was followed by semi-structured interviews with a range of stakeholders. The results of the analysis were used by the researchers and government officials to tailor the content of the recommendations to make them more politically palatable (Buse et al. 2009). In Chapter 10 you will learn some of the methods, such as stakeholder analysis, to help in prospective analysis for policy.

An example of how analysis *of* a policy can help to identify action *for* policy is seen in a study undertaken by McKee et al. (1996) in which they compared policies across a number of high income countries to prevent sudden infant deaths – sometimes called 'cot deaths'. Research had highlighted that many of these deaths were avoidable by putting infants to sleep lying on their backs. The study showed that evidence had been available from the early 1980s but it was some years before it was acted on. The study suggested that statistical evidence seemed to have been of little importance as governments in many countries failed to recognize the steady rise in sudden infant deaths, even though the evidence was available to them. Instead focusing events, such as television programmes which drew media attention, and the activities of NGOs were much more important. The lessons *for* policy depended to some extent on the political system: in federal forms of government, it seemed that authority was diffused, so strong central actions were difficult. This could be overcome by well-developed regional campaigning, and by encouraging NGOs and the media to take up the issue. In one country it seemed that a decentralized statistical service had led to delays in pooling mortality data, so recognition of the problem took longer. The authors concluded that many countries needed to review their arrangements to respond to evidence of challenges to public health.

Summary

In this chapter you have been introduced to definitions of policy and health policy and an analytical framework of context, process and actors (the 'policy triangle'), to help you make sense of the politics which affect the policy making process. You have learned that the policy triangle can be used both retrospectively – to analyse past policy, and prospectively – to help shape existing policy. Many of the concepts you have been introduced to will be expanded and illustrated in the chapters that follow.

References

Anderson J (1975) *Public Policy Making*. London: Nelson.

Buse K, Lalji N, Mohamad I, Mayhew SH, and Hawkes S. (2009) Political feasibility of scaling-up five evidence informed HIV policies: in search of deeper and wider policy commitment. *Sexually Transmitted Infections* 85(Suppl. 2): ii37–ii42. doi:10.1136/sti.2008.034058.

Dye T (2001) *Top Down Policymaking*. London: Chatham House Publishers.

Glaziou P, Floyd K, Korenromp EK et al. (2011) Lives saved by tuberculosis control and prospects for achieving the 2015 global target for reducing tuberculosis mortality. *Bulletin of the World Health Organization* 89573–582. doi: 10.2471/BLT.11.087510.

Howlett M, Ramesh M and Perl A (2009) *Studying Public Policy*. Oxford: Oxford University Press.

John P (1998) *Analysing Public Policy*. London: Continuum International Publishing Group.

Leichter H (1979) *A Comparative Approach to Policy Analysis: Health Care Policy in Four Nations*. Cambridge: Cambridge University Press.

Levine P (2003) *Prostitution, Race and Politics: Policing Venereal Disease in the British Empire*. New York: Routledge.

Lindblom CE (1959) The science of muddling through. *Public Administrative Review* 19: 79–88.

McKee M, Fulop N, Bouvier P, Hort A, Brand H, Rasmussen F, Kohler L, Varasovsky Z and Rosdahl N (1996) Preventing sudden infant deaths – the slow diffusion of an idea. *Health Policy* 37: 117–35.

Ogden J, Walt G and Lush L (2003) The politics of 'branding' in policy transfer: the case of DOTS for tuberculosis control. *Social Science and Medicine* 57(1): 163–72.

Sabatier P and Jenkins-Smith H (1993) *Policy Change and Learning*. Boulder, CO: Westview Press.

Shiffman J, Skarbalo M and Subotic J (2002) Reproductive rights and the state in Serbia and Croatia. *Social Science and Medicine* 54: 625–42.

Shiffman J and Smith S (2007) Generation of political priority for global health initiatives: a framework and case study of maternal mortality. *Lancet* 370: 1370–9.

Walt G (1994) *Health Policy: An Introduction to Process and Power*. London: Zed Books.

Walt G and Gilson L (1994) Reforming the health sector in developing countries: The central role of policy analysis. *Health Policy and Planning* 9: 353–70.

2 | Power and the policy process

Overview

In this chapter you will learn why understanding power is fundamental to making and analysing policy and be introduced to a number of theories which will help you understand the relationship between power and policy. These include explanations of power, its distribution in society and how governments exercise power in making decisions. These theoretical insights help to explain why decision making is not simply a rational process but also the result of struggles between competing groups of actors.

Learning objectives

By working through this chapter, you will be able to:

* differentiate between three dimensions of power and apply each to health policy making
* contrast theories which account for the distribution of power in society and understand their implications for who determines health policy
* define a political system, distinguish between regime types, and understand their implications for participation in policy making
* contrast theories of decision making based on an appreciation of the role of power in the policy process.

Key terms

Authority. Whereas power concerns the ability to influence others, authority concerns the right to do so.

Bounded rationality. Theory that policy makers intend to be rational but make decisions that are satisfactory as opposed to optimal.

Elitism. Theory that power is concentrated in a minority group in society.

Government. The institutions and procedures for making and enforcing rules and other collective decisions. Government is a narrower concept than the state since the state also includes the judiciary, military and other public bodies.

Incrementalism. Theory that decisions are not made through a rational process but by small adjustments to the status quo in the light of political realities.

Path dependency. The process by which decisions taken in one period shape and limit the range of policy choices available to decision makers later.

Pluralism. Theory that power is widely distributed in society.

Political system. The processes through which governments transform 'inputs' from citizens into 'outputs' in the form of policies.

Power. The ability to influence people, and in particular to control resources.

Punctuated equilibrium. Theory which explains why long periods of policy stability are upset by abrupt adjustment, policy reversals and reforms.

Rationalism. Theory that decisions are (and should be) made through a rational process by considering all the options and their consequences and then choosing the best.

Sectional group. Interest group whose main goal is to protect and enhance the interests of its members and/or the section of society it represents.

Sovereignty. Entails rule or control over a geographical area that is supreme, comprehensive, unqualified and exclusive.

State. A set of institutions that enjoy legal sovereignty over a fixed territorial area. The state comprises a wider set of institutions than the government and includes the parliament, judiciary, military as well as other bodies.

Introduction

You will be aware that *power* is exercised as a matter of course in many aspects of your everyday life. In the next chapter you will learn that reforms in many countries aimed at 'rolling back the state' were resisted by various actors. Resistance is not surprising if you think of policy making as a struggle between groups with competing interests, some in favour of change and others opposed to it, depending on their interests or ideas. For example, health economists often wish to limit the professional autonomy of the medical profession so as to control spending and improve efficiency. Yet such reforms are often opposed by doctors, some of whom are concerned that this will usurp their professional *authority* and others because it may affect their income. Policy making is, therefore, often characterized by conflicts that arise when change is pursued which threatens the status quo. The outcome of any conflict depends on the balance of power between the individuals and groups involved, and the processes or rules established to resolve those conflicts. Therefore, understanding policy making requires an understanding of the nature of power, how it is distributed and the manner through which it is exercised.

This chapter outlines several theories which describe the relationship between power and health policy making. It is up to you to decide which are more persuasive since all are somewhat dependent on different views of the world. First, the meaning of *power* is explained. Then, a number of theories concerning the distribution of power are presented – particularly contrasting pluralism and forms of elitism. We then turn to how policy making takes place in *political systems* to explain how the pluralists and elitist theorists may both be right, depending on the policy content and context. Finally we will consider the extent to which decision making is a rational process or one in which reason is sacrificed to power.

This chapter deepens your understanding of the *process* dimension of the policy triangle introduced in Chapter 1, and provides the basis for the more in-depth analysis of agenda setting and policy formulation, implementation and evaluation that follow. The chapter identifies specific *actors* in broad terms, particularly the state and organized interest groups who exercise power through the policy process.

What is power?

Power is generally understood to mean the ability to achieve a desired outcome. In policy making, the concept of power is typically thought of in a relational sense as having 'power over' others. Power is said to be exercised when A has B do something that B would not have otherwise done. A can achieve this end over B in a number of ways. In his theory on how governments control their citizens, Steven Lukes (1974) characterized three 'faces' or 'dimensions' of power: power as decision making; power as non-decision making; and power as thought control.

Power as decision making

'Power as decision making' focuses on acts of individuals and groups which influence policy decisions. Robert Dahl's classic study, *Who Governs?* looked at who made important decisions on contested issues in New Haven, Connecticut, US (Dahl 1961). He drew conclusions about who had power by examining known preferences of interest groups and comparing these with policy outcomes. He found that the resources which conferred power on citizens and interest groups varied, and that these resources were distributed unequally: while some individuals were rich in some political resources, they were likely to be poor in others. Different individuals and groups were therefore found to be able to exert influence on different policy issues. These findings led Dahl to conclude that different groups in society, including weak groups, could 'penetrate' the political system and exercise power over decision makers in accordance with their preferences. While only a few people had direct influence over key decisions, defined as successfully initiating or vetoing policy proposals, most had indirect influence through the power of the vote.

What is meant by political resources? From a long list of potential assets, Dahl singled out social standing, access to cash, credit and wealth, legal trappings associated with holding official office, managing staff and control over information as particularly important in this policy arena. The range of resources at the disposal of actors in health policy is equally diverse, and will be a function of the particular policy content and context.

Power as non-decision making

Dahl's critics argued that his analysis, which focused on observable and contested policy issues, was blind to some important dimensions of power because it overlooked the possibility that dominant groups exert influence by limiting the policy agenda to acceptable concerns. Bachrach and Baratz (1962) argued that 'power is also exercised when A devotes his energies to creating or reinforcing social and political values and institutional practices that limit the scope of the political process to public consideration of only those issues which are comparatively innocuous to A'. Consequently, 'power as agenda-setting' highlights the way in which powerful groups control the agenda to keep threatening issues out of sight. Expressed differently, power as 'non-decision making' involves 'the practice of limiting the scope of actual decision making to safe issues by manipulating the dominant community values, myths and political institutions and procedures' (Bachrach and Baratz 1963). In this dimension of power, some issues remain latent and fail to enter the policy arena.

An example of power as non-decision making can be identified in the health sector. In 1999, an independent committee of experts reviewed tobacco industry documents to assess the influence of the industry on the World Health Organization. Its report revealed that the industry used a variety of tactics, including staging events to divert attention from the public health issues raised by tobacco use and secretly paying 'independent' experts and journalists to keep the focus of the Organization on communicable, as opposed to non-communicable, diseases (Zeltner et al. 2000).

Activity 2.1

Drawing on your personal experience, consider how one person (A) may exercise power over another (B); that is, how one person gets another person to do what they would otherwise not have done.

Feedback

You may have identified three possible ways:

- intimidation and coercion (A uses the stick);
- productive exchanges involving mutual gain (A uses the carrot);
- the creation of obligations, loyalty and commitment (A uses the hug).

There are a range of approaches using power to secure compliance in decision making and non-decision making. We briefly differentiate between 'hard' and 'soft' power as well as the relationship between power and authority. Hard power corresponds to the carrot and the stick and soft to the hug. Soft power involves 'getting others to want what you want' (Nye 2002). Soft power relies on co-opting others by shaping their preferences and is associated with having an attractive and enviable culture, values, ideas, and institutions.

Considerable influence over others can also flow from authority; that is, having the legitimate right to get someone to do what you want. Max Weber (1948) identified three sources of authority. First, *traditional authority* exists where obedience is based on custom and the established way of doing things (for example, a king or sultan has traditional authority). People conform as part of everyday life as a consequence of socialization. For example, pregnant women in rural Guatemala do not question whether the practices and advice of their midwives are evidence-based, but surrender to their authority because of trust that society places in midwives based on their experience and the expectation that they know best (Lang and Elkin 1997).

Second, *charismatic authority* is based on intense commitment to a leader and their ideology or other personal characteristics. Those exercising authority on the basis of charisma, for example, some religious leaders, statesmen (e.g. Nelson Mandela) and health gurus do so on the basis of being perceived as having authority.

Weber's third category is *rational–legal authority*. It is based on rules and procedures. In this case, authority is vested in the office as opposed to the attributes of the particular office holder. As a result, the office holder, irrespective of his/her training or expertise, is *in* authority. Many countries with a history of British colonial rule designate the Secretary or permanent head as the most senior bureaucrat in the ministry of health. The Permanent Secretary is rarely a doctor but instead is a professional manager. While many doctors implement the dictates of the Secretary, they do so on the basis of his/her rational-legal authority rather than on the basis of traditional or charismatic authority. Indeed, given the role that knowledge and expertise play in the health policy process, it may be useful to add a category to Weber's classification (traditional, charismatic, rational-legal) entitled *technical authority*. Patients respect the advice of their doctors (for the most part) on the basis of the technical knowledge that doctors are thought to possess.

This raises the question of what induces people to surrender their personal judgement to authorities and that is where the concept of legitimacy is useful. Authority is considered legitimate if personal judgement is based on trust and acceptance. This is different from being coerced on the basis of threat (e.g. by the police). Legitimate authority occupies the space in the middle of the spectrum between coercion (stick) and persuasion (carrot). Approaches which are based on either too much coercion or persuasion may result in policies which enjoy little popular legitimacy, may not be readily accepted, and may be difficult to implement.

Power as thought control

Steven Lukes (1974) recognized power as decision making and non-decision making, but argued that it is also useful to understand 'power as thought control'. In other words, power can be a function of the ability to influence others by shaping their initial preferences. In this dimension, 'A exercises power over B when A affects B in a manner contrary to B's interests'. For example, poor working Americans voted for President George W. Bush in 2004 in spite of his domestic policies which were not in their interests. Once in office, he gave 2 trillion dollars in tax cuts to the wealthiest Americans and conducted two very expensive wars.

Lukes argues that A gains B's compliance through subtle means. This could include the ability to shape meanings and perceptions of reality which might be done through the control of information, the mass media or through the processes of socialization. Returning to the presidency of George W. Bush, he and his office began using the term 'tax relief' when describing tax cuts for the affluent. As George Lakoff (2004) points out, 'a relief' evokes the necessity of 'an affliction, an afflicted party, and a reliever who removes the affliction and is therefore a hero'. In this metaphor, taxation is the affliction, the President is the hero and anyone standing in the way is the bad guy. Essentially, through framing tax cuts as tax 'relief', the Republicans were subtly able to project their view of the problem (taxes as an unproductive burden) and its solution (tax cuts).

Turning from tax policy to health policy, McDonald's, the fast food company, is reported to spend over two billion dollars annually on advertising and marketing. Its symbolic Golden Arches are reported to be more widely recognized globally than the Christian cross (Schlosser 2001). In China, research suggests that children have been indoctrinated to accept that the company's mascot, Ronald McDonald, is 'kind, funny, gentle and understands children's hearts', thereby subtly conditioning this rapidly growing market of young consumers to think positively about McDonald's products. McDonald's targets decision makers as well as consumers. For example, before a parliamentary debate on obesity in the UK in 2004, the company sponsored 20 parliamentarians to attend the European Football Championships in Portugal.

Activity 2.2

Why might McDonald's invite parliamentarians to watch football at its expense?

Feedback

Without access to internal company documents, one can only speculate on the aims of such largesse. One plausible explanation is that McDonald's hoped to instil in these legislators an association between McDonald's and the company's actions to support increased physical activity as a route to reducing obesity; an association which might displace other associations that the policy makers might have between, for example, the company's products and the risk of obesity.

Lukes argues that the 'thought control' dimension of power is its 'most insidious' form as it dissuades people from having objections by 'shaping their perceptions, cognitions and preferences in such a way that they accept their role in the existing order of things, either because they can see or imagine no alternative to it, or because they see it as natural and unchangeable, or because they value it as divinely ordained and beneficial'.

Wielding such power is routine in policy making – and even encouraged. Joseph Nye (2004) talked of 'soft power as the means to success in world politics' – in which an actor's values, cultures and institutions are the political currencies promoted to get what s/he wants. Nye (2011) argues that in the twenty-first century a form of 'smart power', a variant of soft power, is crucial in wielding influence on the global stage and is likely to come from control over 'cyberspace, the media and narratives' to shape others' values and beliefs.

The largely unregulated market for complementary treatments and tonics may be growing as a result of this form of concealed power. Such treatments are widely used in many countries. In Australia, more than half the population regards vitamins, minerals, tonics or herbal medicine as helpful for treating depression. Surveys in the US suggest that over 50 per cent of respondents who reported anxiety attacks or severe depression had used complementary therapies in the previous 12 months (Kessler et al. 2001). Yet a systematic review of the evidence of the effectiveness of the most popular complementary therapies to treat depression concluded that there was no evidence to suggest that they were effective (Jorm et al. 2002). Meanwhile, adverse reactions to such treatments had doubled in the previous three years (WHO 2004). Arguably, the interests of consumers would be better served if they were to buy items proven to be efficacious.

Activity 2.3

The following describes a classic study of air pollution in the US (Crenson 1971). As you read it consider:

1 Which dimension of power is described?
2 Does the study indicate that power as thought control may have been exercised?

Case Study 2: the un-politics of air pollution

In the 1960s, Matthew Crenson sought to explain why air pollution remained a 'non-issue' in many American cities. He attempted to identify relationships between the neglect of air pollution and characteristics of political leaders and institutions.

Crenson's approach, examining why things do not happen when objectively they should, contrasted with that of Robert Dahl which looked at why they do (1961). Crenson adopted this strategy to test whether the study of political inactivity (or non-decision making) could shed new light on ways of thinking about power.

Crenson began by demonstrating that action or inaction on pollution in US cities could not be attributed to differences in actual pollution levels or to differences in social attributes of the populations in different cities. The study involved two neighbouring cities in Indiana which were both equally polluted and had similar demographic profiles. One of the cities, East Chicago, had taken action to deal with air pollution in 1949, while the other, Gary, did nothing until 1962. Crenson argues that the difference arose because Gary was a single-employer town dominated by U.S. Steel, with a strong political party organization, while Chicago was home to a number of steel companies and had no strong party organization when it passed its air pollution legislation. In Gary, anticipated negative reactions from U.S. Steel appeared to have prevented activists and city leaders from placing the issue on the agenda. Crenson also interviewed political leaders from 51 American cities. These suggested that 'the air pollution issue tends not to flourish in cities where industry enjoys a reputation for power'.

Crenson's major findings were that, first, power may consist of the ability to prevent some problems from becoming issues. Second, that power does not need to be exercised for it to be effective: the mere reputation for power can restrict the scope of decision making. Third, those affected by political power, 'the victims', may remain invisible, because the power or reputation of the powerful may deter the less powerful from entering the policy making arena. He concluded that 'non-issues are not politically random oversights but instances of politically enforced neglect'.

Feedback

1 Crenson's study provides an empirical basis for power as non-decision making.

2 Given that people would probably prefer not to be poisoned by air pollution, the case suggests that people will not necessarily act on their preferences and interests. This raises the possibility that some form of manipulation or indoctrination, i.e. policy making by thought control, was involved, though people were prsumably also concerned to keep industrial jobs in the cities. In other words, non-decision making may well have reflected discussions on the lesser of two evils for the town and reveals the complexity of real-world decision making.

Activity 2.4

From what you have learned so far, provide three simple answers to the question of how a relationship between A and B reveals that A is exercising power over B.

Feedback

A can get B to do what B may not have otherwise done. A can keep issues that are of interest to B off the policy agenda. A can manipulate B in a way that B fails to understand his/her true interests.

So far, you have learned that power is the ability to achieve a desired result irrespective of the means. It concerns the ability to get someone to do what they would not have otherwise done. Dahl, who examined visible decision making, concluded that power is widely distributed in society but was criticized for having failed to identify the true winners and losers – particularly the losers who do not enter the policy arena. Lukes takes the position that power can be exercised in a more subtle manner through keeping issues off the agenda or through psychological manipulation. Common to all these perspectives is the notion that the policy process involves the exercise of power by competing actors to control scarce resources. The manner in which these struggles are resolved depends in large part on who has power in society.

Who has power?

If power concerns the ability to influence others, it raises the question, 'who has the power to impose and resist policies?' There is no correct answer to this question as the distribution of influence will depend on the specific policy content and context. The three 'dimensions' of power suggest different views as to who wields power and how widely it is shared in policy processes. For example, in a country where tobacco constitutes a considerable proportion of the gross domestic product and is a valuable source of government revenue and foreign exchange, the tobacco industry is likely to have more influence over tobacco control policy than the ministry of health and public health and consumer interest groups. Yet, in the same country, industry may have less influence over policy to screen for cancer than, for example, the ministry of health, the medical profession, and patient groups.

Despite the differences that policy content and context exert over the distribution of power in a given policy process, attempts have been made to arrive at general theories. These theories turn on the nature of society and the state. While some theories locate power in society as opposed to the state, all are concerned with the role of the state and the interests which the state is thought to represent in the policy process. The focus is on the state because of the dominant role that it usually plays in the policy process. Theorists differ, however, in two important respects; first, in their assessment of whether the state is independent of society or a reflection of the distribution of power in society (state- and society-oriented respectively); second, in their view of whether the state serves a common good or the interests of a privileged group. You will now learn about how the theories differ and consider the implications of these differences for health policy.

Pluralism

Pluralism represents the dominant school of thought as far as theories of the distribution of power in liberal democracies are concerned. In its classical form, pluralism takes the view that power is dispersed throughout society. No single group holds absolute power and the state arbitrates among competing interests in the development of policy (Dahl 1961).

The key features of pluralism are:

- open electoral competition among a number of political parties;
- ability of individuals to organize themselves into pressure groups and political parties;
- ability of pressure groups to air their views freely;
- openness of the state to lobbying on behalf of all pressure groups;
- the state as a neutral referee adjudicating between competing demands;
- although society has elite groups, no elite group dominates at all times.

For pluralists, health policy emerges as the result of conflict and bargaining among large numbers of groups organized to protect the specific interests of their members. The state selects from initiatives and proposals put forward by interest groups according to what is best for society.

Pluralism has been subject to considerable scepticism for its portrayal of the state as a neutral umpire and for its portrayal of the distribution of power. The major challenge on the first count comes from public choice theorists and on the second from elite theorists.

Public choice

Public choice theorists agree with the pluralists that society is made up of competing groups pursuing self-interested goals but they dispute the claim of the state's neutrality (Olson 1971). They assert that the state is itself an interest group which wields power over the policy process in pursuit of the interests of those who run it: elected public officials and civil servants. To remain in power, officials consciously seek to reward groups with public expenditure, goods, services and favourable regulation in the expectation that these groups will keep them in power. Similarly, civil servants use their offices and proximity to political decision makers to derive 'rents' (that is financial and other illicit benefits) by providing special access to public resources and regulatory favouritism to specific groups. As a result, public servants hope to expand their bureaucratic empires as this will lead to bigger salaries and more opportunities for promotion, power, patronage and prestige. The state is, therefore, said to have an inbuilt dynamic which leads to the further growth and power of government.

Public choice theorists argue that the self-interested behaviour of state officials leads to policy that is captured by narrow interest groups. As a result, policies are likely to be distorted in economically negative ways and are not in the public's interest. Adherents of this school argue that health policies which involve rolling back the state will be resisted by bureaucrats, not because of the technical merits or demerits of the policy, but because bureaucrats favour policies which further entrench their positions and extend their spheres of influence. In Bangladesh, for example, in the late 1990s Ministry of Health and Family Welfare officials resisted proposals to contract out public sector facilities to non-governmental organizations for service delivery as well as a related proposal to establish an autonomous organization to manage the contracting process. Public choice adherents would explain this opposition on the basis of fear of staff redundancies, diminished opportunities for rent-seeking and patronage, and concerns about the diminution of state power and responsibility.

Critics suggest that public choice theory both overstates the power of bureaucrats in the policy process and is largely fuelled by the ideological opposition to escalating public spending and so-called 'big government'.

Elitism

Elitist theorists contend that policy is dominated by a privileged minority. In this view, it is argued that public policy reflects the values and interests of this elite – not 'the people' as is claimed by the pluralists. Elitists question the extent to which modern political systems live up to the democratic ideals suggested by the liberal pluralists. Even in the democratic US, scholars have shown how an elite shapes key decisions. For example, former Presidents, George H.W. and George W. Bush had considerable financial interests in the energy sector as did the latter's Vice-President Dick Cheney who had served as the chief executive officer of the company Haliburton, active in both oil and defence industries. Controversially Haliburton received major contracts to construct and manage military bases on a non-competitive basis during Cheney's tenure in office. In contrast, groups representing small business, labour and consumer interests are typically only able to exert influence at the margins of the policy process.

As far as health policy is concerned, does elitist theory overstate the capacities of the elite to wield power? Certainly, most health policy is considered to be of relatively marginal importance and, consequently, it may be that elitist theories are less useful in accounting for power in health policy. Issues perceived to be of marginal importance are sometimes referred to as 'low politics' – where high politics concerns major ideological, economic and security issues (Walt 1994). Low politics issues often have strong technical components and imply minimal change from the status quo. Nonetheless, you will see many examples in this book which suggest that an elite wields considerable influence even in the relatively mundane realm of day-to-day health policy making.

Elite theorists suggest that power may be based on a variety of resources: wealth, family connections, technical expertise, office or education. Yet what is also important is that for any one member of the elite, power is unlikely to depend on only one source.

According to elite theorists:

- Society is comprised of the few with power and the many without. Only the few who have power make policy.
- Those who govern are unlike those who do not. In particular, the elite comes from the higher socio-economic strata.
- Non-elites may be inducted into the governing circles if they accept the basic consensus of the existing elite.
- Public policy reflects the values of the elite. This may not always imply a conflict with the values of the masses. The elite can manipulate the values of the masses to reflect their own.
- Interest groups exist but they are not all equally powerful and do not have equal access to the policy making process.
- The values of the elite are conservative and consequently any policy change is likely to be incremental.

It would appear that elitist theory is relevant to many countries where politicians, senior bureaucrats, business people, professionals and the military form tight policy circles that become a dominant or ruling class. In some places, the elite may be so few in number that they can be recognized by their family names.

The notion that not all interest groups are equally influential holds intuitive appeal. There is an increasing concentration of ownership in certain industries, for example, tobacco, alcohol, and pharmaceuticals. These powerful groups will likely have more resources and thus more leverage over policy than will public health groups. The following case study highlights the lobbying of some of these groups in the US.

Case Study 3: health care lobbying in the United States

The term 'lobby' as a noun relates to the areas in parliaments where citizens can make demands on legislators and where policy makers meet. The term is also used as a verb, meaning to make direct representation to a policy maker. Lobby and interest groups are similar in that they both attempt to influence policy makers. Lobbyists are hired by various organizations to represent the interests of their clients on a commercial basis.

In 2010, health care lobbyists spent US$521 million to influence US Senators and Representatives, the Executive and other federal agencies at the national level – making it the second largest lobby group after the financial sector in the country (up from US$237 million in 2000). Of this amount, pharmaceutical and health product industries accounted for almost half of spending ($243 million) followed by hospitals and nursing homes ($107 million); physicians and other health professionals ($86 million), and health insurance and managed care companies ($74 million) (Center for Responsive Politics 2010).

Not only have the sums spent on lobbying increased, so too have the number of health sector lobbyists: from 2482 in 2000 to 3220 in 2010. These trends suggest that lobbying is an increasing popular tool to influence health legislation in the American political system (Landers and Sehgal 2004). Some have expressed concern that 'health policy is at risk of being unduly influenced by special interest groups that can bring the most financial resources to the table' (Kushel and Bindman 2004).

There are a number of important elitist frameworks which locate power in specific groups in society. 'Marxism' argues that power is vested in a ruling capitalist class and that this class controls the state. 'Professionalism' draws attention to the power of specific professional groups and the way they wield influence over the policy process. You will learn more about the special position of the medical profession in health policy in Chapter 6. 'Feminism' focuses on the systematic, pervasive and institutionalized power which men wield over women in the domestic and public spheres. Feminist theorists argue that in the most extreme form of patriarchy, women would remain in the private domain (as mothers and wives) while public affairs, such as the state, would be run by and for men. In such patriarchal societies, men would define the problems and their solutions, decide which issues are policy-worthy and which are not. In 1990 the proportion of seats held by women in national parliaments globally was 13 per cent. This figure only increased by one percentage point during the following decade – but had increased to 19 per cent by 2011. It is still the case that only one in five legislators in the world is a woman (UN 2011).

Activity 2.5

As you read the following case study on sex-selective abortions, consider whether or not the claim that health policy in India is captured by men is valid.

Case Study 4: gendered policy implementation

In India, antenatal ultrasound technology, introduced to identify congenital complications and widely available since the early 1980s, has transformed the cultural preference for male progeny into a process through which those who can afford a scan may pre-select males by identifying females during pregnancy and selectively terminating female foetuses. Access to this technology has intensified the 'masculinization' of the sex ratio which has been underway in India since at least the 1960s. The 2011 census revealed a national child (0–6 years of age) sex ratio of 914 females to 1,000 males (whereas one would expect a roughly equal number of girls and boys surviving in a gender-equal society). Some states have higher differentials than others – Punjab, for example, recorded a ratio of 846 girls for every 1,000 boys.

In response to the problem, the federal government passed the Pre-conception and Pre-natal Diagnostic Techniques (Prohibition of Sex Selection) Act in 1994. Little was done to implement the Act until 2001 when an NGO filed a public interest claim with the Supreme Court. The Court directed certain states to take action (seizing machines in clinics without licences) yet there have been few convictions to date. The issue has become all the more urgent with new technologies for sex-selection marketed to Indians by US firms and available over the Internet. Although the law was amended in 2003, it has, nonetheless been argued that there are limits to what the law and the courts can do in face of deep-rooted prejudices against females in general and the status of the girl child in particular.

Feedback

While it is clear that sex discrimination is pervasive in India, some might point to the existence of the 1994 law as proof that women can successfully penetrate the policy process and thereby overcome a patriarchal elite. Feminists would argue, however, that the law was too little, too late, and too poorly implemented. Explaining such failure would require more information on how the problem was framed and who put it on the policy agenda (likely to have been women) and who was responsible for implementation and enforcement, mainly men! But the example points to the limits of policy too – where doctors, clinics and patients collude to undermine government decisions.

Activity 2.6

The following case study is an account of work by Kelley Lee and Hillary Goodman (2002) on the distribution of power in relation to health care financing policy at the international level.

As you read it, make notes of why Lee and Goodman describe the actors as part of a global policy elite and what might account for the success of this global policy network. Also consider why you might argue that the existence of this network is insufficient proof of the existence of a policy elite in health sector reform.

Case Study 5: international health financing reform: dominated by an elite?

In an attempt to demonstrate the impact of globalization on health policy making, Lee and Goodman (2002) undertook an analysis of health care financing reform during the 1980s and 1990s. While it was apparent that a plethora of non-state actors were increasingly involved in the provision and financing of health services, it was less clear whether or not this huge diversity was similarly involved in formulating health policy. Lee and Goodman were sceptical of the claims that globalization had increased the range and heterogeneity of voices in the policy process so they set out to establish who had been responsible for the dominant ideas and content of health care financing policy.

The study began by tracing the significant changes in the content of health financing policy during the period, marked by a transition from strong reluctance to a broader acceptance of private finance for a range of services. The key individuals and institutions involved were identified through a search of the literature. This resulted in a list of individuals who had published in key journals, been frequently cited and/or contributed to seminal policy documents on the topic. The institutional base, source of funding and nationality of these key actors were identified. These individuals were interviewed to elicit their views on the most influential documents, individuals, institutions and meetings in the policy area and their curricula vitae were procured. Finally, the researchers studied records of attendance and presentations at meetings reported by informants to have been critical in the evolution of the policies.

Network maps were developed linking the institutions and individuals. The authors discovered that a small (approximately 25) and tightly knit group of policy makers, technical advisers and academics had dominated the process and content of health financing reform. This group, connected by multiple linkages in a complex network, was based in a small number of institutions led by the World Bank and

USAID. Network members were observed as following a common career progression. Revolving doors circulated members among these institutions, thereby enabling them to occupy various roles as researchers, research and pilot project funders, policy advisers and decision makers.

Lee and Goodman concluded that a global elite had dominated policy discussion through their 'control of the terms of debate through expert knowledge, support of research, and occupation of key nodes' in the network. The authors were less concerned that a small group of leaders had shaped the policy debates, but rather that the group was not representative of the interests at stake: 'the global policy network has been narrowly based in a small number of institutions, led by the World Bank and USAID [but including Abt Associates, a private consultancy firm and Harvard University], and in the nationality and disciplinary background of the key individuals involved'. Lee and Goodman were also concerned that policy did not result from a 'rational convergence of health needs and solutions'. Instead, the elite is described as having exercised its influence on national agendas through both coercive (conditionalities on aid in the context of resource scarcity) and consensual (collaborative research, strategic training of national decision makers and co-option of policy elites) approaches.

Feedback

This case contradicted pluralist claims that globalization was opening up decision making to a wider range of stakeholders and allowing discussion of a broader set of policy ideas.

The group governing the health financing agenda can be portrayed as an elite in that it is small in number, and members have similar educational, disciplinary and national backgrounds. Over a 20-year period, this policy elite is demonstrated to have successfully established an international health financing agenda (a particular set of health care financing proposals) and formulated policies that were adopted in numerous countries. It was able to do this in part because of its control over access to development assistance but more importantly, through its control of technical expertise, expert knowledge and positions, and occupation of nodal points in the network. The existence of this network is not proof that an elite dominates all health reform policy. If it were found that other policy issues in the broader international health policy context were influenced by individuals and institutions which were based in other countries, and staffed by decision makers with different credentials and backgrounds, you might conclude that a form of modified pluralism existed.

A variety of theories that explain the distribution of power in society and the character of the state in policy making have been presented. The differences between them are not trivial in that they carry important implications for analysing who has power and what explains policy change. Some of the discrepancies between theorists can be accounted for by different methodological approaches. Taking into consideration critiques, methodological constraints and new empirical evidence, some of these schools of thought have modified and updated their approaches. Most pluralists now acknowledge that the policy making playing field is not level. They note the privileged position of organized business interests and the role that the media and socialization play in most political systems.

Common to all of these theories is the proposition that understanding policy change requires an understanding of how power is distributed and exercised in society. To some extent, the actual distribution of power will depend on the policy context and content. Issues of great national importance are likely to be made by a power elite, whereas more mundane issues are likely to be influenced by a range of interest groups. What is ultimately useful about the models is that they provide different ways of trying to understand why policy changes or does not, based on who has power over specific issues.

Power and political systems

David Easton's (1965) systems model of policy making provides one approach to simplifying the complexities of political decision making and understanding its key components. A system is a complex whole which is constituted by a number of inter-dependent parts. The system's parts may change as they interact with one another and the wider environment. While these changes and processes of interaction result in a constant transformation within the system, overall they must remain broadly in balance if the system is to survive.

Harold Dwight Lasswell (1936) defined politics as 'who gets what, when, and how'. Consequently, the political system is concerned with deciding which goods, services, freedoms, rights and privileges to grant (and to deny) and to whom they will be granted (or denied). The wider environment (e.g. social context) affects the political system in that it provides opportunities, resources, obstacles and constraints to political decision making. For example, there may be a shortage of nurses. This might provoke action (a policy decision) from the political system to deal with the shortage. Among policy alternatives, the political system may increase the number of nursing places in higher educational facilities, provide monetary incentives such as loans to encourage students to enter the nursing speciality, recruit nurses from other countries, increase the skills of para-medical staff to take on some nursing functions, or do nothing.

Activity 2.7

Identify some of the obstacles and constraints to each of the policy responses to the shortage of nurses proposed above. For example, an increase in the number of nursing places in higher education will require additional funds, will not necessarily attract additional students, and will take a number of years to resolve the problem.

Feedback

1 Providing monetary incentives to nursing students will require additional funds, might be perceived as unfair by other students and disciplines, may be difficult to administer, and may not attract additional students.
2 Recruiting foreign nurses will require additional funds, may require changes to existing foreign worker regulations, and may be resisted by domestic nursing unions, xenophobic groups or patients.
3 Increasing the skills of another cadre of staff to assume nursing functions may result in demand from them to be remunerated as nurses, may require additional funds, and may be resisted by nursing unions.
4 Doing nothing may increase the demands on the political system.

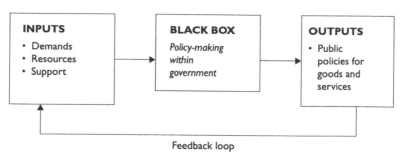

Figure 2.1 Easton's political systems model

Source: Adapted from Easton (1965)

The key processes which the systems model highlights are 'inputs' and 'outputs' and the links between them (Figure 2.1). Inputs take the form of demands and support from the individuals and groups. In the health sector, a demand may be made for higher expenditure on services, free or more affordable care, more convenient services, the right to choice with respect to abortion, and so on. Societal preferences are transformed into demands when they are communicated by citizens to decision makers directly or indirectly through interest groups, lobbyists and political parties. Support comprises action taken by the public to underpin (or oppose) the political system by paying taxes, voting and complying with the law (or not paying taxes, defacing the ballot, and using illicit services – for abortion, for example).

Inputs are fed into policy making to produce outputs which are the decisions and policies of government including legislation, imposition of taxation and budgets. Easton provided relatively few details on how the conversion process takes place and therefore government decision making is considered a 'black box'. Some outputs are obvious and visible, such as a decision by government to train more nurses. Some outputs may be less obvious and even largely invisible. As Bachrach and Baratz (1963) remind us, some decisions may be non-decisions which keep issues off the policy agenda. For example, while some citizens may demand more nursing staff, the government may take no action. Inside the black box a resource allocation decision has been taken without any visible policy making.

The outputs of the policy process are distinguished from their impact. Policy impact relates to the effects of policy decisions on individuals and groups. Ultimately, for example, citizens will be interested in the impact of any policy to address the number of nurses in the health care system and the effect that this has on the quality of care. So, if the policy results in unanticipated consequences (poorer quality nursing or a higher wage bill, for example), affected groups will likely alter their preferences, demands and support in relation to other policy alternatives. These inputs will in turn affect the constraints and opportunities presented to decision makers working within the black box and condition their subsequent approach to the problem. The logic of the systems approach dictates that policy outputs and impacts generate 'feedback' which influences future demands on, and support for, the system – creating a loop. The feedback is characterized as continuous to capture the evolving interdependency among components in the system.

Easton's model explains why political systems are responsive to public pressure. The model also breaks down the policy making process into discrete stages which will be analysed in further detail in subsequent chapters. Its very general nature means that it can be applied to most political systems. Yet, as with any model, its simplification of reality also has some drawbacks.

As a result of the latter two concerns, it is argued that the model fails to explain why governments may employ repression and coercion, as many have at some time, to curb demands. The model is further criticized as it does not account for policy that arises from decision making within private organizations, for example, voluntary industry codes such as on advertising potentially harmful products to children. Furthermore, as already alluded to, the model places too little emphasis on what happens inside the 'black box' of policy making. Are decisions made in a rational way by policy makers or in an incremental manner depending on the exercise of power by interest groups? We will return to these questions later in this chapter.

Despite these shortcomings, the concept of the political system provides an important key to understanding the discrete stages of policy making. Yet before turning to these stages, let us further consider the notion of inputs, in an effort to clarify the relationship between them and the policy making process – specifically citizens' ability to influence the policy process. This relationship hinges on the nature of participation in the political system.

Classifying political systems: participation, benefits and openness

Broadly speaking, citizens can participate either directly or indirectly in the policy process. Direct participation describes attempts to influence policy through face-to-face or other forms of personal contact with policy makers. For example, constituents may meet with their parliamentary representative to discuss options for reducing the length of the local hospital waiting list. Indirect participation refers to actions by individuals to influence the selection of government representatives. This normally takes place by joining political parties, campaigning for particular parties or individuals and voting in elections.

The extent to which people can participate in the political system is partially a function of the culture and nature of the political system – not all political systems are alike. Systems are usually distinguished in terms of who rules, who benefits and how open the systems are.

On the basis of these criteria, five groups of political systems can be distinguished:

- *liberal democratic regimes.* This category is marked by governments that operate with relatively stable political institutions with considerable opportunities for participation through a diverse number of mechanisms and groups: elections, political parties, interest groups, and 'free media'. It includes the countries of North America and Western Europe as well as countries such as India and Israel. Health policy varies considerably from market-oriented in the US to the welfare state in Western Europe.
- *egalitarian-authoritarian.* Characterized by a closed ruling elite, authoritarian bureaucracies and state-managed popular participation (i.e. regimented participation which is less a democratic opportunity than an exercise in social control). Close links often exist between single political parties and the state and its bureaucracies. During the 1970s, Angola, China, Cuba, Mozambique, the Soviet Union, and Vietnam might have been included in this category. These states had the intent to be egalitarian – although the scope and nature of equality were often contested. They had well-developed social security systems and health care was financed and delivered almost exclusively by the state (private practice was banned in some cases) and treated as a fundamental human right. Few such political systems now exist.
- *traditional-inegalitarian.* These systems feature rule by traditional monarchs which provide few opportunities for participation. Saudi Arabia provides an example of this increasingly rare system. Health policy relies heavily on the private sector with the elite using facilities in other countries as the need arises.
- *populist.* These are based upon single or dominant political parties, are highly nationalist and leadership tends to be personalized. Participation is highly regimented through mass movements controlled by the state or a political party. Elites may have some influence on the government either through kinship with the leader or membership of the political party. Many newly independent states of Africa and South America began with populist political systems. Where colonial health services had only been available to the ruling elite, populists attempted to provide health for all as a basic right.
- *authoritarian-inegalitarian.* These political systems have often developed in reaction to populist and liberal democratic regimes. They are often associated with military governments and involve varying degrees of repression. In the mid-1980s, over half the governments in sub-Saharan Africa were military – and many were marked by autocratic personal rule. Health policy reflected the interests of a narrow elite: a

state-funded service for the military while others had to rely heavily on the private sector.

In light of the profound political upheaval at the end of the 1980s associated with the fall of the Soviet Union, the above classification of political systems has been shown to be dated and no clear substitutes have emerged. Francis Fukuyama published a paper in 1989 provocatively entitled 'The end of history?' He claimed that the collapse of communism and the wave of democratization of the late 1980s signalled the recognition of liberal democracy as the superior and 'final form of human government'. Although it is true that some form of democracy is the most common form of political system, Fukuyama's analysis is western-centric, based on values such as individualism, human rights and choice; moreover, it fails to account for the persistence and rise of new forms of political system.

It is apparent that there remain significant differences between political systems and that not all have converged on the Western liberal democratic model. One of the most important features is the extent to which political systems encourage or stifle participation. This in turn has major implications for how health policy is made and whose interest's these policies serve.

Making decisions inside the 'black box'

Now consider contrasting views on decision making presented below with the aim of understanding their implications for health policy making. There has been an ongoing debate between theorists, who portray decision making as a 'rational' process, and others who put forward 'incremental' models. The latter describe a process by which decision makers 'muddle through' in response to the political influences to which they are subjected. Attempts have been made to reconcile these two views. The case of congenital syphilis is employed to illustrate the different approaches to understanding decision making but any health issue could have been used. At the end, the links are made between this debate over decision making and the analysis of power and the role of the state.

Activity 2.9

While reading about the four models (*rationalism; bounded rationalism; incrementalism; mixed scanning*), make a note of whether they aim to be descriptive of the way that decisions are actually made, prescriptive of the way decisions ought to be made (that is, normative), or possibly both. In addition, write down two or three problems inherent in each model.

Rational models of decision making: too idealistic?

It is often assumed that policies are made in a rational way. The rational model of decision making is associated with Simon's (1957) work on how organizations should make decisions. Simon argued that a rational approach involves selecting from among alternatives that option which is most conducive to the achievement of the organizational goal(s). To achieve the desired outcomes, decision makers must work through a number of steps in a logical sequence.

First, decision makers need to identify a problem which needs to be solved and isolate that problem from others. For example, in many countries in sub-Saharan Africa, syphilis rates among pregnant women are over 5 per cent. To isolate the problem, decision makers have to decide whether or not it is a true prevalence or an artifact of improved detection capacity (more sensitive tests), and whether their overriding concern is with the infection of unborn children or with the burden of syphilis in the population more generally.

Second, the goals, values and objectives of decision makers need to be clarified and ranked. For example, would policy makers prefer to reduce the incidence of congenital syphilis by screening all pregnant women (a strategy which might be equitable) or only screen those perceived to be at higher risk – such as sex workers (a strategy which might be more cost-effective in reducing the burden of syphilis in the adult population, but which would take longer to reduce risk for unborn children in the general population)?

Third, decision makers should list all alternative strategies for achieving their goal. Depending on the country, such strategies might include:

* increasing the coverage of ante-natal care, increasing the number of women seeking care early in their pregnancy, training health care providers to deliver effective screening and management of syphilis and strengthening health systems to ensure needed resources are available
* advocating syphilis treatment for *all* women who are pregnant (i.e. presumptive treatment) in high prevalence areas, for example
* targeting presumptive treatment for groups at high risk; or
* controlling genital ulcer disease in the population through, for example, improved access to effective treatment and partner notification strategies.

Figure 2.2 illustrates the relative effect of these options.

The fourth step should involve rational decision makers undertaking a comprehensive analysis of the impact, including unintended consequences, of each of the options. In relation to congenital syphilis, decision makers would need to calculate the reduction in the incidence of syphilis as well as the costs associated with each of the

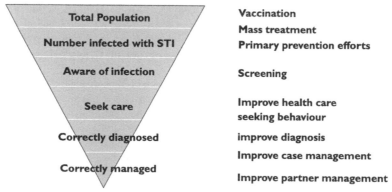

Figure 2.2 Inverted public health pyramid for prevention and care of people infected with syphilis

Note: The inverted pyramid represents from top to bottom the number of people covered by the interventions – with the interventions listed in the right-hand column

Source: Adapted from Schmid (2004)

alternatives (some of which have been listed above). It can be quite complex to quantify the extent to which the intervention meets the objective and the related costs.

Fifth, each alternative and its set of consequences would need to be compared with the other options. Finally, policy makers would choose that strategy which maximizes their values and preferences as far as goal attainment is concerned while minimizing the costs (so that other objectives can be pursued as well). By working through this logical and comprehensive process, a rational decision is taken in that the means are selected which most effectively achieve the policy aim.

It is extremely unlikely that decision makers involved in establishing a policy undertake the steps described above to arrive at their policy decision. The failure to adhere to such a rational process can be explained by the difficulties that many analysts of decision making find in the approach which essentially *prescribes* how policy *ought* to be made rather than *describing* how it is *actually* made in the real world.

One challenge to the rational model lies in the area of problem definition. The precise nature of the problem is not always clear-cut. For example, in relation to congenital syphilis, is the problem one of trying to bring down the overall rate of syphilis in the general population (which includes, of course, pregnant women), or is it one of trying to improve screening and treatment facilities for pregnant women so as to improve child survival?

The rational model has also been criticized in relation to specifying values and objectives. Whose values and aims are to be adopted? No organization is homogeneous and different parts of an organization may pursue different, if not competing, objectives based on differing values. For example, Zafrullah Chowdhury's (1995) analysis of the formulation of an Essential Drugs Policy in Bangladesh drew attention to the conflicting responses of the World Bank to the policy. The Bank's Industry and Energy Unit in Dhaka objected to the policy while its Population and Health Unit provided whole-hearted support to the government.

A third concern lies with the assumption that all possible strategies can be considered. Many contending policy alternatives may be foreclosed by prior investments, commitments and political realities (see discussion of '*path dependency*' below). For example, a congenital syphilis policy aiming to increase ante-natal services in rural areas by relocating doctors to serve in rural facilities would likely face considerable resistance from the medical association.

A fourth, rather obvious, shortcoming relates to its impracticality. In the real world, the problem of gathering information on all alternatives will face budget and time constraints. Allocating sufficient time and money to collect all the relevant data on all possible options to make every decision would not be justified or sanctioned in most organizations.

Others provide a different kind of critique of the model which contests the very idea of understanding the world in a 'rational' manner. In this view, decision makers have a subjective understanding of problems and their solutions – in effect, they create the meaning of the problem and fix it in a manner which corresponds to their values or worldview. As Edelman (1988) has argued, policy makers may 'construct' problems so as to justify solutions and in so doing a policy may be a success as a political device even if it fails to address or ameliorate a problem in the sense that 'the operation was a success, but the patient died'. Years after claiming that Britain was in moral breakdown, a former British Prime Minister admitted that his analysis of the problem had been misguided, but contended that 'the speech was good politics but bad policy' (Blair 2011).

Simon (1957) answered some of these criticisms by arguing that the rational model provides an idealized approach; describing the way that policy ought to be made rather than how it is done in practice. Later, he proposed 'bounded rationality' as a model of the practice of policy making in the real world. Acknowledging the complexities of rational choice and the costs and incompleteness of information facing decision makers, Simon suggested that, in practice, they simplify decision making in two ways. First, they find routine ways to deal with recurrent problems so as not to have to assess each problem in a comprehensive manner. As a result, many policies are not subject to exacting scrutiny. Second, decision makers do not aim to achieve optimal solutions to problems, but rather to find solutions or choose strategies that meet satisfactory standards through what is termed 'satisficing' (March and Simon 1958). Consequently, Simon argues that decision makers are deliberately rational, but are subject to real-world constraints which limit their ability to make perfectly rational choices. In terms of congenital syphilis policy, decision makers adhering to the bounded rationality model would behave as rationally as possible within the constraints of time, information and ability to recognize the consequences of every possible solution – working, for example, with estimates of affected populations, including estimates of the number of sex workers in a certain area, how many clients they typically have sex with, how many pregnant women will seek ante-natal services and when they will likely do so, how much resistance front line staff will mount to undertaking screening, etc.

Incremental models of decision making: more realistic; but too conservative?

Charles Lindblom (1959) proposed an alternative account of decision making which he entitled 'muddling through'. According to Lindblom, decision makers 'muddle' in the sense that they take incremental steps from the initial situation by comparing only a small number of possible alternatives which are not very different from the status quo. Lindblom argues that decision makers will test the political waters in deciding whether or not to pursue a given course of action. The test of a good policy is not whether it maximizes or even satisfices the values of the decision makers (as was the case with the rational and bounded rational models), but whether it secures the agreement of the various interests at stake. If opposition is too strong, an option closer to the status quo will be tested. Subsequent attempts at policy change will again seek to compare options which may challenge the status quo, but only in a marginal way. For Lindblom, the decision making process is marked by mutual adjustment by the affected stakeholders.

Lindblom argued that muddling through not only better describes actual decision making, but it also provides a better recipe for taking policy decisions, in that damaging policy mistakes can be avoided by taking *incremental* steps whose effects can be assessed before taking the next one. Moreover, it is argued that it provides a more democratic and practical approach to finding more 'sensible politics' than the hierarchical, centrally coordinated approaches promoted by the rationalists. For example, as a result of compromise and muddling through, health sector budgets tend to increase modestly each year rather than shift dramatically.

To return to the example of congenital syphilis policy, incremental decision making would eschew bold policy initiatives which attempted to eliminate the condition. Instead, decision makers might proceed initially by piggy-backing ante-natal syphilis screening onto routine HIV testing in ante-natal settings. If this intervention were broadly accepted by AIDS activists, health workers and women attending ante-natal clinics, decision makers might then take another incremental step by pursuing a policy of allocating some additional resources to increase the number of pregnant women attending ante-natal clinics. If, however, AIDS activists baulked at attempts to highjack 'their' services, or health workers would not accept the additional workload, decision makers would likely explore other incremental steps, such as expanding dedicated syphilis screening programmes.

'Path dependency' and institutional 'stickiness' have been used to explain incremental change. Path dependency refers to the tendency of antecedent factors and previous decisions to limit the range of choices available thereafter, and thereby set a specific trajectory for public policy. For example, the training curricula for nurses cover a given set of functions and competencies. A policy which seeks to broaden the range of functions to include some of those performed by doctors will be limited by the training received by earlier cohorts of nursing staff. As a result, those seeking to alter nursing functions would likely muddle through in an incremental manner as they do not have a huge degree of discretion to radically alter the policy of nursing practice in the short term.

Others have argued that incrementalism in policy making is largely a function of the inertia inherent in the institutions established to govern society – particularly those set up by government. Institutions, as you learned in Chapter 1, can be thought of as the 'rules of the game' governing how things are done. It is argued that institutions are resistant to change – or 'sticky' – as a result of political gridlock among interest groups or the failure to appreciate the availability of alternatives. Taking the example of nurse competencies, rapid policy change might be resisted by institutions set up to train physicians and nurses, associations set up to promote their interests as well as patient groups – even if managers and politicians would like to see change. All of these institutions would need to be convinced of the benefits of change – something that would take time and resources.

While the incremental model presents a more realistic account of decision making than does the rational one, it too has been the subject of criticism. One critique of the model revolves around its inability to explain how radical decisions are taken. If decision making involves small exploratory steps from the existing policy, how can one account for policies that involve fundamental reforms of an entire health care system? In addition to this limitation to its descriptive capacity, are concerns about its prescriptive or normative position on policy making. In effect, incrementalism advocates a conservative approach to decision making. Policy makers are discouraged from pursuing strategies which result in goal maximization if these are found to run up against *vested interests*. Given that change is most likely to be resisted precisely where it is most needed, incrementalist approaches are unlikely to foster innovation or significant progress, and are likely to be unfair as they favour those with more power. Incrementalism, in theory and practice, fails to address the unequal distribution of power among interest groups or to tackle the possibilities that bias excludes certain items from policy consideration.

Lindblom rejected this criticism and argued that a succession of minor steps could amount to fundamental change (Lindblom and Woodhouse 1993). For example, advocates of a particular policy could over time whittle away at political opposition towards a longer-term goal. Others have been more sceptical, arguing that in practice the approach does not deal with what will guide the incremental steps. These 'may be circular – leading to where they started, or dispersed – leading in many directions at once but leading nowhere' (Etzioni 1967).

Punctuated equilibrium

Others, such as Baumgartner and Jones (1991) have observed that over the long term, policy is not marked so much by incremental change as by long periods of little change, which are then ruptured by quite fundamental reform. It is argued that *vested interest* groups or governing elites – termed policy monopolies – convincingly articulate a view of a problem and its solution, and establish a set of policy responses and political institutions to address the problem. Working through these institutions, policy monopolies manage to retain policies in stable equilibrium for long periods. However, at times, this equilibrium is punctuated as a result of external (contextual) shocks bringing about quite far-reaching change. Such exogenous shocks may come about as a result of the ascendency of new governing coalitions or major changes in market conditions. The '*punctuated equilibrium*' model has been used to explain the tendency for policy stasis and abrupt change in relation to a number of health policy issues in the US including pesticide control, auto safety and drug abuse (Baumgartner and Jones 1993). Taking a long-term view of efforts to control polio, malaria and tuberculosis, Shiffman et al. compared the ability of the rational, incremental and punctuated equilibrium models to explain why political priority emerged for these diseases and policy change ensued (Shiffman et al. 2002). The authors concluded that the punctuated equilibrium model corresponded most closely with policy governing these diseases. In each of these cases, long periods of stability were ended when three factors converged: widespread concern with the threat posed by the disease; perceptions that control was feasible; and the formation of a transnational coalition advocating action.

Mixed-scanning approach to decision making: the middle way

Attempts have been made to combine the idealism of the rational-comprehensive approach with the realism of the incremental models while overcoming the unrealistic requirements of rationalism and the conservative slant of incrementalism. In particular, Amitai Etzioni proposed a 'mixed-scanning' model of decision making which was based on weather forecasting techniques (1967) in which broad scans of an entire region are coupled with images of selected areas of turbulence. Etzioni claimed that mixed scanning was not only a desirable way of making decisions but also provided a good description of decision making in practice. Mixed scanning would involve a wide sweep of the problem as a whole and more detailed analysis of a select component of the problem. Etzioni drew a distinction between major and minor decisions. In his view, with respect to major decisions, policy makers undertake a broad analysis of the area without the detailed analysis of the policy options as suggested by the rationalists. More detailed reviews are conducted of options in relation to less important steps which might lead up to or follow from a fundamental decision. Mixed scanning is thought to overcome the unrealistic expectations of rationalism by limiting the details required for major decisions, while the broad view helps overcome the conservative slant of incrementalism by considering the longer-run alternatives.

Applying the mixed-scanning model to health policy making might identify the following practice which exists in some countries. On the one hand, ministries of health periodically undertake exercises aimed at estimating and quantifying the overall burden of disease associated with major disease categories which provide the basis for attempts to prioritize specific disease programmes and establish broad targets for resource allocation across competing expenditure categories. On the other hand, disease-specific programme managers undertake more detailed analysis of the options available in relation to funding specific interventions. Neither exercise is comprehensive. However, in many countries, decision making proceeds in a much less structured way, either through unplanned drift or in response to the pressure of time, resources or political pressures or opportunities – including major financial grants from external sponsors.

Global health policy making can also be characterized by the mixed scanning approach. The growing burden of non-communicable diseases – and the future costs they would impose – dawned on the international community toward the end of the first decade of this century. Yet the challenge of non-communicable diseases is vast – not only the range of conditions but also the risk factors – particularly those that are structural in nature such as poverty. In response, the World Health Organization undertook a broad scan and selected cancer, cardiovascular, respiratory diseases and diabetes as the top non-communicable diseases for attention. More detailed strategies address each of these, including on diet, alcohol, tobacco control, and so on.

Feedback

Compare your answers with those in Table 2.1. Most people like to think that they are rational and prize the use of rationality in decision making. The rational model of decision making proposes that a series of logical steps is undertaken so that the best option can be identified and selected. Rational models serve mainly prescriptive purposes as there are many constraints to practising rationality in the real world. Bounded rationalism acknowledges that decision makers intend to be rational but, given information uncertainties and the costs of knowledge, reach a decision that 'satisfices'. Incremental models explicitly take power into account and provide a largely descriptive account of how policy makers 'muddle through' in response to complex political pressures. While critics claim that incrementalism is biased in favour of the status quo, a series of small steps can cumulatively result in major changes and small steps may serve to guard against major policy disasters. Mixed scanning has been proposed as a middle ground. Mixed scanning provides a relatively accurate account of decision making in the real world – even if the distinction between major and minor decisions remains conceptually murky.

Table 2.1 Decision making theories compared

Theory/model	Major proponent	Descriptive vs prescriptive	Criticisms
Rationalism	Simon	Prescriptive	Problematic definition Problematic, who sets goals? Many options foreclosed Impractical/impossible to collect data
Bounded rationalism	Simon	Prescriptive and descriptive	Problematic definition Problematic, who sets goals? Many options foreclosed
Incrementalism	Lindblom	Mainly descriptive Claims for prescription	Does not explain major policy change/reform Inbuilt conservative bias
Mixed scanning	Etzioni	Prescriptive and descriptive	Distinction between fundamental and routine decisions not clear

Summary

This chapter has introduced theories to enable you to apply the concept of power in relation to policy making. Power was defined and the three ways that it is exercised were illustrated. The debate on how power is distributed in society with pluralists and elitists occupying two extreme positions was introduced. In practice, the distribution of power will depend on the policy issue, its significance and the political system in which the policy is being made. A generalized account of how decision making takes place in any political system was also introduced. Although there has been a long debate concerning the manner in which policy decisions are made between rationalists, on the one hand, and incrementalists, on the other, the role that power plays in decision making is incontrovertible. The rational view has often been described as prescriptive (setting out how policies ought to be made) and the incremental view as descriptive (describing how policy is made). Much health policy making is likely to be characterized by mixed scanning and/or muddling through. Understanding the interests of various actors and the manner in which they wield power is therefore intrinsic to an understanding of the policy process and essential for any attempt to influence that process.

References

Bachrach P and Baratz MS (1962) The two faces of power. In Castles FG, Murray DJ and Potter DC (eds) *Decision, Organisations and Society.* Harmondsworth: Penguin.

Bachrach P and Baratz MS (1963) Decisions and nondecisions: an analytical framework. *American Political Science Review* 57: 641–51.

Baumgartner FR and Jones BD (1991) Agenda dynamics and policy subsystems. *The Journal of Politics* 53(4): 1044–74.

Baumgartner FR and Jones BD (1993) *Agendas and Instability in American Politics.* Chicago: University of Chicago Press.

Blair T (2011) Blaming a moral decline for the riots makes good headlines but bad policy. *The Guardian.* 20 August 2011. Available at: http://www.guardian.co.uk/commentisfree/2011/aug/20/tony-blair-riots-crime-family (accessed 25 September 2011).

Center for Responsive Politics (2010) Available at: http://www.opensecrets.org/lobby/indus. php?id=H&year=2010.

Chowdhury Z (1995) *Essential Drugs for the Poor.* London: Zed.

Crenson M (1971) *The Unpolitics of Air Pollution.* Baltimore, MD: The Johns Hopkins University Press.

Dahl RA (1961) *Who Governs? Democracy and Power in an American City.* New Haven, CT: Yale University Press.

Easton D (1965) *A Systems Analysis of Political Life.* New York: Wiley.

Edelman M (1988) *Constructing the Political Spectacle.* Chicago: University of Chicago Press.

Etzioni A (1967) Mixed scanning: a 'third approach' to decision making. *Public Administrative Review* 27: 385–92.

Fukuyama F (1989) The end of history? *National Interest.* Summer, 3–18.

Jorm AF, Christensen H, Griffiths KM and Rodgers B (2002) Effectiveness of complementary and self-help treatments for depression. *Medical Journal of Australia* 176(10 Suppl.): S84–95.

Kessler RC, Soukup J, Davis RB, Foster DF, Wilkey SA, Van Rompay MI and Eisenberg DM (2001) The use of complementary and alternative therapies to treat anxiety and depression in the United States. *American Journal of Psychiatry* 158(2): 289–94.

Kushel M and Bindman AB (2004) Health care lobbying: time to make patients the special interest. *American Journal of Medicine* 116(7): 496–7.

Lakoff G (2004) *Don't Think of an Elephant! Know Your Values and Frame the Debate*. White River Junction, VT: Chelsea Green.

Landers SH and Sehgal AR (2004) Health care lobbying in the United States. *American Journal of Medicine* 116(7): 474–7.

Lang IB and Elkin ED (1997) A study of the beliefs and birthing practices of traditional midwives in rural Guatemala. *Journal of Midwifery and Women's Health* 42(1): 25–31.

Lasswell HD (1936) *Politics: Who Get What, When, How*. New York: McGraw-Hill.

Lee K and Goodman H (2002) Global policy networks: The propagation of health care financing reform since the 1980s. In Lee K, Buse K and Fustukian S (eds) *Health Policy in a Globalising World*. Cambridge: Cambridge University Press, pp. 97–119.

Lindblom CE (1959) The science of muddling through. *Public Administrative Review* 19: 79–88.

Lindblom CE and Woodhouse EJ (1993) *The Policy-Making Process*, 3rd edn. Englewood Cliffs, NJ: Prentice-Hall.

Lukes S (1974) *Power: A Radical Approach*. London: Macmillan.

March JG and Simon HA (1958) *Organizations*. New York: John Wiley and Sons.

Nye JS (2002) *The Paradox of American Power: Why the World's Only Superpower Cannot Go it Alone*. Oxford: Oxford University Press.

Nye JS (2004) *Soft Power: The Means to Success in World Politics*. New York: Public Affairs.

Nye JS (2011) *The Future of Power*. New York: Public Affairs.

Olson M (1971) *The Logic of Collective Action: Public Goods and the Theory of Groups*, rev. edn. Cambridge, MA: Harvard University Press.

Schlosser E (2001) *Fast Food Nation: The Dark Side of the All-American Meal*. Boston: Houghton Mifflin.

Schmid G (2004) Economic and programmatic aspects of congenital syphilis control. *Bulletin of the World Health Organization* 82(6): 402–9.

Shiffman J, Beer T and Wu Y (2002) The emergence of global disease priorities. *Health Policy and Planning* 17(3): 225–34.

Simon HA (1957) *Administrative Behaviour*, 2nd edn. New York: Macmillan.

United Nations (2011) *The Millennium Goals Report*. New York: United Nations. Available at: http://mdgs.un.org/unsd/mdg/Resources/Static/Data/2011%20Stat%20Annex.pdf.

Walt G (1994) *Health Policy: an Introduction to Process and Power*. London: Zed Books.

Weber M (1948) *From Max Weber: Essays in Sociology*. London: Routledge and Kegan Paul.

WHO (2004) *Guidelines on Developing Consumer Information on Proper Use of Complementary and Alternative Medicine*. Geneva: WHO.

Zeltner T, Kessler DA, Martiny A and Randera F (2000) *Tobacco Company Strategies to Undermine Tobacco Control Activities at the World Health Organization*. Geneva: WHO.

The state and the private sector in health policy

3

Overview

This chapter introduces you to two of the most important actors in health policy – the state and the private for-profit sector – although in some situations other actors play influential roles. The chapter traces the changing roles of these two sectors in health policy and thereby provides the context to understanding the content and processes of contemporary health policy making.

Learning objectives

After working through this chapter, you will be better able to:

* understand why the state is at the centre of health policy
* describe and account for the changing role of the state in the past few decades, and what this has implied for the state's role in health policy
* identify a range of private sector organizations with an interest in health policy
* explain how the private sector increasingly influences health policy.

Key terms

Company. Generic term for a business which may be run as a sole proprietorship, partnership or corporation.

Corporation. An association of stockholders (shareholders) which is regarded as a 'person' under most national laws. Ownership is marked by ease of transferability and the limited liability of stockholders.

Decentralization. The transfer of authority and responsibilities from central government to local levels.

Industry. Groups of firms closely related and in competition in a particular sector of the economy due to use of similar technology or producing similar products.

Multinational corporation. Business which controls operations in more than one country, even if it does not own them but operates through a franchise.

New public management. An approach to government involving the application of private sector management techniques.

Private sector. That part of the economy which is not under direct government control.

Privatization. Sale of publicly owned property to the private sector.

Regulation. Government intervention enforcing rules and standards (e.g. in the private sector).

Transnational corporation. Business which owns branch companies in more than one country.

Introduction

This chapter concerns the central yet changing role of the state in health policy. The state is typically a central focus of policy and policy analysis. This is in part the result of its omnipresence and, in part, because it does more than any other body to decide what public policies should be adopted and implemented. Policy decisions of governments extend deeply into people's lives from the relatively trivial to the life-changing. Depending on where you live, the state may, for example:

- decide whether or not divorcees are allowed a second child (allowed in Shanghai but not in the rest of China);
- prohibit private medical practice (Cuba);
- prohibit commercial sex work (116 countries);
- determine the age at which sex-change therapy is allowed (currently 10 years in Australia);
- determine whether or not emergency contraception is available over-the-counter (not available in Austria but available in the UK).

The state may also:

- subject people of different race, ethnicity, or religion to different laws;
- imprison suspected terrorists indefinitely without charge (France) or suspend protections of the Geneva Conventions for enemy combatants (the US).

For much of the twentieth century the state played a dominant role in the economies of most countries: airlines were owned and operated by the state, as were other utilities such as railways, water, electricity, and telephones. Many governments presided over 'command and control' economies in the context of five-year development plans. In many newly independent countries, the government also became the major employer. For example, in Tanzania, the government's workforce grew from 27 per cent of those formally employed in 1962 to over 66 per cent in 1974 (Perkins and Roemer 1991). By the 1980s things began to change; states were 'rolled back' and the private sector was encouraged to enter fields that once had been the preserve of the state – including health care. This shift has had implications both for the content of health policy as well as the actors participating in the health policy process.

In this chapter, you will chart the changes to the roles of the state and private market. The activities of different branches of government in the policy process are explored in greater detail in Chapter 4. The chapter begins by outlining state involvement in health and presents arguments which justify its prominent role. You will then learn why disillusion with the monopoly role of the state has grown over the past three decades and why this has given impetus to a worldwide movement of health sector reform. The emergence of the private for-profit sector in health services is highlighted and three ways that it increasingly affects health policy are illustrated.

The role of the state in health systems

By the early 1980s, the state had assumed a leading place in health care finance and in service delivery in most countries. In addition, it played the central role in allocating resources among competing health priorities and in regulating a range of activities which impinge upon health. To take just one example, think of the role that states might play with respect to the regulation of health care service delivery. Mills and Ranson (2005) have identified a wide range of regulatory mechanisms which have been applied in low and middle income countries.

To regulate the quantity and distribution of services, the state has:

* licensed providers (in all countries) and facilities (increasingly common for hospitals);
* placed controls on the number and size of medical schools (common), controlled the number of doctors practising in certain areas, and limited the introduction of high technology;
* provided incentives for health professionals to practise in rural areas.

To regulate prices of services, governments have:

* negotiated salary scales;
* set charges;
* negotiated reimbursement rates (many social insurance schemes).

To regulate quality of health services, governments have:

* licensed practitioners;
* registered and accredited facilities;
* required providers to establish complaints procedures;
* required provision of information for monitoring quality;
* controlled training curricula;
* set requirements for continuing education.

In addition to the finance, provision and regulation of health services, most states have assumed a range of public health functions, for example, they do the following:

* ensure safe water and food purity;
* establish quarantine and border control measures to curb the spread of infectious diseases;
* regulate roads and workplaces to reduce the threat of injuries;

- legislate to curb environmental and noise pollution;
- set standards for food labelling, the level of lead in petrol, and tar and nicotine in cigarettes;
- regulate and license industries as well as oblige them to adopt different technologies on public health grounds.

You could likely add to the above list which is meant to illustrate the state's deep and wide involvement in health and health policy in the early twenty-first century. This raises the question of how such growth has been justified.

Activity 3.1

The following reviews the rationale for the engagement of the state in health. While reading through the section, makes notes as to the main reasons for such involvement in the health system.

Economists have focused on 'market failure' as the principal reason for a pronounced role for the state in health care finance and provision. Efficient markets depend on a number of conditions. These are often not met because of specific characteristics of health and health services. First, the optimal amount of health services will not always be produced or consumed because the externalities (costs and benefits) are not taken into consideration by consumers or producers. For example, childhood immunization rates in the UK decreased in the 2000s because of parents' decisions. These related to the perceived risks and benefits of protecting their children, as opposed to the benefits of protection of others by reducing the pool of susceptible children. Second, the market will fail to provide many so-called 'public goods' because of the lack of incentives to do so. Public goods are those that are 'non-rival' in consumption (consumption by one person does not affect consumption of the same good by others) and 'non-excludable' (it is not possible to prevent a consumer from benefiting by making them pay), for example, control of mosquito breeding or research knowledge. Third, monopoly power may lead to overcharging. Monopolies could be established by the medical profession, the drug industry or a hospital in a given catchment area. However, some economists argue that the lack of efficient health care markets provides relatively weak justification for state delivery of health services (except in relation to public and preventive health services) as market failure could be dealt with through regulation.

Another argument in favour of a strong state role hinges around the 'information asymmetry' between consumer and providers. Consumers are at a disadvantage and private providers are in an unusually strong position to take advantage of this imbalance through profit seeking and over-treatment. Another characteristic of the health care market is that the need for health care is uncertain and often costly. This provides an argument in favour of insurance. However, experience suggests that private insurance markets do not work well in health. Both of these reasons provide compelling support for state involvement.

Yet it is unlikely that these economic arguments can account entirely for the prominent role of the state in health. If any philosophical principle were invoked, it would likely be related to equity or fairness and the concern that some individuals will be too poor to afford health care, and require the support and protection of the state. This touches on the wider debate on the ethical underpinnings of a health care system.

There are those who argue that health services should be treated similarly to other goods and services for which access depends on ability and willingness to pay. Others argue that access to health care is a right of all citizens, irrespective of their income or wealth.

In practice, the precise role of the state in health service finance and provision has varied significantly between countries, depending on whether or not private markets have developed for insurers and for providers and whether or not the state has taken responsibility for providing some services for the whole population (e.g. India and Zambia) or catered more for the poor (e.g. Mexico and Thailand). Nonetheless, what was uniform across all countries was an expansion of the role of the state in health during the twentieth century, with the state assuming the central and primary responsibility for health services and thereby taking the centre stage for health policy making.

Feedback

The main justifications for state involvement are:

* market failure;
* information asymmetry between consumer and provider;
* need for care uncertain and often costly;
* to achieve equity of access to care.

The critique of the state

Considerable disaffection with the expanded role of the state mounted during the 1980s and led to a reassessment of its appropriate role in the health sector. This happened in the context of a global economic recession, escalating government indebtedness and spiralling public expenditure. Conservative governments came to power which questioned what they saw as bloated and inefficient public sectors presiding over important areas of the economy. Reforms were introduced in many countries which involved liberalizing trade, selling off publicly owned industries, deregulating utilities and private industry, and curbing public expenditure. Tapping into widespread dissatisfaction with state administrations generally, which were often viewed as distant, undemocratic, unresponsive, unaccountable and even corrupt, the idea of 'rolling back' the state spread among high income countries and later to middle and low income countries. International financial institutions, such as the World Bank and the International Monetary Fund, pressured governments to reduce their deficits, and control public expenditure by implementing what were termed 'structural adjustment programmes'. In return for targeted loans and grants, governments promised to reform their economies, principally by privatization and by reducing the involvement and responsibility of the state, particularly in service provision.

The 1980s were marked by a global turn in favour of the market, with a concomitant scepticism about the merits of pursuing equity through government action. The collapse of the Soviet Union at the end of the decade further discredited the notion of centrally planned, state-controlled economies. Anti-state, pro-market philosophy was promoted around the world by international agencies and private foundations. They, often rightly, claimed that the public sector provided patronage instead of service, employment rather than goods and services, and used office to secure political support. As proof, they pointed to poorly performing, costly and overstaffed bureaucracies, providing inadequate service in disintegrating facilities.

These trends were reflected in the health sector and led to a movement for health sector reform (Roberts et al. 2004). The state was widely regarded as having failed to provide services for everyone, despite rising levels of expenditure. Political pressures had resulted in public finance of health services which were not cost-effective while more cost-effective services were not widely provided. The political demands of the economic elite and the self-interest of urban-based bureaucrats resulted in a disproportionate allocation of resources to urban tertiary facilities at the expense of basic services for the bulk of the population. Poor management decreased the efficiency of services and resulted in problems such as lack of continuous drug supplies. In many low income countries, inadequate finance meant poor equipment, poorly paid staff, leading to poor quality care. Public providers were often absent from their posts (sometimes attending illegal private practice), poorly motivated, seen as unresponsive and charging patients illicit fees for services that governments proclaimed were freely available to all. Those people who required publicly financed services failed to access them while those who were politically connected were able to capture this state subsidy. Many, including the poor in the poorest countries, were in practice relying heavily on the private sector – often facing catastrophic payments to do so.

Reinvention of government and health sector reform

Given the widespread problems experienced in the sector, it is not surprising that the idea and narrative of reform were seized upon so readily. Yet the means for reform were greatly influenced by the prevailing ideology of the appropriate role for the state in the delivery of public health services. The state was to be slimmed down, health provision was to be made more efficient by introducing competition and decentralizing decision making, and the private sector was to be afforded a much larger role (Harding 2003).

Neo-liberal economic thinking was brought to bear to understand the root causes of the malaise in the health sector and greatly influenced prescriptions on the appropriate role for the state. Two theories stand out: public choice and property rights. *Public choice*, discussed in Chapter 2, deals with the nature of decision making in government. It argues that politicians and bureaucrats behave like other participants in the political system in that they pursue their own interests. Consequently, politicians can be expected to promote policies which will maximize their chances of re-election while bureaucrats can be expected to attempt to maximize their budgets because budget size affects bureaucrats' rewards either in terms of salary, status or opportunities to engage in corruption. As a result of these perverse incentives, the public sector is deemed to be wasteful and not concerned with efficiency or equity. *Property rights* theorists explained poor public sector performance through the absence of property rights. They argue that in the private sector, owners of property rights, whether owners of firms or shareholders, have strong incentives to maximize efficiency of resource use as the returns to investment depend upon efficiency. In contrast, such pressure does not arise in the public sector; staff may perform poorly at no cost to themselves, resulting in a poorly performing systems overall. Civil servants, it is argued, have few reasons to do well because they cannot benefit personally from goal performance, unlike in a business. Both theories draw attention to the interests and therefore incentives which motivate state officials and how these affect the policies that they pursue.

Beliefs based on these theories gave rise to proposals to curb the state – to radically contain public expenditure – but also to introduce 'new public management' in those areas of the health sector which were not privatized. It was 'new' in the sense that it sought to expose public services to market pressures by establishing 'internal markets' within the public sector. Internal markets were established by forcing public providers (e.g., general practitioner groups or hospitals) to compete for contracts from public purchasers, contracting out service provision by competitive tendering (for hospital catering and cleaning services, for example) and devolving significant decision making to subordinate organizations, particularly making hospitals more autonomous, and to lower levels of government. These reforms involved the creation of purchasing agencies and the introduction of contractual relationships between purchasers and providers within the public sector.

In addition to reforms within public administration, new mechanisms to finance health care were put on the policy agenda (such as out-of-pocket fees for service use), restrictions on private providers were lifted, diversity of provider ownership in the health sector was promoted, and efforts were made to improve the accountability of providers to consumers, patients and communities.

Decentralization, another popular reform, aimed to transfer the balance of power within the state. In one form, functions held by the ministry of health were transferred to newly established executive agencies which assumed management responsibility at the national level. The ministry could then focus its efforts on policy and oversight. In other cases, authority was transferred to district or local levels. Decentralization distributes power from the ministry of health to other organizations.

Although the state was slimmed down in many countries in the course of such reforms, it is almost universally agreed that the state ought to (and often does) retain a variety of functions. On the one hand, governments need to 'steward' the sector. Stewardship involves safeguarding population health by developing policy, setting and enforcing standards, rationing and setting priorities for resource allocation, establishing a regulatory framework, and monitoring the behaviour of providers. On the other hand, governments need to 'enable' – whether that is enabling the private sector to deliver quality services or ensuring the fair financing of service provision through tax or mandatory insurance in high income countries and targeting public expenditure towards the poor in low and middle income countries. These functions were characteristics of 'good governance', and were proposed to overcome lack of transparency, accountability and weak legal systems. For example, transparency required open competition for public contracts; accountability demanded effective financial accounting and auditing, but also penalties for corruption; and they both had to be framed by a predictable, independent and competent judicial system.

The World Bank was highly influential in promoting these reforms in low income countries, both through policy advice and through conditions attached to loans and grants. While these reforms were nothing short of revolutionary in their intent, they had mixed results. Although most governments embraced reform, at least rhetorically, few managed successfully to implement them. Implementation also sometimes resulted in unanticipated consequences (see Chapter 7). For example, while user fees for public services were introduced primarily to raise resources, they were not very successful in this regard but often had a negative impact on the use of services. Arrangements to protect the poor from charges were difficult to administer. In China, reforms resulted in fewer people being covered by health insurance. While over 70 per cent of the population had some form of health insurance in 1981 (including almost half of the rural population), by 1993 the level had fallen to 21 per cent, with 7 per cent coverage of the rural population. These reforms were eventually reversed and, as a result, by 2011, 95 per cent of the population was once again covered by basic medical insurance. In the UK, the Conservative government introduced the Public Finance Initiative (PFI) in the early 1990s. It was a scheme for the construction and management of public infrastructure such as hospitals influenced by property rights thinking. The idea was that the private sector would build, own and operate new facilities, and lease them back to the state for a defined period. The theory was that the cost to the state would be reduced since private owners would have incentives to build and operate the facilities more efficiently than the state because of their ownership stake. PFI schemes in the NHS have had mixed success. Many have tied NHS hospitals into long-term, unnecessarily costly and inflexible deals with the private sector. Others have produced new facilities that might never have been built through conventional public sector procurement.

Activity 3.2

Make a list of some of the health reforms which have been discussed or introduced during the past decade in your country. See if you can find reference to each of the reforms listed above and, if possible others, using Table 3.1. Depending on your general knowledge of health reform in your country, you may need to do some research. If you live in a low or middle income country, one approach to gathering the information would be to consult the World Bank's website where you can search for analytic or project lending reports (staff appraisal reports) for your country. If you live in a high income country, you can refer to the European Observatory on Health Systems and Policies (www.euro.who.int/observatory) which covers a number of countries outside of Europe as well, or the Organization for Economic Cooperation and Development (OECD) (www.oecd.org).

Table 3.1 Health reform checklist

Health reform	Yes	No
Liberalizing laws on private providers		
Introducing user fees and strategies to exempt poor		
Introducing community-based insurance		
Introducing social health insurance		
Creation of purchasing agencies		
Introducing contractual relationships and management agreements between purchasers and providers		
Decentralizing health services		
Decentralizing hospital management		
Encouraging competition and entry of more diverse providers		
Giving patients more choice over where they are treated and the nature of their care		
Paying providers for services delivered		
Paying providers for performance (e.g. according to achievement of quality standards)		

Feedback

It is not likely that you ticked 'yes' to all reforms, as the content of reforms differ across countries. Nevertheless, it is likely that you identified a number of them, as virtually no health system has remained untouched by such reforms.

The health care reform movement highlights the power of ideas and ideology in policy change. Yet reforms have provoked significant resistance. Some opposition was philosophical and ideological in nature. Many questioned the lack of evidence upon which reforms were based as well as the imposition of 'blueprints' developed by international experts without due consideration of national and local context (Lee et al. 2002). In fact, reforms were more often resisted on the basis of the costs that they imposed on the incomes and interests of those actors who benefited from the prevailing system. Consequently, successive rounds of reforms were rolled out unevenly across countries, with considerable evidence of limited progress and poor results, leaving the process largely unfinished in many countries (Roberts et al. 2004). Part of the failure of reform programmes rested on the disproportionate emphasis placed on the technical content of reform at the expense of understanding the politics of the reform process.

Yet reforms continue to be announced. For example, despite a very difficult financial situation and historically high levels of performance, in 2010, the Coalition government in the UK announced further radical organizational changes to the English NHS designed to turn the publicly financed system into a fully fledged provider market on the grounds that greater patient choice and competition were the best way to continue improving the service (Department of Health 2010). The changes proposed succeeded in mobilizing opposition from a wide range of political, professional and public actors and were regarded by many as a distraction from managing the system.

The for-profit sector and health policy

The assault on the state in the 1980s and 1990s provided an opportunity for the private for-profit sector to become more engaged in health policy. While the private sector was already providing health services in many countries, it was usually overlooked in relation to its influence on health policy and regulation. This is surprising because it is difficult to identify health policies in which the private sector does not have an interest or play some role. But what exactly is the for-profit sector and how is it involved in health policy? The following provides a brief overview of the types of private sector actors in health and differentiates the three main ways that the private sector is involved in health policy.

What is the private sector?

The private for-profit (or commercial) sector is characterized by its market orientation. It encompasses organizations that seek to make profits for their owners. Profit, or a return on investment, is the central defining feature of the commercial sector. Many firms pursue additional objectives related, for example, to social, environmental or employee concerns but these are, of necessity, secondary and supportive of the primary profit interest. In the absence of profit, and a return to shareholders, firms cease to exist.

For-profit organizations vary considerably. The sector consists of firms which may be large or small, domestic or multinational. In the health sector there are single doctor's surgeries and large group practices, pharmacies, generic drug manufacturers and major research and development pharmaceutical companies, medical equipment suppliers, logistics companies, management consultancies and private hospitals and nursing homes.

When thinking about the role of the commercial sector in health policy, it is often useful to broaden the scope of analysis to include some organizations that are registered as not-for-profit in their legal status. These may have charitable status but are established to support the interests of a firm or industry. These may include business associations or trade federations. For example, both PhRMA (American Pharmaceutical Manufacturers Association) and BIO, the biotechnology industry organization, are engaged in various health policy processes to promote the economic interests of their member firms.

A wide range of industry-funded think tanks, 'scientific' organizations, advocacy groups (such as patient groups) and even public relations firms working for industry are actors engaged in the health policy arena. For example, the tobacco company, Philip Morris, established the Institute of Regulatory Policy as a vehicle to lobby the US federal government and delay the publication of a report by the Environmental Protection Agency on environmental tobacco smoke (Muggli et al. 2004). The International Life Sciences Institute (ILSI), established in 1978, was envisioned by its first President as a mini-World Health Organization. It describes itself as a 'Global Partnership for a Safer, Healthier World' which employs strategic alliances to bring scientific solutions to public health issues, particularly in areas such as diet, tobacco and alcohol. While it is at pains to present itself as a scientific body, its first President served simultaneously as a Vice-President of the Coca-Cola Company and it is predominantly funded by the food industry. It has gone to great lengths to conceal the commercial sponsorship of its research and publications, and present itself as scholarly and independent (James 2002).

Industry also organizes and supports patient groups to influence health policy decisions of governments. For example, 'Action for Access' was set up by Biogen in 1999 to lobby the UK National Health Service to provide interferon beta for multiple sclerosis patients (Boseley 1999). Many mental health patient advocacy groups are supported by the pharmaceutical industry in the US. As one trade industry publication put it, such groups help drug companies to 'diffuse industry critics by delivering positive messages about the healthcare contributions of pharma companies to legislators, the media, and other key stakeholders' (Cox 2002). In some health policy debates, public relations firms play important roles. Firms are employed to put across industry views, through the media or other means, as apparently disinterested third parties with the aim of influencing policy.

Looser groups supported by industry can also be influential in the health policy process. ARISE (Associates for Research into the Science of Enjoyment), promotes the pleasures of smoking, alcohol, caffeine and chocolate. With support from companies such as British American Tobacco, Coca-Cola, Philip Morris, RJR, Rothmans, Miller Beer and Kraft, it publishes articles that promote and advocate consumer freedom in relation to those substances and deride the necessity of public regulation. One publication called *Bureaucracy against Life: The Politicisation of Personal Choice* attacks the European Community for 'paternalistic' restriction of individual choice in connection with 'the alleged dangers associated with alcohol, tobacco, caffeine and an increasing range of foods'.

Activity 3.3

Look at the business section of a national or international newspaper. Find examples of each of the types of commercial organizations listed below with a linkage to a health issue (either due to the goods or services they manufacture, promote, distribute, sell or regulate). Provide one or two examples of each category of commercial entity, the health issue in which they have an interest, what they manufacture, distribute, sell, or promote, and the relationship of these goods or services to health (either positive or negative). Also, see if you can find any references to less formal commercial organizations – this may be more difficult. You may need to scan newspapers for a few days to get an example of each type of organization.

The types of organization to consider are:

- Small firm
- Multinational corporation or transnational corporation
- Business association
- Professional association
- Think tank
- Patients' group
- Commercial scientific network
- Public relations firm
- Loose network.

Feedback

It should be evident that a wide range of organizations associated with the private sector are interested and involved in health policy in your country. It may also be evident from the business news that these organizations vary tremendously in relation to their size (by staff, sales or market capitalization – value on the stock exchange), organizational form and interest in particular health policies.

What makes the private sector a powerful actor in health policy?

Power is the ability to achieve a desired result. Resources often confer power and, on that basis, the power of some industries and firms may be obvious to you. Of the top 100 'economic entities' in the world, 63 are countries, but 37 are firms when measured by revenues. Figure 3.1 compares the market value of ten of the largest companies in the world, ten leading pharmaceutical firms, with the gross national income of those low income countries for which there was data in 2010. Note how the firms dwarf the size of the collective economies of the poorest countries. The revenue of the top 50 pharmaceutical firms amounted to over US$590 billion in 2010 – marking a major increase over the past decade (from US$296 billion in 2002). The increase came about in part due to consolidation in the industry which makes individual firms much larger and more powerful than in the past (Cacciotti and Clinton 2011). Big pharma only constitutes one element of the private sector with health interests. Firms representing the makers of snacks, drinks and cigarettes were active in the run-up to the first ever UN General Assembly meeting on non-communicable diseases as they saw their estimated worldwide sales of over US$2 trillion at stake. Contrast the magnitude of

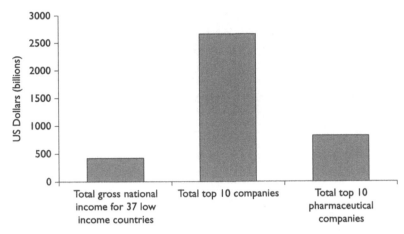

Figure 3.1 Market capitalization of largest companies (2011) compared with the gross national income of 37 low income countries (2010)

Sources: World Bank (2011); DeCarlo (2011)

corporate sales with the annual budget of WHO: approximately US$2 billion – a figure which has remained stagnant in real terms for years.

Firms provide governments with tax revenues, some are major employers in the economy, and governments gain influence in international affairs on the coat-tails of their large corporations and are therefore interested in their success. In many sectors, firms have specialist knowledge which governments rely on in making policy. For these reasons, small and large businesses are often important actors in policy debates.

How is the private sector involved in health policy?

In Chapter 1, a distinction between public and private policy was made. You learned that the private sector develops policy related to health – whether it is a firm setting down rules for its staff (e.g., on sick leave) or an industry federation establishing policies for its members (e.g., in relation to environmental pollution). This is one way that the private sector is involved in health policy, through self-regulation. You will now explore private health policy making in further detail looking at two mechanisms – self-regulation and co-regulation – as well as consider how the private sector engages with public policy.

Self-regulation

Self-regulation concerns efforts by private companies to establish their own rules and policies for operating within a specific domain. For example, rules governing how to design, categorize, produce and handle particular goods and services are routinely adopted by groups of companies and industries. Self-regulation ranges from codes of conduct on advertising (which, for example, might restrict advertising of unhealthy products to children) to standards governing voltages within medical equipment.

One can distinguish between two types of self-regulation. First are those which attempt to regulate what are termed private 'market' standards and, second, the regulation of 'social standards'. In the case of market standards, aspects of products, process and business practice are subject to self-regulation for the purpose of facilitating commerce. Common standards support business by reducing transaction costs, ensuring compatibility, and creating fair competition for all firms in the market. Companies may support self-regulation in relation to codes of conduct on advertising: for example, agreeing to restrict advertising of unhealthy products to children.

Self-regulation through social standards is generally undertaken in response to concerns raised by consumers, shareholders, or to the threat of impending public regulation which may be more onerous. Initiatives include corporate social responsibility, voluntary codes and reporting initiatives, and some corporate philanthropic programmes. These initiatives sometimes govern social issues that are already subject to (often ineffective) statutory regulation.

Company and industry-wide codes of conduct represent one increasingly prominent form of self-regulation through social standards. Voluntary codes cover a variety of corporate practices that are important determinants of health. Depending on your line of work, you may be aware of voluntary codes which cover such aspects as occupational health and safety, wages and hours, minimum age of work and forced labour. The promise and perils of voluntary self-regulatory codes are set out below to allow you to judge whether or not they are good substitutes for public regulation.

It is relatively easy to understand why firms and industries adopt voluntary codes governing social issues. First, by doing so, firms are often able to generate public relations material and improve their corporate image. Second, early adoption of a code can differentiate a firm from a competitor and thereby increase its market share. Third, adoption of codes in response to consumer or shareholder demand permits firms to demonstrate that they listen, which may, in turn, boost sales and investment. Depending on the issue, codes can be used to stave off consumer boycotts and also public regulation. As you can see, there is a market logic to codes.

Codes can also be good for society. First, the introduction of a standard by one firm or a group of firms can compel other firms to adopt similar standards so as to prevent the loss of market share. By pulling up the laggards, leading firms can ratchet up standards across an industry. Second, in some contexts, compliance with voluntary codes may be more effective than compliance with statutory public regulation. The theory is that companies adopt codes so as to gain market share and comply with them so as not to lose the confidence of their consumers/shareholders. Third, codes are promoted as curbing government expenditure on public regulation.

At first glance, codes appear to benefit all but closer inspection reveals some weaknesses in this form of private policy making. One analyst concludes that 'corporate codes of conduct are treated with disdain and largely dismissed by knowledgeable and influential opinion leaders among various stakeholder groups, as well as by outside analysts and the public-at-large' (Sethi 1999).

Activity 3.4

Based on your general knowledge of codes, take the following test to see if you can deduce why Sethi made such pessimistic remarks:

1 Do codes typically:

(a) enunciate general principles; or

(b) provide specific standards (i.e. quantifiable and measurable indicators)?

2. Do codes typically:

(a) focus on concerns of consumers in high income countries (e.g. child labour, or pesticide residue on organic fruit); or

(b) focus on concerns of local employees (e.g. right to collective bargaining, pesticide exposure)?

3 Is code compliance likely to be:

(a) divorced from reward structure, operating procedures, or corporate culture; or

(b) linked to internal reward structures in the company (are there incentives to ensure that the code is implemented)?

4 Do companies typically make public:

(a) mainly those aspects of the findings which are favourable; or

(b) the process by which they seek to comply with the code and the findings related to the code?

5 Is reporting of code implementation typically:

(a) handled internally by the company; or

(b) subject to external scrutiny?

Feedback

While there are undoubtedly exceptions to the rule, Sethi (1999) concludes that codes typically comprise lofty statements of intent, are largely responsive to consumer pressure and therefore highlight issues in consumer-sensitive industries (e.g. clothing) while ignoring many others, and that companies tend to lack the means to communicate compliance with the code in reliable and believable ways. The correct answers are all (a).

A review of voluntary codes of pharmaceutical marketing concluded that they lacked transparency and public accountability because consumers were not involved in monitoring and enforcement, they omitted major areas of concern, and lacked timely and effective sanctions (Lexchin and Kawachi 1996). Similarly, a former Executive Director of WHO argued that self-regulation in the case of tobacco manufacturing and smoke-free policies 'failed miserably' (Yach 2004).

Another problematic aspect of voluntary codes relates to their reliance on company 'commitment' to stakeholders. Undertaking to voluntarily uphold a particular principle is qualitatively distinct from being held accountable under law to ensuring specific rights, for example, of people affected by company operations. As a consequence, patchwork self-regulation results in 'enclave' social policy which governs select issues and groups of workers at a specific point in their working lives (e.g. only those workers in a specific plant and only while they hold their jobs). Some fear that these self-regulatory efforts will erode societal commitment to universal rights and entitlements.

In summary, an increasing number of self-regulatory mechanisms are being adopted by the business community in areas which affect health. Private actors are involved in policy formulation, adoption and implementation, often without reference to state actors. While private policy may promote health, it may also have negative impacts. Consequently, the need for public regulation remains.

The private sector and public policy

In the following chapters you will learn more about how the government makes and implements public policy – and you will read many examples that illustrate the involvement of the private sector in the process. The private sector is often affected by public policy and, as a result, may attempt to influence the content of such policy. The private sector wields influence in a number of ways. Firms will often provide finance to political parties and to political campaigns in the hope that once those parties and politicians are in office, they will be more responsive to demands that firms may make in the policy process.

Private organizations will also lobby for or against particular policies. Influence can also be wielded through corporate participation in government committees and working groups. Moreover, corporate executives also compete for public office, and, if successful, may take positions in line with business interests. Large corporations may also take legal action to shape public policy. For example, in 2011, five tobacco companies filed a lawsuit against the US Food and Drug Administration over its requirement to include graphic depictions of the harms of smoking on all cigarette packs. The manufacturers claimed that being forced to put disturbing images on their packs violated their free speech rights and forced them to become a 'mini-billboard for the government's antismoking campaign' (http://legaltimes.typepad.com/files/motion-for-summary-judgment.pdf).

Co-regulation

Co-regulation presents an apparent 'third way' between statutory regulation and self-regulation. It may be viewed as public sector involvement in business self-regulation. The idea is that public and private sectors will negotiate an agreed set of policy or regulatory objectives. Subsequently, the private sector will take responsibility for implementation of the provisions. Monitoring compliance may remain a public responsibility or may be contracted out to a third party – sometimes a non-governmental watchdog. Co-regulatory initiatives often involve public, private and civil society actors working in partnership.

Co-regulation is relatively new, with limited experience at the national and regional levels. For example, in the UK, the Advertising Standards Authority has a range of sanctions against misleading advertisements which is backed up by statutory regulations of the Office of Fair Trading which can secure a High Court injunction to prevent a company publishing the same or similar advertisements. In other words, the statutory backing gives the self-regulatory code teeth. The European Union is also experimenting with co-regulation particularly with respect to the Internet, journalism and e-commerce.

The Public Health Responsibility Deal in England is a distinctive form of co-regulation. It was established by the Coalition government in 2010 to tap into the potential for businesses and other organizations to improve public health and tackle health inequalities through their influence over food, alcohol, physical activity and health in the workplace (Department of Health 2011). Businesses signing up to the Responsibility Deal commit to take action to improve public health. This action is expressed as a series of negotiated pledges signed by individual firms covering food, alcohol, physical activity and health at work that are intended to complement government action. For example, one of the specific pledges in relation to alcohol developed by industry and approved by the Department of Health is as follows: 'We will ensure that over 80% of products on shelf (by December 2013) will have labels with clear unit content, NHS guidelines and a warning about drinking when pregnant.' The Responsibility Deal is based on the assumption that encouraging businesses to become leaders in their sector will bring about progress faster than government regulation.

Summary

In this chapter you have learned why the state is considered the most important actor in policy making. While it is important to understand the role of the state in policy making, an analysis focused entirely on the state is no longer sufficient. This is because the role of the state has changed and the private sector now features more prominently in health policy making – either independently or in association with the state. The increasing number and profile of public–private partnerships in the health sector reflect these changes and is a subject of discussion in Chapter 8.

References

Boseley S (1999) Drug firm asks public to insist NHS buy its product. *The Guardian*. 29 September.

Cacciotti P and Clinton J (2011) 12th *Annual Pharma Exec 50*. Available at http://pharmexec.findpharma.com/pharmexec/article/articleDetail.jsp?id=719596&pageID=1&sk=&date (accessed 1 September 2011).

Cox T (2002) Forging Alliances Advocacy partners, *Pharmaceutical Executive*. September.

DeCarlo S (2011) The world's 25 most valuable companies: Apple is no longer on top. *Forbes*. Available at: http://www.forbes.com/sites/scottdecarlo/2011/08/11/the-worlds-25-most-valuable-companies-apple-is-now-on-top/ (accessed 1 September 2011).

Department of Health (2010) *Equity and excellence: liberating the NHS*. Cm 7881. London: The Stationery Office.

Department of Health (2011) *The Public Health Responsibility Deal*. London: Department of Health.

Financial Times (2000) *Human Development Report 2000*. FT500, 4 May.

Harding A (2003) Introduction to private participation in health services. In Harding A and Preker AS (eds) *Private Participation in Health Services*. Washington, DC: The World Bank, pp. 7–74.

James JE (2002) Third-party threats to research integrity in public–private partnerships. *Addiction* 97: 1251–5.

Lee K, Buse K and Fustukian S (eds) (2002) *Health Policy in a Globalising World*. Cambridge: Cambridge University Press.

Lexchin J and Kawachi I (1996) Voluntary codes of pharmaceutical marketing: controlling promotion or licensing deception? In Davis P (ed.) *Contested Ground: Public Purpose and Private Interest in the Regulation of Prescription Drugs*. New York: Oxford University Press, pp. 221–35.

Mills AJ and Ranson MK (2005) The design of health systems. In Merson MH, Black RE and Mills AJ (eds) *International Public Health: Disease, Programs, Systems and Policies*. Sudbury, MA: Jones and Bartlett.

Muggli ME, Hurt RD and Repace J (2004) The tobacco industry's political efforts to derail the EPA report on ETS. *American Journal of Preventive Medicine* 26(2): 167–77.

Perkins D and Roemer M (1991) *The Reform of Economic Systems in Developing Countries*. Cambridge, MA: Harvard University Press.

Roberts MJ, Hsiao W, Berman P and Reich MR (2004) *Getting Health Reform Right: A Guide to Improving Performance and Equity*. Oxford: Oxford University Press.

Sethi PS (1999) Codes of conduct for multinational corporations: an idea whose time has come. *Business and Society Review* 104(3): 225–41.

World Bank (2011) *World Development Indicators Database*. Available at: http://siteresources.worldbank.org/DATASTATISTICS/Resources/GNIPC.pdf (accessed 1 July 2011).

Yach D (2004) Politics and health. *Development* 47(2): 5–10.

4 Agenda setting

Overview

This chapter looks at how issues are identified as a matter of concern for policy making. Why do some issues gain attention to the extent that action is likely to be taken? According to the simple 'stages model' of the policy process introduced in Chapter 1, problem identification is the first step in the process of changing and implementing policy. However, it can be surprisingly difficult to explain how and why some issues become prominent in the eyes of policy makers and others recede from view. In terms of the health 'policy triangle', also set out in Chapter 1, the explanation most often relates to changes in the policy context which enable the policy actors concerned to change policy by persuading others that action should be taken. Objective conditions, such as changes in disease patterns, rarely straightforwardly determine the health policy agenda. The focus in this chapter will be mainly on government policy making and why governments choose to act on some issues but not on others. The chapter also looks at the range of interest groups that contribute to agenda setting, paying particular attention to the role of the mass media since they often play an important part in shaping issues so that they are more or less likely to find their way onto the policy agenda.

Learning objectives

After working through this chapter, you will be better able to:

* define what is meant by the *policy agenda*
* understand different explanations as to how issues get onto the policy agenda and how certain issues get priority for policy development over others
* compare the respective roles of a range of interest groups in setting the policy agenda.

Key terms

Agenda setting. Process by which certain issues come onto the policy agenda from the much larger number of issues potentially worthy of attention by policy makers.

Feasibility. A characteristic of those issues for which there is a practical solution.

Legitimacy. A characteristic of those issues which policy makers see as appropriate for government to act on.

Policy agenda. List of issues to which an organization, usually the government, is giving serious attention at any one time with a view to taking some sort of action.

Policy stream. The set of possible policy solutions or alternatives developed by experts, politicians, bureaucrats and interest groups, together with the activities of those interested in these options (e.g. debates between researchers).

Policy windows. Points in time when the opportunity arises for an issue to come onto the policy agenda and be taken seriously with a view to action.

Politics stream. Political events such as shifts in the national mood or public opinion, elections and changes in government, social uprisings, demonstrations and campaigns by interest groups.

Problem stream. Indicators of the scale and significance of an issue which give it visibility.

Support. A characteristic of those issues to which the public and other key political interests want to see a response.

What is the policy agenda?

The word 'agenda' can be used in a number of different ways, for example, to describe the formal sequence of business to be conducted at a meeting. At other times, people are accused of having a 'hidden agenda', meaning that they have ulterior motives for their actions. In relation to public policy making, the term agenda means something rather different, namely:

> the list of subjects or problems to which government officials and people outside of government closely associated with those officials, are paying some serious attention at any given time ... Out of the set of all conceivable subjects or problems to which officials could be paying attention, they do in fact seriously attend to some rather than others.
>
> (Kingdon 2010)

Activity 4.1

List some of the health-related subjects or problems that you are aware of to which the government in your country has recently paid serious attention. If you cannot remember any, have a look at the news reports for the last few months to see which health issues and policies are mentioned. This may provide an indication of the issues on, or near the agenda.

Feedback

Out of the potentially wide range of health and related issues that the government could be attending to, there is usually a shorter list of 'hot' topics actively under discussion and thus on the agenda. For example, the government could be concerned about combating non-communicable diseases such as diabetes, reducing trends in sexually transmitted disease, providing care for frail older people, improving the recruitment and retention of nurses in hospitals, boosting the immunization rate in remote rural areas, or deciding whether nurses should be able to prescribe essential drugs.

Obviously the list of problems under active consideration varies from one section of the government to another. The president or prime minister will be considering major items such as the state of the economy or relations with other countries. The minister and ministry of health will have a more specialized agenda which may include a few 'high politics' issues, such as whether a system of national health insurance should be established, as well as a larger number of 'low politics' issues such as whether a particular drug should be approved for use and, if so, whether or not it should be paid for as part of the publicly financed health care system.

Why do issues get onto the policy agenda?

Sometimes it is obvious why policy makers take particular issues seriously and then act upon their understanding of them. For instance, if a country is invaded, the government will rapidly recognize this as a problem requiring a government response. It will then act to mobilize the armed forces to attempt to repel the invader. But this sort of appreciation and reaction to a crisis are not typical of most policy making. Most policy making is, as Grindle and Thomas (1991) put it, 'politics-as-usual changes': a response to routine, day-to-day problems that need solutions. Given that there are always more such problems being publicly discussed than government has time, energy and resources to give them, where does the impetus for change or response to a particular problem come from when there is no crisis?

Agenda setting in 'politics-as-usual' circumstances

Early explanations of what constituted a public problem, as against something that individuals and families would have to deal with themselves, assumed that problems existed purely in objective terms and were simply waiting to be recognized by government acting in a rational manner, for example, because the problems threatened the well-being of the population and the role of the government was to protect the population (see Chapter 2 for more on the rational model of policy making). According to this explanation, governments would actively scan the horizon and the most 'important' issues would become the subject of discussion followed by policy attention (e.g. in health terms, government would focus on the diseases responsible for the greatest share of illness, death and disability). A more sophisticated variant of this approach was to argue that what got onto the policy agenda was more a function of long-term changes in socio-economic conditions which produced a set of problems to which governments had to respond eventually, even if there had been no systematic assessment of potential policy problems. From this perspective, countries with ageing populations will have to respond eventually to the implications for retirement pensions, health services, long-term care, transport, and so on.

Later political scientists and sociologists emphasized the importance of power and ideas rather than the more rational process of problem identification and discussion (see Chapter 2 for more on power). Ideas matter because recognizing something as a problem for government to respond to involves defining what is 'normal' in a society and thus what is an unacceptable deviation from that position (Berger and Luckman 1975). This perspective draws attention to the ideologies and assumptions within which governments operate and how they shape what is defined as an issue for government attention as well as how it is regarded. The manner and form in which problems are understood and described (or 'framed') are important influences on how they will eventually be tackled by policy makers (Cobb and Elder 1983). So, for example, if the problem of people with mental illness is largely 'framed' by the media in terms of the risk they pose to themselves, this will have quite different consequences for the way in which mental health enters the policy agenda than if the problem is articulated as one of protecting the public from the threat of violence from people with mental illness. In neither scenario are the prevalence and incidence of mental illness central to the question of whether the issue will get taken seriously and the priority it will receive. This perspective recognizes that not everyone will necessarily agree on how a phenomenon should be framed (i.e. what sort of a problem is this?) and whether it should be a matter for government action. Important policy actors can clash and compete in attempting to persuade government not only to put an issue on the agenda but also in the way they wish to see it presented and dealt with. For example, rival 'frames' are apparent in the way that HIV/AIDS is conceived. Rushing (1995) identifies three different conceptions:

• archaic – HIV/AIDS as a punishment for moral failings attracting stigma;
• metaphorical – HIV/AIDS as something to be fought against as in a 'war';
• medical scientific – a range of conceptions from fatal to chronic disease, virus to sexually transmitted infection, etc.

Rushing notes how these 'frames' have affected the response over time. For example, the first two conceptions tend to be associated with discriminatory and exclusionary approaches to tackling HIV/AIDS.

There are a number of theoretical models of agenda setting that attempt to make sense of these processes. Two of the most prominent and widely used are described now.

The Hall et al. model: legitimacy, feasibility and support

This approach proposes that only when an issue and likely response are high in terms of their *legitimacy, feasibility* and *support* do they get on to a government agenda. Hall and colleagues provided a simple, quick to apply model for analysing which issues might be taken up by governments (Hall et al. 1975).

Legitimacy is a characteristic of those issues with which governments believe they should be concerned and in which they have a right or even obligation to intervene. At the high end of a spectrum of legitimacy, most citizens in most societies would expect the government to keep law and order and to defend the country from attack. There would be more debate about the role of government in other issues such as whether it was necessary for the government to own hospitals to ensure that care was provided equitably.

Activity 4.2

Briefly list those health-related government policies and programmes that are generally regarded as highly legitimate.

Feedback

Probably the most widely accepted role for government in relation to health is to act to reduce the risk of infectious disease becoming established and spreading through the population. Another is regulating air and water pollution. Even in these areas, there is usually some debate about the precise nature and limits of government action.

However, there are many other areas where legitimacy is contentious. Legitimacy varies greatly from country to country and changes over time. Things that were not seen as the domain of government regulation in the past (e.g. control of smoking in workplaces) are now increasingly accepted as legitimate and vice versa (e.g. relaxation of laws prohibiting homosexual activity in many countries). Typically, in times of perceived external threats, the public and politicians are more willing to curb individual liberties because they believe that such actions will protect the community from worse harm.

Feasibility refers to the potential for implementing the policy. It is defined by prevailing technical and theoretical knowledge, resources, availability of skilled staff, administrative capability and existence of the necessary infrastructure of government. There may be technological, financial or workforce limitations that suggest that a particular policy may be impossible to implement, regardless of how legitimate it is seen to be. If a potential policy cannot be shown to pass a test of feasibility, it is unlikely to find its way onto the policy agenda.

Activity 4.3

Which policies would you like to introduce into the health system in your country but which are likely to face major feasibility problems?

Feedback

You may have made all sorts of suggestions. One common one is to try to achieve geographical equity of provision and use of health services since this commonly encounters the reluctance of health care professionals to work in 'less desirable' areas such as remote, rural locations. Another common feasibility problem relates to health care financing in low income countries. Their governments may wish to introduce more public finance into their health care systems to improve coverage but frequently lack robust tax systems to raise the revenue because so many people work in the informal sector of the economy.

Finally, *support* refers to the elusive but important issue of public support for government, at least in relation to the issue in question. Clearly, more authoritarian and non-elected regimes are less dependent on popular support than democratic governments but even dictatorships have to ensure that there is some support among key groups, such as the armed forces, for their policies. If support is lacking, or discontent with the government as a whole is high, it may be very difficult for a government to put an issue on the agenda and do anything about it (see Easton's model of the political system in Chapter 3).

Thus, the logic of Hall and colleagues' model is that governments will estimate whether an issue falls at the high or low end of the three continua of legitimacy, feasibility and support. If an issue has high legitimacy (government is seen as having the right to intervene), high feasibility (there are sufficient resources, personnel, infrastructure), and high support (the most important interest groups are supportive – or at least not obstructive), then the odds of the issue reaching the policy agenda and faring well subsequently are greatly increased.

Of course, this does not rule out more tactical reasons for putting an issue onto the policy agenda. Sometimes, governments will publicly state their position on a particular issue to demonstrate that they care, or to appease donors who demand a response as a condition of aid, or to confound the political opposition, even when they do not expect to be able to translate their concern into a policy that could be implemented because it has low feasibility and/or support.

The Kingdon model: 'policy windows' and three 'streams' within the policy process

John Kingdon's (2010) approach focuses on the role of policy 'entrepreneurs' inside and outside government who take advantage of agenda setting opportunities – known as *policy windows* – to move items onto the government's formal agenda. The model suggests that the characteristics of issues combine with the features of political institutions and circumstances, together with the development of policy solutions, in a process that can lead to the opening and closing of 'windows of opportunity' for shifting an issue onto the agenda. He conceives of policy emerging through three separate, continuous 'streams' of activity or processes: the *problem stream*, the *policy stream* and the *politics stream*. Policies are only taken seriously by governments when the three streams run together (Figure 4.1). Kingdon's 'windows' are the metaphorical launch 'windows' in a space mission. Blast-off can only occur when the all the conditions are favourable.

The *problem stream* refers to the perceptions of problems as public matters requiring government action and is influenced by previous efforts of government to respond to them. Officials learn about problems or socio-economic conditions through indicators, feedback from existing programmes and pressure groups, or sudden, focusing events such as crises. Indicators may include routine health statistics, for example, showing an increase in childhood obesity or a return of TB to a population previously free of the disease. However, such facts rarely if ever 'speak for themselves' and lead directly to action (see Chapter 9 for more on the links between research and policy), though governments can use the definition, timing of release and interpretation of official statistics (e.g. on unemployment) to attempt to shape the policy agenda.

The *policy stream* consists of the ongoing analyses of problems and their proposed solutions together with the debates surrounding these problems and possible responses. In this stream of ideas, a range of possibilities is explored and, at times, may be progressively narrowed down or promoted. For an idea or solution to get to the surface, it must be technically feasible, consistent with dominant social values, be capable of handling future feasibility constraints (such as finance and personnel), be publicly acceptable and resonate with politicians.

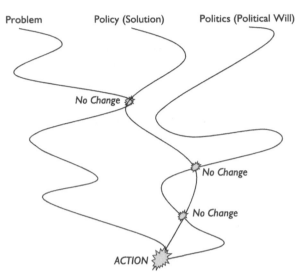

Figure 4.1 Kingdon's three stream model of agenda setting

Source: Adapted from Kingdon (2010)

The *politics stream* operates quite separately to the other two streams and is comprised of events such as swings of national mood, changes of government and campaigns by interest groups.

Kingdon identifies visible and hidden participants affecting the coming together of the streams. The visible participants are organized interests which highlight a specific problem, put forward a particular point of view, advocate a solution and use the mass media to get attention. Visible participants may be inside or outside government. For example, a new president or prime minister may be a powerful agenda setter because he/she has only recently been elected and is given the benefit of the doubt by the electorate. Other highly visible participants include UN 'goodwill ambassadors' for particular issues such as Carla Bruni, the wife of French President Nicolas Sarkozy, who became a goodwill ambassador for the Global Fund to Fight AIDS, Tuberculosis and Malaria in 2008, focusing on the elimination of mother-to-child transmission of HIV. The hidden participants are more likely to be the specialists in the field – the researchers, academics and consultants who work predominantly in the policy stream – developing and proposing options for solving problems which may get onto the agenda. They also include business lobbyists. Hidden participants may play a part in getting issues onto the agenda, particularly if they work with the mass media. Increasingly, universities, which are competing with one another for research funds, encourage their staff to promote their research findings in the mass media. This may mean that some academics shift from hidden to more visible roles in the agenda setting process.

According to Kingdon's model, the three streams flow along different, largely independent channels until at particular times, which become *policy windows*, they flow together, or intersect. This is when new issues get onto the agenda and policy is highly likely, but not guaranteed, to change. As a result, policies do not get onto the agenda according to some logical series of stages. The three streams flow simultaneously, each with a life of its own, until they meet or align, at which point an issue is likely to be taken seriously by policy makers. The meeting of the streams cannot easily be engineered or predicted.

Activity 4.4

Suggest possible reasons why the three streams might meet, leading to a problem moving onto the policy agenda. Locate each possible reason in one of Kingdon's three 'streams'.

Feedback

The main reasons why the three streams might converge and open a policy 'window' include:

- the activities of key players in the *political stream* who work to link particular policy 'solutions' to particular problems and at the same time create the political opportunity for action. These people are known as *policy entrepreneurs* since this is the political version of the activity of bringing buyers, sellers and commodities together on which commerce thrives;
- media attention to a problem and to possible solutions (*problem* or *policy streams* influencing the *politics stream*);
- a crisis such as a serious failure in the quality or safety of a service or other unpredictable event (*problem stream*);
- the dissemination of a major piece of research (*problem or policy stream*);
- a change of government after an election or other regular, formal landmarks in the political process (e.g. budgets) (*politics stream*).

Thus, in reality, participants in the policy process rarely proceed from identification of a problem to seeking solutions. Alternative courses of action are generated in the policy stream and may be promoted by experts or advocates over long periods before the opportunity arises (the policy window opens) to get the issue they relate to and their solutions onto the agenda.

The two general models you have just read about are useful because they can be applied to a wide range of public policy areas, including health. They should be able to help explain why a particular issue is on the policy agenda, or why it has not reached the policy agenda.

Activity 4.5

Read the following case study based on Reich (1994), which describes getting an essential drugs policy onto the policy agenda in Bangladesh. Apply the two models of agenda setting to this case study to explain the events that took place.

Case Study 6: getting the issue of an essential drugs policy onto the policy agenda in Bangladesh

Lieutenant-General and Army Chief of Staff HM Ershad seized power in a military coup in Bangladesh in 1982. Within four weeks of the coup he had established an expert committee of eight to confront widely discussed problems in the production, distribution and consumption of pharmaceuticals. Less than three months later, the Bangladesh (Control) Ordinance of 1982 was issued as a Declaration by Ershad. The main aim of the Ordinance was to halve the 'wastage of foreign exchange through the production and/or importation of unnecessary drugs or drugs of marginal value'. The drugs policy was to be applied to both private and public sectors and created a restricted national formulary of 150 essential drugs plus 100 supplementary drugs for specialized use which could be produced at relatively low cost. Over 1,600 products deemed 'useless, ineffective or harmful' were banned.

The formulation of the drugs policy was initiated by a group of concerned physicians and others with close links to the new president, without external consultation and discussion. The Bangladesh Medical Association was represented by one member of its pharmaceuticals sub-committee, but its General-Secretary was not officially involved because of his known connections to a transnational pharmaceutical corporation. The pharmaceutical industry was not represented at all on the expert committee. It was argued that its presence would distort and delay policy change. Once the policy was on the agenda and had been promulgated, the industry both domestic and transnational launched an advertising campaign against the drugs list.

Among the physicians on the committee was a well-known doctor and hero of the fight for independence, Zefrullah Chowdhury, who had established the Gonoshasthaya Kendra (GK) health care project soon after independence in 1971. Among other activities, GK manufactured essential generic drugs in Bangladesh. Production had begun in 1981 and by 1986 GK Pharmaceuticals Ltd was producing over twenty products. Later Dr Chowdhury was accused of promoting the interests of GK Pharmaceuticals through the committee.

Feedback

Applying the Hall et al. model

The policy of essential drugs had *legitimacy* because Ershad's government was new and new policies were both expected and allowed. Further, there was a strong case for limiting the number of drugs imported both because many were deemed ineffective and because they wasted scarce foreign currency which a poor country like Bangladesh could ill afford.

It was *feasible* to introduce radical change because it could be done by passing an Ordinance from the President: it did not require a long parliamentary process. Its passage was made more feasible by keeping opposition to a minimum by acting quickly. In addition, there were virtually no financial implications for the government. If anything, this policy would reduce public drug expenditure.

Support was more difficult: there was considerable resistance from health professionals, from multinational pharmaceutical firms and initially from national drug companies. But, as the people and national industries gained (through lower prices and greater local production), so support for the policy grew. In addition, as a dictator, Ershad was able to ignore initial opposition since he did not need parliamentary support for his policy to be enacted.

Applying the Kingdon model

The problem of ineffective and expensive drugs had been floating in the *problem stream* for some time, but without any action being taken. However, in 1982, a new president took over, eager to win popular support by showing his willingness to act on recognized problems that affected many people (change in the *politics stream*) and to propose solutions that appealed to nationalistic sentiments (*policy stream*). The most obvious losers included foreign pharmaceutical companies which were unlikely to be widely supported within Bangladesh. A small group of Bangladeshi health professionals, chaired by a celebrated doctor with an interest in health projects and the local pharmaceutical industry, had been highly concerned about the pharmaceutical issue for some time before Ershad took power. Some of its members were hidden participants in the *policy stream*, collecting information and monitoring the situation, and others were visible participants, advocating change explicitly. They recognized an opportunity to get an essential drugs policy on the agenda when the government changed and had close links to the new president. The technical feasibility, public acceptability and congruence with existing values were all judged to be favourable, and so the three streams came together, putting an essential drugs policy on the policy agenda.

Agenda setting and policy change under crisis

You have seen that a perceived crisis is one reason why policy 'windows' open. Policy making in times of crisis is different from ordinary, business-as-usual policy making. For example, it is easier to get radical policies seriously considered in times of crisis than other times. A crisis exists when important policy makers perceive that one exists, that it is a real and threatening set of circumstances where failure to act could lead to even more disastrous consequences. Events that do not have all these characteristics are not likely to be considered a crisis. However, where the gravity of the situation is confirmed by pressure from outside government, such as a dramatic fall in the price of a key export crop, and the government has access to corroborating information from its own experts, then the chances are that the government will see the problem as a crisis, and pay it serious attention. This may or may not, in turn, lead to an actual change of policy.

Many examples of new policies moving onto the agenda occur in times of economic crisis. Radical reforms in macro-economic, trade, labour market and social welfare policy in New Zealand after 1984 were prompted by a conviction on the part of the incoming Labour government, its principal advisers in the Treasury and influential segments of the business community that the country was on the brink of economic collapse. This justified a radical change in the issues on the policy agenda, particularly policies favouring the free market in many areas of national life that had been discussed by hidden participants for some time earlier. The reforms included major changes to the operation of the public health care system, including splitting the public part of the system into purchasers and providers (see Chapters 3 and 7 for more on this kind of thinking). It is unlikely that the cascade of changes to the economy and the public services would have occurred without the impetus of a strong sense of economic crisis coupled with a change of government.

Since crises are defined by the intersection of 'objective' conditions and perceptions of the gravity of those conditions, there is always scope for interest groups and governments to heighten the sense of crisis in order to pave the way for changes they particularly want to introduce. One interpretation of the change strategy for the UK National Health Service (NHS) of the Blair government between 1997 and 2005 was that it comprised identifying problems and solutions, but also engendering a strong sense that the NHS was in grave crisis – that without reform it could not continue in its present form and would have to be abolished and replaced with something quite different. Thus the Blair government identified the quality of cancer services and long waiting times as major problems threatening the very existence of a tax-financed, universal system. The government also used scandals of poor clinical quality at particular hospitals as a rationale for general changes to the regulation and oversight of clinicians. The Coalition government that followed used a similar, if disputed (Appleby 2011), assessment of relatively poor health care outcomes to put further major NHS changes on the agenda (Secretary of State for Health 2010).

Non-decision making

While both crisis and politics-as-usual models are useful for helping explain how issues come onto the policy agenda and are acted upon, or why eventually they are not (because they may lack legitimacy, feasibility or support or because the three policy 'streams' do not come together in favourable circumstances to provide a 'window of opportunity'), observable action provides an incomplete guide to the way all policies are decided. In other words, you need to think about the possibility of *non-policy making*, or *non-decision making* when thinking about what gets onto the public policy agenda (see Chapter 2 for a fuller discussion of this).

According to Bachrach and Baratz (1963), the power to keep things off the policy agenda is as important as the power to push certain issues onto the government's agenda. For instance, those with enough power (e.g. economic elites) are not only capable of stopping items reaching the agenda; they are also able to shape people's wishes so that only issues deemed acceptable and non-threatening to their interests are discussed, never mind acted on.

Activity 4.6

Until the 1970s, stopping smoking was widely seen as almost entirely an individual matter (except for deterring children from smoking). As a result, there was not even discussion about the possibility of limiting where smoking could take place in the health interests both of smokers and non-smokers.

Do you think the lack of discussion of smoking bans in the 1970s is an example of non-decision making through force, prevailing values or avoidance of conflict on the part of Western governments?

Feedback

The main reason for non-decision making related to the prevailing values of the time, which, in turn, were supported by the tobacco industry and its advocates who attempted to manipulate the flow of information reaching the public (e.g. on passive smoking) as well as mounting libertarian arguments against regulation of smoking. In addition, governments were reluctant to face conflict with the tobacco industry and court public unpopularity. This anticipation of conflict with the industry and with voters kept the issue off the agenda for many years.

Another example of non-decision making relates to the fact that the often radical 'market' reforms of many health care systems in the 1990s rarely if ever challenged the monopoly control exercised by the medical profession over who can and cannot initiate treatment and prescribe drugs for patients. While many previous assumptions as to how health care systems should be organized and directed were overturned (e.g. privatization of public hospitals and competition between providers), the fundamental interests of the dominant occupational group prevented any concerted debate about opening medical work to other professions.

Who sets the agenda?

In the rest of this chapter you will explore how the main actors in the policy process, particularly the government and the media, put issues on the policy agenda. Since you will be moving on to consider government policy making in the next chapter, and the business community, the medical profession and other interest groups are covered in Chapters 3 and 6, more time will be spent here on the role of the media than any of the other actors in agenda setting. Furthermore, in most circumstances, the media's primary role in policy making is likely to be in helping to set the policy agenda by shaping and structuring issues rather than in other aspects of the process. However, it must be recognized that business interests can be very influential in keeping issues off the policy agenda or delaying them reaching the agenda (see above). They frame public health issues in ways that favour their interests, for example, portraying them as matters of individual responsibility rather than societal action.

Activity 4.7

From what you know, how would you say alcohol and its use and misuse are framed by the alcohol industry in contrast to how the same issues are presented by public health advocates in order to shape the policy agenda?

Feedback

The alcohol industry and its lobbyists tend to frame alcohol consumption as a much valued, enjoyable part of everyday life and alcohol abuse as harmful use by a small group of susceptible or ignorant individuals. Public health practitioners would tend to frame alcohol as a powerful legal drug that causes extensive social harm and which should be tackled through population-wide measures rather than by targeting individuals. They would tend to favour government regulation (e.g. raising the price of drinks through taxation) while the industry would tend to favour voluntary codes encouraging responsible drinking (e.g. by putting sensible drinking advice on posters advertising alcoholic drinks).

More recently, in the field of international health and development, private charitable donors have also come into the reckoning as agenda setters, particularly in relation to poor countries and their governments due to the resources they control. The Bill and

Melinda Gates Foundation, for instance, is increasingly recognized as both influencing the process and, in some cases, setting the global health agenda through the size of its budget. The Foundation has advocated and invested in ambitious strategies to eradicate polio and malaria rather than supporting more conventional prevention and control programmes. Critics argue that the Foundation is inappropriately altering the international priority given to different diseases and responses.

Governments as agenda setters

Governments, particularly those of large, wealthy countries, can be very influential in setting the policy agenda. For example, PEPFAR, US President George W. Bush's initiative to combat the global epidemic of HIV actively promoted its 'ABC' ('abstinence, be faithful and condom use') strategy for HIV prevention within the international public health community and high prevalence countries, particularly in sub-Saharan Africa, in the face of criticism from many experts and activists. It was able to do so because of the large sums of money it was making available for HIV prevention and the conditions it applied to the use of these funds.

Within their own countries, governments are plainly crucial agenda setters since they control or at least shape the legislative process and often initiate policy change. The detailed institutional arrangements within different countries (see Chapter 5) affect the power of government (the executive) to set and control the agenda. For example, in parliamentary systems where the government is drawn from the political party or parties with a majority of the seats, political parties usually set the agenda for their term of office in advance by publishing relatively detailed election manifestos and promising to implement the changes set out in the manifesto if elected. This is one of the more obvious ways in which elected governments can attempt to set the agenda. However, being in the manifesto only increases the likelihood of an issue getting onto the agenda and being acted on, it is not a guarantee of action. For example, political activists writing the manifesto may not give enough weight to the feasibility of what they have proposed.

In the United States, the committees of the Congress (the lower House of Representatives) have the right to bring proposals to a vote by the legislature. The President as leader of the executive cannot do so. By contrast, in the British Parliament, the government (the executive) largely initiates and controls this process, giving the government much greater influence over the policy agenda and eventual legislation.

As there are always more issues competing for attention than governments can attend to at any one time, do governments pursue an active programme of issue search – looking for items to go on the policy agenda? Hogwood and Gunn (1984) argue that governments *should* do so because they need to anticipate problems before they occur in order to minimize any adverse consequences or avert a potential crisis. Perhaps the most obvious reasons for engaging in issue search lie in the external environment such as demography, technology, and so on. In almost all countries, the growing numbers and proportion of older people in the population have to be taken into account in setting health policy in areas such as paying for services, long-term care of frail people and the management of chronic diseases. New solutions become available to old problems such as linking patients' records kept by different providers. New problems begin to assume clear contours such as the potential effect of climate change on agrarian economies and on public health. As well as serving the elected government of the day, one of the functions of a responsible civil service is to provide reports identifying and drawing future policy issues to the attention of ministers, such as the effects of global warming.

However, there is no guarantee that the government of the day will wish to respond to what it may perceive to be a long-term issue that its successors can deal with.

The mass media as agenda setter

How far and in which circumstances do the mass media guide attention to certain issues and influence what we think about? How much influence do they have on policy makers in their choice of issues of political concern and action? In the past, the role of the media tended to be underestimated in policy making. However, the mass media have had a major influence over many years on governments' policy agendas through their ability to raise and shape, if not determine, issues and public opinion which, in turn, influences governments to respond. The arrival of the Internet in the 1990s and a range of electronic social media in the 2000s have made this process even more apparent. They have enabled the rapid dissemination of information and images, and the mobilization and channelling of public opinion to governments in ways that they cannot easily predict or control, but which they may have to respond to in some way. Electronic media such as more conventional websites, blogs, social networking sites like Facebook and different forms of messaging from SMS to Twitter are now used by governments, interest groups and the public in more and more different ways to raise issues, critique policies and justify positions. For instance, in the UK government if an e-petition reaches more than 100,000 signatures, it will be sent to Parliament which will decide if the issue should be debated in the Lower House.

In many respects, intelligent use of new media has lowered the cost of entry into policy debate. A good example is Avaaz (meaning 'voice' in several languages) which has used the Internet since 2007 to organize political campaigns on the issues its millions of members (almost 10 million in 172 countries in 2011) judge to be important. Each year, Avaaz sets overall priorities through all-member polls and tests ideas for specific campaigns using weekly polls of 10,000 members drawn at random. Issues that find a strong response at 'tipping-point moments of crisis and opportunity' become large-scale campaigns. Avaaz claims that hundreds of thousands of its members can take part in signing petitions, funding media campaigns and direct actions, emailing, calling and lobbying governments, and organizing protests within days or even hours (http://www.avaaz.org).

There are two basic types of mass media: print and electronic. They serve a range of vital functions: they are sources of information; they function as propaganda mechanisms; they are agents of socialization (transmitting a society's culture and instructing people in the values and norms of society) and they serve as agents of legitimacy, generating mass belief in, and acceptance of, dominant political and economic institutions such as democracy and capitalism. They can also criticize the way societies and governments operate, bringing new perspectives to the public.

The way the media function is affected by the political system. In some countries newspapers and television stations are entirely state-owned and censor themselves, fearing government reprisals for covering issues in an inappropriate way, thereby prejudicing their impartiality. In others, media are notionally independent of the state, but editors and journalists are intimidated, jailed, expelled or worse. The Internet and satellite broadcasting are less easy for individual regimes to influence or undermine but are less accessible in poorer countries than television and radio which are easier to control. Even in liberal democracies, the mass media may be controlled in subtle ways. Governments, increasingly concerned about their image in the media, can favour certain more cooperative broadcasters over others, giving them exclusive news stories and advance warning of policy announcements to boost their viewer numbers in return for generally favourable coverage. Most mass media organizations in Western democracies are part of large conglomerates with a wide range of media interests in many countries. Some of the best known are owned by business magnates, such as Silvio Berlusconi (who has also been Italian prime minister) and Rupert Murdoch. Their personal political values and commercial goals often shape the orientation of the news reporting and political commentary provided by their television channels and newspapers without the proprietors necessarily having to direct their journalists on a day-to-day basis. Most commercial media are also dependent to some degree on advertising. Taken together, the pattern of ownership and the requirements of advertisers tend to mean that in most countries the majority of newspapers and television stations tend to adopt broadly right-of-centre, pro-capitalist, political positions. Advertisers and commercial interests can also, on occasions, influence the content of media directly, for example, through the sponsorship of newspapers and the placement of articles in the press apparently written by neutral journalists but intended to promote the industry's interests (e.g. enthusiastic reports of the latest pharmaceutical innovation).

Despite being largely controlled by the state and major commercial interests, the media can, sometimes, put an issue on the policy agenda which researchers or interest groups unconnected with the state or business are trying to promote. Occasionally, they act like pressure groups by running campaigns on unjustly neglected issues. One of the most notable in the UK was the *Sunday Times'* successful campaign in the 1970s to win higher compensation for children with birth defects after their mothers had taken the tranquillizer, thalidomide to control their nausea in pregnancy. The newspaper's researchers succeeded in showing that the risk of congenital malformations had been foreseeable (Karpf 1988).

Campaigns can also be more blatantly populist and be designed to win readers such as the UK *Daily Mail's* campaign against speed cameras in the 2000s. The campaign portrayed the research on injury reduction as severely flawed and, instead, appealed to the cynicism of the readers by focusing on the government revenue raised by the cameras in fines, much to the disappointment of public health experts trying to reduce traffic-related injuries and deaths.

There have been calls for the mass media to become more responsible in their coverage of public health issues. Research in the UK on media coverage of health issues shows that the amount of news coverage of a topic is unrelated to the risk posed to the public health (Harrabin et al. 2003) and, indeed, the diseases with the lowest risk to population health frequently received the highest level of coverage and vice versa. For example, coverage of vCJD, or mad cow disease in humans, bore no relationship to its extreme rarity. Yet, as the same research showed, politicians changed their priorities in response to media coverage rather than on the scientific evidence of what was in the best interest for public health.

Nevertheless, the extent of media influence on government policy makers is open to question. First, policy makers have many different sources of information and can use the media themselves to draw attention to a particular issue. Often, the contents of government press releases will be reported verbatim by busy journalists. Second, it is difficult to separate different strands of influence on what gets onto the agenda. The media are both part of the process itself and outside it, and they are not alone in shaping the agenda. Mostly, the media highlight movements that have started elsewhere – that is, they help to delineate an issue, but they do not necessarily create it. For example, in the late 2000s, the mass media in most European countries helped raise concern about the need for government action to protect the population from the potential harm of an impending pandemic of swine 'flu. Yet, when it became apparent that the outbreak was less severe than predicted, the media in some countries switched their attention to highlighting government overreaction in the shape of unused vaccine stocks. They also accused the pharmaceutical industry of exaggerating the pandemic threat for profit. At each stage, the media were following events while shaping their interpretation.

Third, policy makers are less likely to be moved to action by a single media account. Concerted action by the press may make a difference, but in a competitive media environment, there is unlikely to be a unified view of an issue and the news media particularly are always looking for novelty.

Just as there are examples of the media inspiring policy shifts, so there are clear examples of politicians and their officials resisting media pressure to change policy. The controversy over the combined mumps, measles and rubella (MMR) vaccine in the UK is a good example of the latter. It showed how the mass media can provide a misleading picture of the relative weight of scientific evidence on a public health issue. While the vast majority of scientific evidence indicated that the MMR vaccine did not cause any significant harm, the sceptics' voices were heard relatively loudly in the mass media, perhaps because they injected drama and controversy into what could have been a relatively dull public health discussion (Boyce 2007).

So, there are no simple answers to questions such as: how much do the mass media influence public opinion and/or policy makers? The content of the policy issue, the political context and the process by which the debate unfolds and the policy issue is decided, all have a bearing on how influential the media will be.

In low and middle income countries, the influence of the media on policy makers is less easy to discern. Journalists, editors, broadcasters and producers are members of the urban elite, and generally have close ties with policy makers in government. Where media are owned directly by government, there is unlikely to be much critical analysis of gaps in government policies. Policy circles tend to be smaller in many low and middle income countries, and those journalists who are perceived as threatening a political regime are often the first to be arrested when repression strikes. Although this is changing, the independence of the mass media remains vulnerable to political whim and to the need to attract income. For example, in high income countries consumer advertising revenue, which is not present to the same extent in other countries, gives the mass media considerable financial independence of governments, but not necessarily independence from commercial interests.

The presence or absence of democracy also appears to be important in the influence of the media on agenda setting in low and middle income countries. Sen (1983) compared the role of the media in reporting food shortages and famines in China and India since World War II and the impact on governments' responses. In 1959–61, China suffered a massive famine due to crop failures. Between 14 and 16 million extra deaths occurred but the mass media remained silent. India, on the other hand, despite being a similarly poor country at the time, had not experienced a famine since independence in 1947 despite years with great food problems. Sen argued that India could not have famines because India was a democracy with a free press, unlike China:

> Government cannot afford to fail to take prompt action when large-scale starvation threatens. Newspapers play an important part in this, in making the facts known and forcing the challenge to be faced. So does the pressure of opposition parties.
>
> (Sen 1983)

In China, there were few ways of challenging the government to act to avoid the catastrophe and the famine could be kept hidden. Ironically, during the same period, communist China was far more committed to distributing food at public expense to guarantee some food for all than India. In normal times, this avoided the widespread malnourishment and non-acute hunger observed in India.

Priorities and the policy agenda

The focus of this chapter up to now has been on how topics get onto the public policy agenda of a particular country government or international agency. However, it is one thing for an issue to get onto the agenda, quite another for it ultimately to be acted upon. For the latter to happen, the issue and related policy proposals need to achieve a position high on the agenda. Just as there are inevitable limits on the number of issues to which any government is giving serious attention at any time, so there are finite resources available for subsequent action such as money, staff, expertise and time. According to the rational model of the policy process often associated with the application of economic principles to decision making, priorities (the position of an issue on the agenda) should be set according to the balance of costs and benefits likely to be produced by pursuing particular policies in relation to that issue. However, you saw in Chapter 2 that the policy process does not necessarily proceed in this way. For example, despite an international, shared body of knowledge about public health issues and potential responses, the policy agendas and priorities within those agendas of different countries can differ substantially.

Aware of this phenomenon, American political scientist, Jeremy Shiffman carried out a series of studies in the 1990s and 2000s to try to explain why the priority given to the issue of reducing maternal mortality differed across countries. He explained these differences in terms of efforts by international agencies to establish a global norm about the unacceptability of maternal death; the agencies' provision of financial and technical resources within countries; the degree of cohesion among national safe motherhood policy promoters; the presence of national political champions to promote the cause; the availability and strategic use of credible evidence to show policy makers that a problem existed; the generation of clear policy options indicating that the problem was surmountable; and the organization of attention-generating events to raise the national visibility of the issue (Shiffman 2007).

Shiffman and his colleague, Stephanie Smith then took their work to the international level to try to explain why the global Safe Motherhood Initiative to reduce maternal mortality launched in 1987 had not received much attention and remained a relatively low international public health priority. Shiffman and Smith (2007)) developed a framework based on four elements: (1) the strength of the actors involved and their cohesion; (2) the power of the ideas used to portray the issue; (3) the way that the political context either inhibited or enhanced support for the issue; and (4) the characteristics of the issue itself (see Table 4.1).

The Safe Motherhood Initiative was hampered in all four respects. In relation to the power of the interest groups most involved with maternal mortality, Shiffman and Smith found that, among other things, they were divided over the intervention strategy that should be adopted, reducing their credibility with international and national political leaders. There were no strong guiding organizations or leaders who could engineer consensus, and civil society organizations were weakly mobilized.

At the level of ideas, the contrasting approaches to 'framing' the issue of maternal mortality led to confusion. For example, some viewed it as a human rights issue, others in terms of its adverse economic consequences, yet others as harming children and

Table 4.1 Shiffman and Smith's framework of determinants for understanding the political priority of different global health initiatives

	Description	*Factors shaping political priority*
Actor power	The strength of the individuals and organizations concerned with the issue	1. Policy community cohesion: the degree of coalescence among the network of individuals and organizations that are centrally involved with the issue at the global level
		2. Leadership: the presence of individuals capable of uniting the policy community and acknowledged as particularly strong champions for the cause
		3. Guiding institutions: the effectiveness of organizations or coordinating mechanisms with a mandate to lead the initiative
		4. Civil society mobilization: the extent to which grassroots organizations have mobilized to press international and national political authorities to address the issue at the global level
Ideas	The ways in which those involved with the issue understand and portray it	5. Internal frame: the degree to which the policy community agrees on the definition of, causes of, and solutions to the problem
		6. External frame: public portrayals of the issue in ways that resonate with external audiences, especially the political leaders who control resources
Issue characteristics	Features of the problem	7. Credible indicators: clear measures that show the severity of the problem and that can be used to monitor progress
		8. Severity: the size of the burden relative to other problems, as indicated by objective measures such as mortality levels
		9. Effective interventions: the extent to which proposed means of addressing the problem are clearly explained, cost effective, backed by scientific evidence, simple to implement, and inexpensive
Political contexts	The environments in which actors operate	10. Policy windows: political moments when global conditions align favourably for an issue, presenting opportunities for advocates to influence decision makers
		11. Global governance structure: the degree to which norms and institutions operating in a sector provide a platform for effective collective action

Source: Adapted from Shiffman and Smith (2007: 1371)

families. In some countries, the issue of child survival generally took precedence over that of mothers though not without controversy. There was also confusion over whether maternal mortality or maternal health should be the focus, what the appropriate interventions should be and how the issue related to other women's health concerns such as reproductive health.

In terms of issue characteristics, Shiffman and Smith argued that maternal mortality failed to become a priority because maternal death was not as common as other causes of death (e.g. from communicable diseases), was difficult to measure, and there was no single, simple intervention that was readily available to avert maternal deaths. The evidence supporting interventions was also weaker than for other competing health programmes.

In relation to the global policy context, potential policy 'windows' opened periodically, but the safe motherhood policy community was not well placed to take advantage of them. For instance, there was no single or obvious 'home' within United Nations organizations for safe motherhood.

Despite these difficulties, a potentially very important 'policy window' opened in 2000 with the promulgation of the Millennium Development Goals. MDG 5 was the reduction of the global maternal mortality ratio by 75 per cent over 1990 levels by the year 2015. Influenced by MDG 5, countries such as the UK increased their allocation of development resources to maternal health (e.g. from £0.9 million in 2001/02 to £16.2 million by 2005/06). It seems that the greater priority resulting from the MDGs and the merging of the Safe Motherhood Initiative into a broader partnership for maternal, newborn and child health, was beginning to pay off in terms of attention and resources for this issue. By 2010 it was being suggested that global maternal mortality rates were beginning to decline although some countries had made little progress (Hogan et al. 2010). Overall, progress has been slow.

Activity 4.8

What is notable about Shiffman and Smith's approach to explaining the political priority given to maternal mortality both within countries and at the international level from the perspective of the 'rational' approach to policy making described in Chapter 2?

Feedback

Only part of the explanatory framework relates to the influence of objective data such as indicators of the scale of the problem of maternal death and the (cost) effectiveness of potential interventions to reduce it which, according to the rational approach to policy, should be central to deciding on priorities. Instead, the main factors contributing to the priority given to maternal death as a public health issue are social and political, relating to the inter-relationships between the main organizations operating in the field, the wider political context, and the way that influential people and agencies view and project the issue.

Summary

You have learnt how agenda setting is not a clear-cut part of the policy process. There are many actors involved and it is not necessarily dominated by government though governments are normally central to agenda setting. The policy agenda may change at times of crisis or through 'politics-as-usual', but in both cases, certain factors will be important. A crisis will have to be perceived as such by the most influential policy elites, and they will have to believe that failure to act will make the situation worse. In 'politics-as-usual' many different reforms may compete for policy makers' attention and which one reaches the policy agenda will depend on a number of different factors, including who gains and who loses in the change. Objective indicators of the nature of a problem and evidence about possible solutions play a part, but far from fully explain why some issues get onto the policy agenda and attract high priority. The prominence of an issue is a product of how well actors in the relevant policy community work together, construct a persuasive account of the issue and its solution, and take advantage of opportunities to draw attention to the issue. Timing is also important, and issues may be around for a while before all three 'streams' ('problem', 'policy' and 'politics') come together, and an issue is propelled on to the policy agenda.

The media can be important for drawing attention to issues and encouraging governments to act but this is more likely in relation to 'low politics' issues. On major, or 'high politics' topics (such as economic policy or threats to national security), the media tend to shape and structure issues rather than bringing them to attention in the first place.

References

Appleby J (2011) Does poor health justify NHS reform? *BMJ* 342: 310–11.

Bachrach P and Baratz MS (1963) Decisions and nondecisions: an analytical framework. *American Political Science Review* 57: 641–51.

Berger PL and Luckman T (1975) *The Social Construction of Reality: A Treatise on the Sociology of Knowledge.* Harmondsworth: Penguin.

Boyce T (2007) *Health, Risk and News: The MMR Vaccine and the Media.* New York: Peter Lang.

Cobb RW and Elder CD (1983) *Participation in American Politics: The Dynamics of Agenda-Building.* Baltimore, MD: Johns Hopkins University Press.

Grindle M and Thomas J (1991) *Public Choices and Policy Change.* Baltimore, MD: Johns Hopkins University Press.

Hall P, Land H, Parker R and Webb A (1975) *Change, Choice and Conflict in Social Policy.* London: Heinemann.

Harrabin R, Coote A and Allen J (2003) *Health in the News: Risk, Reporting and Media Attention.* London: Kings Fund.

Hogan M, Foreman KJ, Naghavi M, Ahn SY, Wang M, Makela SM, Lopez A, Lozano R, and Murray CJL (2010) Maternal mortality for 181 countries, 1980–2008: a systematic analysis of progress towards Millennium Development Goal 5. *The Lancet,* 375: 1609–23.

Hogwood B and Gunn L (1984) *Policy Analysis for the Real World.* Oxford: Oxford University Press.

Karpf A (1988) *Doctoring the Media.* London: Routledge.

Kingdon J (2010) *Agendas, Alternatives and Public Policies,* updated 2nd edn. Harlow: Longman Classics.

Reich M (1994) Bangladesh pharmaceutical policy and politics. *Health Policy and Planning* 9: 130–43.

Rushing W (1995) *The AIDS Epidemic: Social Dimensions of an Infectious Disease.* Boulder, CO: Westview Press.

Secretary of State for Health (2010) *Equity and Excellence: Liberating the NHS.* Cm 7881. London: The Stationery Office.

Sen A (1983) The battle to get food. *New Society* 13 October: 54–7.

Shiffman J (2007) Generating political priority for maternal mortality reduction in five developing countries. *American Journal of Public Health* 97: 796–803.

Shiffman J and Smith S (2007) Generation of political priority for global health initiatives: a framework and case study of maternal mortality. *Lancet* 370: 1370–9.

5 Government and the policy process

Overview

The previous chapter showed how issues get onto the policy agenda through processes not necessarily controlled by government. This chapter focuses on the roles of government in the formulation and shaping of policy, and how much influence it has on the policy process. While policy formulation usually involves taking account of a wide variety of interests, albeit driven by the ideological assumptions of the government in power, the way this happens is dependent on the type of government institutions or constitution of a country. You will look at the role of the government bodies most frequently assumed to be directly involved in forming and carrying out policies: the legislature; the executive; the bureaucracy; and the judiciary. In terms of the framework for policy analysis introduced in Chapter 1, the focus in this chapter is on a particular set of official 'actors' within the policy process and their relationships. In terms of the 'policy stages' model also discussed in Chapter 1, the main focus is on policy formulation with some reference to policy implementation.

Learning objectives

After working through this chapter, you will be better able to:

- describe the main bodies involved in government policy making – the legislature, the executive, the bureaucracy and the judiciary – and their roles
- understand how they relate to one another differently in different types of government system and how these relationships shape how policy is made
- understand the special characteristics of government policy making in the health sector
- understand how different parts of government (e.g. different ministries) and different levels (e.g. national, regional and local) require active coordination if policies are to be successful
- describe the organization of the health system of your country and be aware that the official chart of its organization may not reflect the true pattern of power and influence in the system.

Key terms

Bicameral/unicameral legislature. In a unicameral legislature, there is only one 'house' or chamber, whereas, in a bicameral legislature, there is a second or upper chamber, the role of which is to critique and check the quality of draft legislation promulgated by the lower house. Normally, only the lower house can determine whether draft legislation becomes law.

Bureaucracy. Comprises the public officials, often known as civil servants, whose job it is to advise ministers (the executive) on how best to take forward their policy goals and then to manage the process of policy implementation.

Executive. Leadership of a country (i.e. the president and/or prime minister and other ministers). The prime minister/president and senior ministers are often referred to as the cabinet.

Federal system. The sub-national, state or provincial level of government is not subordinate to the national government but has substantial powers of its own which the national government cannot take away.

Institutions. The 'rules of the game' determining how government and the wider state operate. Institutions can be formal structures and procedures, but also informal norms of behaviour that may not be written down.

Judiciary. Comprises judges and courts which are responsible for ensuring that the government of the day (the executive) acts according to the laws passed by the legislature.

Legislature. Body that enacts the laws that govern a country and oversees the executive. It is normally democratically elected in order to represent the people of the country and commonly referred to as the parliament or assembly. Often there will be two chambers or 'houses' of parliament.

Parliamentary system. The executive are also members of the legislature and are chosen on the basis that the majority of the legislature supports them.

Presidential system. The president or head of state is directly elected in a separate process from the election of members of the legislature.

Proportional representation. Voting system designed to ensure that the proportion of votes received by each political party equates to their share of the seats in the legislature.

Unitary system. The lower levels of government are constitutionally subordinate to the national government, and receive their authority from central government.

Government and public policy

Chapter 2 introduced a range of different ways of understanding public policy based on underlying notions of the distribution of power in society. The 'pluralist' perspective assumed that politics transmitted the preferences of citizens to which governments responded appropriately. And, in contrast, the 'elitist' perspective emphasized inequalities, particularly in economic power between groups and the ability of powerful groups to ensure that policy decisions favoured them. An alternative approach is to seek to explain the formulation and implementation of public policies by reference to the characteristics of the government and wider state system. This approach sees individual politicians and bureaucrats as actors driven by their ideas and their self-interest, but also sees the organization of government as a set of structures and rules that shape the policy process (Evans et al. 1985). The latter are referred to by political scientists as *institutions* – that is, the norms and procedures of government such as the electoral system, who has the right to initiate legislation, the relations between the legislature and judiciary (see below), the rules governing lobbying of political representatives by agents of interest groups, the way in which specific interest groups are consulted by government, and so on. A focus on *institutions* tends to draw attention to the obstacles and limits on policy change since structures and procedures, particularly constitutions, tend to change less frequently than, for example, the distribution of support between political parties. A focus on institutions also tends to emphasize how they constrain policy development processes and thinking, keeping them to well-worn paths so that decisions in the past limit the room for manoeuvre in the future. This phenomenon is known as *path depend-ency*. It has been used extensively to explain why the US has never managed to introduce universal health insurance despite much popular support (Steinmo and Watts 1995).

This chapter explores policy making in government systems mainly focusing on democ-racies where there are periodic opportunities for the people to change their leaders.

Characterizing government systems

Two features of government systems have a major effect on their ability to make and implement policy: *autonomy* and *capacity* (Howlett et al. 2009). In this context, *autonomy* means the ability of government institutions to resist being captured by self-interested groups and to act fairly as an arbiter of social conflicts. The government system may not be neutral in a political sense (after all, it serves governments of different ideological complexions), but, if it is autonomous, it operates with some objective regard to improving the welfare of the whole country not just responding to and protecting the interests of sections of the community. *Capacity* refers to the ability of the government system to make and implement policy. It springs from the expertise, resources and coherence of the machinery of government. For example, it is essential that a govern-ment is able to pay its civil servants on time and keep corruption in check. At a more sophisticated level, it helps if individual ministries respect the fact that their decisions and behaviour can have major implications for other arms of government, and they refrain from self-interested actions. The different forms of government system have implications for the autonomy and capacity of government policy making.

Federal versus unitary systems

All governments operate at a variety of levels between the national and the local (for example, public health systems frequently have national and regional levels of adminis-tration). However, there is an important, basic distinction between *unitary* and *federal* systems which cannot be overlooked when thinking about policy change in health systems. In the former, there is a clear chain of command linking the different levels of government so that lower levels are strictly subordinate to higher levels. In France, for example, the national government has potentially all the decision making powers. It can delegate these powers to lower levels of government, but can also take these powers back relatively easily. China, Japan and New Zealand are similar. The UK has a largely unitary system in which local government derives its powers from central government, but Scotland, Wales and Northern Ireland were granted their own powers over most of their domestic affairs, including health services, under legislation passed by the national parliament in London in 1999. There are elected bodies with varying decision making powers in the devolved countries separate from the national parliament in London, so that the UK is now somewhere between a unitary and federal state.

In fully federal systems, there are at least two separate levels of government within the country with power shared between them. In other words, the sub-national level of government is not subordinate to the national level but enjoys a high level of freedom over those matters under its jurisdiction. Central government cannot remove these freedoms without the consent of the sub-national tier which normally means rewriting the constitution of the country. For example, Australia, Brazil, Canada, India, Nigeria and the US are all federal countries. In Canada, for instance, the health system is the responsibility of the provinces, not the federal government, though the latter contributes some of the funding for health services. This leads to lengthy negotiations and disputes between the two levels of government about who pays for what and what decision rights each level of government has and should have.

Indeed, federalism is widely regarded as a major reason for the relative inability of governments in these countries to bring about major, nation-wide policy changes in the health sector except when circumstances are highly favourable. A further complication is that federal and sub-national governments may be controlled by different political parties with different values and goals. Furthermore, elections at one or the other level rarely coincide, so policy development processes that require lengthy negotiations between the affected interests can be disrupted by a change of government at either level. So, typically, unitary government systems are associated with far more rapid policy change and less need to compromise when formulating policy. However, this does not necessarily mean that policies developed in this way will be implemented on the ground as their architects at national level intended (as you will see in Chapter 7). Even in unitary systems with relatively few constitutional obstacles to legislative change, the underlying conditions for fundamental system reform rarely occur. These are typically a combination of a government with a high level of authority (e.g. a strong parliamentary majority) and the political will to incur the risks of major change (i.e. reform must be sufficiently central to its policy agenda) (Tuohy 2004).

Majoritarian versus proportional electoral systems

Another basic distinction between government systems relates to the rules governing parliamentary elections. In *majoritarian* systems, typically, candidates from different political parties compete for votes within electoral districts, sometimes known as constituencies. The candidate with the most votes represents the district in parliament, and political parties aim to win as many such contests as possible so as to have the most seats in parliament. In contrast, under *proportional representation*, the number of seats gained by each party is related to its share of the national vote (though different systems do this to differing degrees) and the aim of political parties is to maximize total votes. This difference between these two systems can affect the policies promoted by parties to the electorate. Under proportional representation, the goal is to appeal to a wide range of potential voters whereas under the majoritarian, which is often referred to as the 'first past the post' system, parties may tailor their policies to the issues affecting particular constituencies within the country.

Relations between the legislature, executive and judiciary

Another feature of each country's government system affecting how public policy is formulated concerns the relations between the legislature or parliament, the executive and the judiciary. The *legislature* is the body which represents the people, enacts the laws that govern the people and oversees the *executive* which is the leadership of the country (i.e. the president and/or prime minister and other ministers, commonly referred to in democracies as 'the government of the day' or the cabinet). The *judiciary* is primarily responsible for ensuring that the government of the day acts within the laws passed by the legislature and adjudicates on the inevitable disputes that occur in the interpretation of laws in practice. Typically, in *parliamentary* systems, the executive is chosen by the legislature from among its members (i.e. ministers are members of the parliament or assembly and are generally from the party or parties that can command a majority in the parliament). The executive remains in office as long as it has majority support among the legislators. Typically, in *presidential* systems, such as the US, the executive in the shape of the president and his team is separate from the legislature, elected separately by the public and need not have the support of the majority of members of the legislature to govern.

These differences have major implications for the way in which policy is developed. In presidential systems, the executive (the president and senior colleagues) can propose policy but the approval of the legislature (the majority of whose members may not even be from the same political party) is required for the policy to become law. As a result, the US president, for example, frequently has to offer concessions to the legislature in one area of policy in return for support in another. In the US system, the president has to rely on the legislature (the House of Representatives) to initiate legislation, and members of the legislature can play an active part in designing and amending policies. This means that the policy development process is more open than in parliamentary systems and there is more room for interest groups to exert influence and for complex bargaining to occur between interests and their representatives.

In parliamentary systems, while there may be some dispute and bargaining over policies within the governing political party or coalition, this usually takes place behind the scenes and the executive can normally rely on its majority in the legislature to obtain support for the measures it wishes to enact. Where the executive does not have an outright majority in the legislature, as happens more often in countries with systems of proportional representation, where there may be a larger number of political parties and coalition governments are more common, it has to compromise in order to get policies through the legislature. This makes the policy process slower and more complex, but not as difficult as policy making in presidential systems. Policy making is still ultimately centralized in the executive in all types of parliamentary systems which usually allows more rapid and decisive action to be taken by government.

Activity 5.1

As well as the separation of powers between the executive (the president and his or her staff) and the legislature (the two Houses of Congress), which other parts of the governmental system make major policy change (e.g. reform of the financing of the health care system) more difficult in the US than in many other countries?

Feedback

The US system is also federal so the individual states will have to be persuaded to support any major change in domestic policy. This explains why presidents of the US tend to spend quite a lot of time and energy on defence and foreign policy where their power is less restricted and they can act on behalf of the entire nation.

The position of the judiciary also affects the government policy process. In federal systems and/or those based on a written constitution, often including a statement of human rights, there is typically an autonomous judiciary such as the US Supreme Court, charged with adjudicating in the case of disputes between the different tiers of government and with ensuring that the laws and actions of the government are consistent with the principles of the constitution. The US Supreme Court has frequently challenged the laws of individual states: in the 1950s, it enforced the civil liberties of black people by overturning legislation in the southern states which would have segregated schools between black and white. In countries like Britain without a written constitution, though independent of government, the courts are more limited in what they can do to constrain the executive in the protection of the rights and liberties of individual citizens and, again, policy making is easier.

Real-world government systems are built of combinations of the features discussed above so that the effects of one feature may be mitigated by another. Thus, a country such as New Zealand has a unitary, parliamentary system with only one parliamentary chamber (see below) that tends to concentrate power, but members of parliament are elected by proportional representation, thereby giving a wider range of political opinion a say in who is elected. The introduction of proportional representation in 1996 was principally a popular reaction to the previous majoritarian system that was blamed for producing violent policy swings between successive governments. There was a desire among the public to make it harder for a new government to abolish what its predecessor had put in place.

Activity 5.2

Imagine that you are a national minister of health wishing to introduce a major change into a health care system such as user fees for patients to use public hospitals. List the different considerations you would have to take into account if you were trying to introduce such legislation in a federal, presidential system versus a unitary, parliamentary system. Make two lists of factors.

Feedback

Your notes might look something like those presented in Table 5.1.

You will immediately see that the larger number and greater complexity of the considerations which the minister of health in a federal, presidential system will have to take into account compared with his counterpart in the unitary, parliamentary system. Thus, US President Barack Obama faced many formal and informal institutional obstacles in his quest to widen health care insurance coverage and lower its cost. As

Table 5.1 Federal-presidential and unitary-parliamentary systems compared

Federal, presidential system	Unitary, parliamentary system
Which level of government is responsible for which aspects of health policy? Is this change within the jurisdiction of national government? If so, does national government control all the necessary resources to bring about the change?	Has the intended reform been discussed in the governing political party or parties? Is it in the election manifesto or coalition agreement? What does the governing political party or parties think about the intended reform? Are they broadly supportive? If not, are the majority of members of the legislature from the government party or parties likely to be in support? Has the government got a majority in the legislature (parliament) to enact the changes? If not, can the government get sufficient votes from other parties?
Is the national legislature likely to support the changes? If not, what concessions might be made either in health or in other areas of policy to win the necessary support? Are these concessions worth making for this reform? What are the odds of the proposed legislation passing through the national legislature without substantial amendment? If the government will be dependent on the support of states or provinces to bring about the changes, which state or provincial governments are of the same political persuasion as the national government? What concessions to the states/provinces could the government make in health or other areas of policy without undermining its position with its supporters in order to obtain sufficient support for the health reforms, particularly from states/provinces governed by opposition parties? For example, will national government have to fund the changes in their entirety to have any chance of getting them accepted? What view are the courts likely to take to the reforms?	What concessions, if any, will be needed to get a majority in support of the reforms?

a result, the original reform bill included many concessions to opponents of reform and further concessions had to be made throughout the process (Hacker 2010).

Note that Table 5.1 does not cover the implementation of the proposed changes, simply the ability of the minister and the government to get the reforms accepted and into law within the various legislative bodies. The officials and health professionals at lower levels in both systems of government may not agree with parts of the reforms, and may have considerable ability to resist or change the direction of policy. This is one of the central issues in policy implementation (see Chapter 7).

Political parties

In liberal democracies (i.e. where people are free to set up political parties and put themselves forward for election without executive and judicial interference), as opposed to one party states, political parties sit somewhere between wider societal actors such as pressure or interest groups (see Chapters 3 and 6) and the institutions of government, in that members of the executive and legislature are frequently drawn from one or another of the main political parties. Parties produce manifestos and policy documents on which they campaign at elections. So parties can directly affect the outcomes of elections and what follows. However, voters tend not to vote on the basis of specific policies, but are invited to support a broad package of measures designed to maximize the party's appeal. The detail of which policies reach the government agenda and how they are developed subsequently is outside the direct control of the party and the voters (see Chapter 4). Of course, a government in office has to be careful not to move too far away from what it promised its party members, supporters, funders (e.g. from business or trade unions) and the voters at the election, even if circumstances change, otherwise it will jeopardize its future support, but it is not required to follow party policy in every detail. Indeed, circumstances may change and once in office politicians may find that turning manifesto promises into coherent policy is far more difficult technically and politically than they had envisaged while in opposition.

The evidence suggests that political parties have a modest direct effect on policy, their greatest contribution being at the early stages of policy identification – but a larger indirect effect through influencing the staffing of the legislature and executive (and sometimes the judiciary).

In single or dominant party systems one political party formulates all or most policies and it becomes the task of the government to find the best ways of implementing them. There is no clear cut or simple separation between the party and the executive or legislature. Both the latter can be criticized by the party to the extent that ministers and members of parliament can be removed for not responding with sufficient zeal to the party's views.

The role of the legislature

In the overwhelming majority of countries, the constitution states that the decisions of the legislature are the expression of the will of the people (i.e. there is popular sovereignty) and that the legislature is the highest decision making body. Most have three formal functions: to represent the people; to enact legislation; and to oversee the executive (the prime minister or president and ministers). Legislatures in democracies are generally composed exclusively of elected members (known as deputies, senators, or members of parliament). Three-fifths of the countries in the world have *unicameral* or single chamber legislatures; the rest have *bicameral* arrangements with two chambers or houses that are typically elected and composed differently. Generally, the job of the upper house is to review and refine draft legislation that has started out in the lower house and thereby contribute to better policy and law making. In presidential systems, as we saw earlier, the legislature has autonomy from the executive and, on occasions, can make policy. In parliamentary systems, the task of the legislature is primarily to hold the government to account on behalf of the public for its performance rather than to initiate most policy. Legislators can identify problems in draft legislation and request changes.

In fact, in a range of different government systems, legislatures are increasingly regarded as bodies that rubber-stamp decisions taken elsewhere and even struggle to hold the executive to account. For example, in most parts of Africa, legislatures in the period after independence were largely regarded as bodies that approved the decisions of an authoritarian executive (Healey and Robinson 1992). However, while legislatures remain relatively weak, there are some positive trends (Barkan et al. 2010). Bills are increasingly scrutinized and often amended before being passed into law. More effective oversight of the executive also appears to be emerging in some countries, supported by a greater involvement of civil society in the political process especially in countries with large urban areas (see Chapter 6).

Efforts have been made in a number of countries to strengthen the role and influence of the legislature, principally by ensuring that members of parliament have the powers, staff and other resources to investigate and critique the activities of the executive and to develop alternatives to government policies. In the UK, a system of cross-party parliamentary select committees was introduced in 1979. There is a House of Commons (lower house) select committee for each government department, examining three aspects: spending, policies and administration. Select committees have powers to summon witnesses, including government ministers and senior civil servants, to appear to answer members' questions. These departmental committees have a minimum of 11 members, who decide upon the line of inquiry and then gather written and oral evidence. Findings are reported to the House of Commons and published. The government then usually has 60 days to reply to the committee's analysis and recommendations.

Activity 5.3

What obstacles do national legislatures (i.e. parliaments and assemblies) typically face in influencing government policy making and in holding the executive to account?

Feedback

Five main reasons are usually given for the difficulties faced by legislatures in fulfilling their functions. The relative importance of each depends on the country in question, but most are related directly or indirectly to the power of the executive:

1 increasingly strong political party discipline, controlling the activities of members and reducing criticism of the executive;
2 the ability of the executive to use its powers of patronage (i.e. the ability to offer or withhold opportunities for promotion into ministerial and other positions) to control potentially dissident members of the legislature;
3 the shift of much political and policy debate from the parliamentary debating chamber to the mass media (e.g. to the set-piece television interview or debate between party leaders);

4 the expansion of government activities and their delegation to a range of specialized agencies so that many decisions can be taken by bureaucrats and special advisers far from parliament without the need for new laws or legislative debate;

5 the increasing influence of supra-national bodies such as the European Union (EU), the International Monetary Fund (IMF) or the World Trade Organization (WTO) that limit or remove issues from domestic legislative politics (see Chapter 8).

Although some legislatures rarely propose new laws and others struggle to fulfil their three main functions, they survive because they have great symbolic value, upholding the ideal of democratic representation of the public. Also, particularly in presidential systems, they can block the proposals of the executive by right. In parliamentary systems, legislators can scrutinize and delay legislation, but where a government has a parliamentary majority and reasonable party discipline, it will prevail over opponents. Only where there is no clear majority and the government is dependent on several smaller parties do individual legislators have opportunities to shape policies directly. This is one of the arguments in favour of proportional representation.

If even the legislature does not have a great deal of say in policy formulation, who does?

The influence of the executive

As you have seen, in most countries with multi-party systems and even more in one party states, most of the power to initiate and make policy lies with the executive – the elected politicians who become prime minister or president and their ministers or immediate advisers. This group is usually called 'the cabinet'. The executive is generally more powerful in parliamentary than presidential systems, though this depends on the constitution of the country in question. The elected and appointed members of the executive are supported by the bureaucrats or civil servants who both advise ministers and take direction from them. There is debate about the relative influence on policy of elected officials and bureaucrats. It depends strongly on the country and the period studied as well as the nature of the policy issue at stake. In some countries, the senior level(s) of the bureaucracy are political appointees liable to change as the government changes, thereby blurring the distinction between political and bureaucratic influence on policy. In others, the civil service is permanent, politically neutral and separate from elected politicians. In the latter system, there has been a trend towards ministers appointing their own political advisers in addition to the ministry civil servants to give political, presentational and policy advice to ministers, including helping write political speeches.

Compared with the legislature, the executive or cabinet has far greater informational, financial and personnel resources. The cabinet has the authority to govern the country and usually has the ultimate authority to initiate policies. Crucially, it can generally choose when to introduce draft laws to the legislature, though not in all presidential systems. In parliamentary systems, as long as the government has majority support in the legislature, there can be few limits on the power of the executive. In presidential systems, the executive has to convince the legislature to approve its proposed measures where these involve legislation. However, there are still wide areas of policy where the executive has discretion, particularly in relation to defence, national security and foreign policy where legislation is rarely needed for action. Frequently, once the budget has been approved by the legislature, the executive has a great deal of control over the detail of how public resources are used.

The role of the chief executive

If the executive is very powerful, does this power emanate from the collective decision making of the cabinet, or from the strength of the prime minister or president who occupies a position similar to the chief executive of a private corporation? In those low and middle income countries where political leadership can be personal and unaccountable – where constitutional checks on the executive rarely operate – most major policy decisions will be made by the chief executive.

Sometimes, decision making is in the hands of a small group of ministers chosen from among the cabinet by the chief executive because they closely identify with the chief executive's goals and methods. There has been increasing discussion in parliamentary systems, especially in the UK, about the rise of a more authoritarian style of decision making of prime ministers. It started with Margaret Thatcher, the Conservative Prime Minister in the 1980s, and continued under Labour governments from 1997 to 2010. Observers noted that the prime minister and immediate staff were increasingly the key policy initiators with most of the cabinet and the civil service relegated to managing the detail of implementation. Just as Prime Minister Margaret Thatcher launched a major review of the management and organization of the National Health Service (NHS) in 1987 during a television interview without consulting any of her cabinet colleagues, so too Prime Minister, Tony Blair, made a major announcement on air in 2000. Without warning the rest of his cabinet or civil servants, he announced that he intended to bring the UK's level of health care spending up to the EU average as a share of national income. This sudden, personal commitment led to a review of the sources and level of spending on the NHS, and decisions to increase NHS spending to unprecedented levels over a five-year period (Wanless and the Health Trends Review Team 2002).

Thus, individual political leadership does matter, even in the complex and inter-connected contemporary world which constrains national governments in many ways (as you will see in Chapter 8). One of the most striking examples of the impact of con-trasting leadership decisions concerned government policy on AIDS in South Africa and Uganda in the late 1990s and early 2000s. Both countries had a very high prevalence of HIV. In South Africa, President Thabo Mbeki denied the link between HIV and AIDS as part of a national political struggle over the control of information and resistance to Western dominance of science (Schneider 2002). His government refused to support the purchase of anti-retroviral drugs for the treatment of people with AIDS. In Uganda, President Yoweri Museveni was widely credited with a quite different policy of openly discussing AIDS and inviting all groups to help develop a national response to the epidemic. Although the wider political environment in Uganda particularly favoured such a stance (e.g. there was no major tourist industry to be harmed by openness), the President himself contributed decisively to the direction of policy (Parkhurst 2001).

The contribution of the bureaucracy

The appointed officials who administer the system of government are referred to as civil or public servants. Although referred to as 'servants' of the politicians, their role extends beyond simply serving to managing policy processes in many areas of policy. There are far too many functions for the executive to discharge, so they delegate many to bureaucrats to carry out in their name. Civil servants also have influence because of their expertise, knowledge and experience. While ministers and governments may come and go, most of the bureaucrats remain to maintain the system of government. Even in countries such as the US and most of Latin America where top civil servants change when the ruling government changes, most public servants' jobs are unaffected. In countries like Australia, the UK and New Zealand, there is a strong tradition of civil service neutrality and independence of politicians. New governments and new ministers are clearly dependent on their officials for information, if only until they are familiar with what is happening in their field of responsibility and with the detail of how the system of government works. However, they may also be suspicious of officials who until recently had served a government led by their opponents and less likely to accept their views on policy options. In such situations, they tend to rely on their own political advisers who play increasingly important roles as the eyes and ears of the minister.

The power of the bureaucracy vis-à-vis politicians differs from country to country, over time and from sector to sector. For instance, in France, Japan, Korea and Singapore, the civil service traditionally has high status, a neutral professional ethos and a clear mandate to provide independent advice to politicians. After a long period of training, civil servants form a homogeneous, well-informed group and pursue a lifelong career in government.

Activity 5.4

How does the civil service in your country compare with those discussed in the preceding paragraph? You might want to structure your answer by writing a few sentences in answer to the following questions:

- What is the social status of civil servants?
- How well is the civil service paid?
- What special training do civil servants receive?
- How expert are they in different policy fields?
- Is being a civil servant a secure career or more like any other job?
- Does the civil service have a tradition of providing neutral, independent advice to ministers or is it more an extension of the executive?
- Do senior positions in the civil service change when the government changes?
- How do you think your civil service could be improved, particularly in relation to the health system?

Feedback

Clearly, the way the civil service operates varies from country to country. To answer these questions, you will most likely have had to do some research of your own. If you find that there are important gaps in your knowledge, you need to consult reference books and/or government publications to complete your description. There may be a department of central government or an agency that controls the civil service with a website, or there may be descriptions in books on government in your country that discuss the civil service.

Looking around the world, it becomes apparent that countries like Korea with strong bureaucracies are exceptional. In many countries, particularly poorer ones, with low wages, corruption and lack of infrastructure, bureaucracies often do not have the capability to deal with the problems the country faces. In such settings, the executive and its political supporters tend to use the government machinery and policy to pursue their own interests, at the expense of the needs and well-being of the majority of the population. In other words, the government lacks the twin features of *autonomy* and *capacity* discussed earlier in the chapter.

Even in countries with a much better equipped civil service, the power of the bureaucracy depends on its internal organization within a particular sector. Thus, if in the health sector, there are a small number of institutions and a small number of officials in each body who have some decision making power independent of politicians, bureaucrats will tend to be influential in certain health policy processes. By contrast, if there are a large number of agencies, each with some authority, no one group of officials is likely to be influential on a specific issue and politicians will most likely have more direct influence over a wider range of policy areas.

Similarly, the influence of the civil service on policy formation also depends on the extent to which it has a monopoly over advice reaching ministers. Thus, in Australia, the UK and New Zealand where traditionally the professional, politically neutral civil service was the main source of advice to ministers, governments have acted in the past 30 years to widen the range of sources of advice to ministers, for example, by developing policy and strategy units within government staffed by a mixture of political advisers and hand-picked civil servants, and by opening up civil service posts to outside applicants. One approach is to recruit successful entrepreneurs to advise on the reform of government itself as well as its policies. In this way, the boundaries between the civil service and the political sphere, together with other walks of life such as business and academia, have been deliberately blurred, and political appointees have grown in number and influence within the government process.

Finally, the influence of the bureaucrats depends on the type of policy at issue. Major policies (macro-economic policy, for example), and/or those with a high profile and ideological significance (i.e. 'high' politics) are more likely to be driven by the senior politicians and their personal advisers. If the civil service opposes such a policy direction, then, if the government persists, the civil service role will be confined to ensuring that the wishes of the government are implemented. By contrast, on issues of 'low politics' – dealing with technical problems relating to the day-to-day working of government such as the details of hospital reimbursement systems – civil servants tend to have much greater influence in shaping the issue and offering solutions.

The position of the ministry of health

The bureaucracy is not a seamless organization. It is divided into departments or ministries, as well as other agencies with specific functions. Indeed, specialization is a feature of bureaucracies. Each of these organizations will have its own interests and ways of operating. Most obviously, the ministry of finance is responsible for ensuring that resources are allocated between different ministries in line with government priorities whereas an individual ministry, such as health, is responsible for ensuring that the needs of the health sector are properly represented when decisions are made. Some conflict of view is inevitable as each ministry argues for what it regards as its proper share of the government's budget. In addition, different ministries relate to different 'policy communities' or 'policy networks' (i.e. more or less organized clusters of groups inside and outside government in a particular sector trying to influence government policy, see Chapter 6), which can vary in complexity and scale, thereby shaping the way ministries function. Furthermore, individual ministries are internally divided, often along functional, technical or policy lines. Thus, a ministry of health might have divisions relating to the main contours of the health system such as hospitals, primary health care and public health or the main diseases such as malaria, tuberculosis and HIV, as well as medical, nursing and other professional advisory departments which cut across these divisions. Each division tends to pursue its own interests and ideas in relation to policy formulation and implementation. There are also likely to be regional or district levels of the ministry or separate health authorities which may not play a large part in policy identification and formulation, but are important for policy implementation, depending on the extent of decentralization in the government system (more on this in Chapter 7).

Ministries of health play an essential function in governing and steering health systems. This function is sometimes referred to as *stewardship* or overall system oversight, which 'encompasses the tasks of defining the vision and direction of health policy, exerting influence through regulation and advocacy, and collecting and using information' (WHO 2000: xiv). Ministries shape and maintain the policy and regulatory framework within which health services are paid for and delivered. These frameworks, often in the form of legislation, define the respective roles, responsibilities and accountabilities of the ministry and other health system agencies.

The roles and responsibilities of ministries of health vary depending on how decentralized the health system is, particularly in systems paid for from taxation (ministries generally have more regulatory and fewer planning and resource allocation roles in systems based on social or private insurance). The following are some of the usual responsibilities:

- Advising the minister of health and the wider government on how to respond to the health problems facing the country currently and in the future, including priorities and targets for action and spending, and the institutional framework within which the actors in the health system operate.
- Developing, implementing and enforcing legislation and related regulations.
- Negotiating the operating and capital budgets for the public system with the ministry of finance in tax-financed systems, or ensuring the financial viability of the insurance funds in social insurance-based systems so that the financial risks of health care are shared across the population.
- Defining which services are covered by the public system and setting prices for goods and services (particularly in social insurance systems).
- Allocating resources (money, staff, equipment, facilities) to different parts of the country and/or services through strategies and plans.
- Planning the future workforce and subsidizing training.
- Setting standards and regulating the quality of care at organizational and individual professional levels.
- Monitoring health and health system performance according to goals of equity, efficiency, acceptability, responsiveness, etc.
- Providing infrastructural services such as for information technology, payment of physicians, etc.
- Coordinating action with other ministries and agencies that have roles to play in protecting health (e.g. in transport, agriculture and food).
- Generating appropriate information and research evidence to support all the above activities.
- Engaging in international cooperation to improve health policy and outcomes, for example, through the World Health Assembly (see Chapter 8).

Ministries have differing status. Where in the informal hierarchy of ministries does the ministry of health usually sit? In low and middle income countries, the health ministry is often seen as low down in the hierarchy, well behind the ministries of finance, defence, foreign affairs, industry, planning and education, despite having a relatively large budget because of the workforce, health centres and hospitals which it may pay for.

Activity 5.5

Why do you think that the ministry of health and health policy are often relatively low down the hierarchy of status and attention in low and middle income countries? Do you think that this is always justifiable?

Feedback

Explanations for the low status include the fact that such countries frequently face very pressing economic problems, the solutions to which are generally seen as lying in reforming and stimulating the economy rather than investing in health. The economists in dominant ministries of finance frequently regard spending on health as 'consumption' (i.e. current spending which produces only current benefits) and tend not to see it as 'investment' (i.e. spending now to produce a stream of benefits into the future) to which they would give higher priority. Their approach traditionally has been to try to restrict consumption as far as possible in favour of investment in fields such as infrastructure (roads, harbours, drainage schemes) with a view to making longer-term economic gains. However, it is increasingly being recognized that wisely targeted spending on health improvement (e.g. HIV prevention) can be a worthwhile investment, especially in countries with low life expectancy, and should be seen as part of economic policy since a healthier workforce is highly likely to be more productive (Commission on Macroeconomics and Health 2001).

Despite these insights, it is still true to say that health issues tend to come to the attention of the cabinet mostly at times of crisis (see Chapter 4). Although there may be crises about epidemics of disease such as cholera, malaria, TB, AIDS or SARS, economic crises are more likely to force discussions about health issues such as how to pay for expensive medicines or new technologies against a background of falling government revenues. It is very common in such circumstances to see intensive discussion of proposals to introduce user fees into free clinics. Often, these fees are very unpopular, but more importantly, blanket fee increases tend to reduce access among the neediest groups in society.

Relations with other ministries

In all countries, not just those where the ministry of health is of low status, other ministries whose policies affect health tend to be absorbed in their own sectoral policy issues rather than concerned to contribute to a government-wide set of health policies. Thus, departments responsible for sectors such as natural resources, agriculture and education, most notably, have their own goals to pursue and are accountable for meeting them. As a result, they may not give high priority to the human health implications of their decisions. Many countries set up inter-sectoral (cross-departmental) bodies in the

1970s for the development and implementation of health policy (e.g. a national health council in Sri Lanka) or across the whole of government (e.g. the Central Policy Review Staff in the UK) in response to a growing awareness of such problems. In the 1990s, many countries set up national committees or task forces in an attempt to respond to the HIV epidemic in a coherent way across all relevant agencies of government. Despite these continuing efforts, most policies tend to be pursued sectorally, reflecting the overriding structure of separate government ministries. Typically, ministries of agriculture continued to promote crops (e.g. tobacco) and forms of husbandry (e.g. intensive stock rearing) with the sole aim of maximizing profits without serious consideration of the potentially negative effects on the natural environment and nutrition. Many governments today continue to strive for more integrated or 'joined up' institutions and processes for policy formulation and implementation but fragmentation within the policy process is far easier to identify than to rectify. In many ways, it is perpetuated by other objectives such as raising the level of expertise within government which can lead to greater specialization and greater need for better systems of coordination.

Activity 5.6

Which government policy decisions in your country would have been different if their health implications had been taken into account properly?

Feedback

Your answer will obviously be specific to your country and your experience. Typically, policies such as large environmental projects (e.g. dams or highways) are not thoroughly assessed for their health consequences either directly or indirectly. For example, better and faster roads, unless well engineered with a view to reducing pedestrian injuries and deaths, can have major adverse consequences, especially for children. Such effects are often not well understood or not weighed in the balance against other costs and benefits. If they were, policy decisions might be different. Another example of policy that might well have been different if the health implications had been taken into account relates to government subsidies for the production of tobacco in a number of low and middle income countries. The costs of the negative health effects of consuming locally produced tobacco can outweigh the economic gains from production and exports.

While health should not always be the predominant goal of government decisions, since there are many other objectives that contribute to the well-being of populations and to better health (e.g. higher educational attainment), it is important for the full range of consequences of major policy decisions to be taken into account as far as possible. In the late 1990s, international agencies such as the Organization for Economic Cooperation and Development (OECD) promoted a more 'outcomes focused' approach to government policy making as a way to encourage better coordination of the actions of different ministries and agencies, and greater attention to all the outcomes of policies (OECD 1997). The idea is that all ministries should be required to show how they are contributing to improving the outcomes which the government values most, such as improving literacy and infant health, by the actions they take in their individual sectors. So, in principle, under such a system of reporting and accountability, the ministries of education and health should be more likely to take into account the interdependence of their activities since children's health is important for their educational attainment and vice versa. Similarly, the ministry of transport would be required to report its contribution to child health by demonstrating that its road schemes were designed to protect pedestrians as well as ensure the smooth flow of traffic. All government policies would be subject to health impact assessment (HIA) which is a means of assessing the health impacts of policies, plans and projects in diverse economic and policy sectors using quantitative, qualitative and participatory techniques. While rational, this cross-sectoral approach to policy analysis complicates the policy formulation and implementation processes.

Professional versus other sources of advice

A notable feature of ministries of health lies in the relatively high status of their principal advisers and of the health professionals they are trying to influence with their advice. They employ and purchase technical advice from doctors, nurses, pharmacists and other professionals. In many countries, the divisional heads are mostly health professionals, particularly doctors. Potential conflict between high status professionals and other bureaucrats is clearly possible. If the head of the ministry is a doctor, there may be some dissonance between professional and other goals. For example, the permanent head may be reluctant to initiate reforms which threaten the clinical freedom of doctors. There may be a tendency in policy thinking to see medical care as the main means of health improvement to the neglect of public health measures such as immunization or better water supplies.

Activity 5.7

Now that you have read about the main elements in systems of government, prepare a description of the government system in your country. The following questions will help you organize your account:

1 How many political parties are there? How do elections work (i.e. is there a form of proportional representation or a majoritarian system)? Do the parties prepare manifestos setting out what they would like to do if they were to be elected to government? Were their views presented through television, radio, newspapers, the Internet, Twitter, etc.? Does the current government have its political party office separate from the government? Is the current government made up of one or more political parties?
2 Is the system of government unitary or federal, i.e. are there regions or provinces which have substantial freedom to organize their own affairs (e.g. in health services) or are all the main decisions taken at national level and simply carried out at lower levels?
3 Is the national legislature uni- or bi-cameral? Are all members elected or are some appointed? If so, who appoints them? How much influence does the legislature have compared with the executive (cabinet)? Can its members question or challenge the decisions of the president and/or prime minister?
4 Who makes up the executive? If there is a president and a prime minister, what are their respective roles? Is the executive entirely separate from the legislature or do members of the executive have to come from the legislature? How strong

is the chief executive (president or prime minister) compared with other ministers in the executive?

5 What are the powers of the judiciary in relation to the actions of the executive and legislature? How independent are the judges of the governing party or parties? Is there a written constitution? Is it enforced by the courts?

6 How are public servants recruited and what is their role? How influential are civil servants on the actions of the elected government?

7 Overall, what sort of government system would you say you have in your country? Refer to the types of political regimes described in Chapter 2.

Feedback

If you find that there are important gaps in your knowledge, you need to consult reference books and/or government publications to complete your description. The United Nations also publishes information on the government systems of countries around the world.

Activity 5.8

Now that you have an understanding of the wider government system in your country, it is time to sketch out the main organizations of government that relate to the health system. The following questions should help you structure your account:

1 Is there a minister of health at national level or is the portfolio shared with other areas of policy? What is the scope of the relevant minister's responsibilities? Is the minister responsible for health in the cabinet? Is the post regarded as an attractive one for politicians?

2 Is there a national ministry of health or is health part of another ministry? How does it relate to the minister and to the legislature? What are its responsibilities? Where do its resources come from? How is the ministry staffed (i.e. by generalists, specialists or a mix) and how is it organized internally? Is there a hierarchy of national, regional, district and local functions and activities in the ministry, or does the ministry just operate at national level (e.g. setting the general direction of policy)?

3 Are there other national organizations relevant to health policy (e.g. official bodies responsible for training, quality improvement, information, etc.)? What does each do? How do these bodies relate either to the minister or ministry of health?

4 If there are advisers or experts from international agencies involved at national level, what do they do and how do they relate to the ministry of health?

5 How is the health system organized below the national level? Who owns the provider organizations? Is the clinical workforce employed by these organizations or contracted privately?

6 How do you think each of the organizational features you have described above affects the way that health policy decisions are made and implemented?

7 How does the wider government system which you summarized in the previous activity shape the way that the ministry of health and health system operate?

You will probably find it helpful to draw a diagram of how the different bodies relate to one another. This is known as an *organogram* or organizational chart. It is a convenient way of summarizing a lot of organizational information relatively simply. Typically, the chart shows lines of authority and accountability between different levels in a hierarchy. Arrows can also be used to show how resources and information flow between bodies, as well as consultative and advisory relationships.

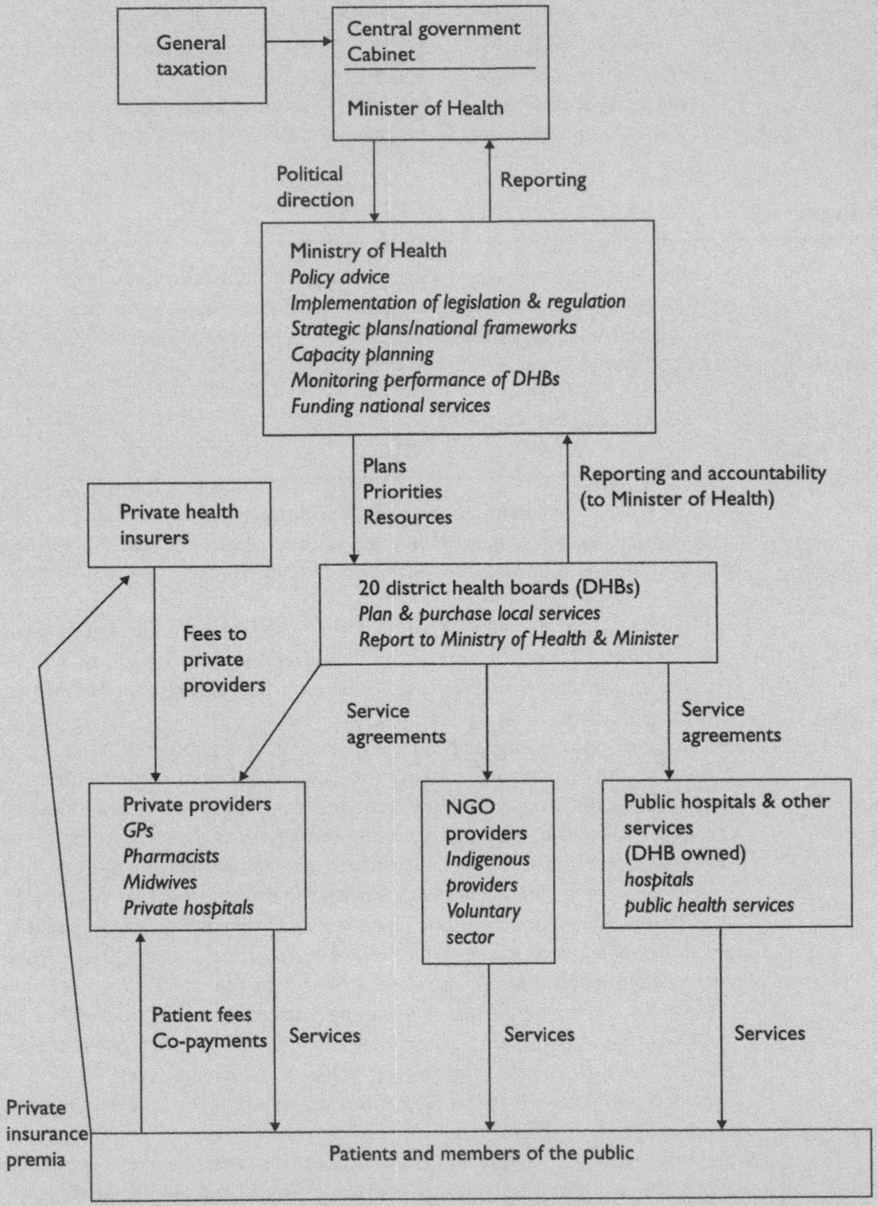

Figure 5.1 Organogram of New Zealand's health system, 2011

Source: Adapted and simplified from New Zealand Ministry of Health. *Structure of the Health and Disability Sector.* 9 March 2011. URL: http://www.health.govt.nz/new-zealand-health-system/overview-health-system/structure-health-and-disability-sector

Figure 5.1 is an example of an organizational chart for the health system of New Zealand. Some of the detail has been removed to make it clearer to see the leadership role of the ministry of health. There are a number of national bodies at arm's length from the ministry with specialized functions as well as a series of advisory committees serving the minister of health (e.g. the National Health Committee advises on the prioritization of new technologies and services) that have not been shown for simplicity.

Feedback

Clearly your answer to these questions will depend on your country of choice.

It is important to be aware that organization charts are a highly abstract picture of the system and can be misleading. The way a system works in practice may not correspond very closely to the way it is presented formally on an organizational diagram. The organizational chart perhaps most closely reflects the idealized rational model of the policy process (see Chapter 2). One of the aims of this book is to show that while this may be an aspiration, it is rarely an accurate depiction of the policy process. The previous chapter on how issues get onto the policy agenda, and the following two chapters on the role of interest groups and on policy implementation, show that the health policy process is strongly influenced by groups outside the formal decision making structure of the health system. In addition, the hierarchical, 'top-down' way in which systems are typically represented often fails to capture the way in which front-line staff can play a critical role in whether, and if so, how policies developed at higher levels are implemented (see Chapter 7).

Summary

Although most countries have legislatures which ostensibly make policy, their main function is normally one of debate and scrutiny of proposals coming from the executive. In most sectors of policy, the executive (ministers) and the bureaucracy (civil servants) usually have the resources and position to control what gets on to the policy agenda and is formulated into policy, with the legislators in a subsidary role, particularly in parliamentary systems. Where politicians change frequently, a permanent bureaucracy may have very significant power in policy formulation, but, in general, politicians initiate the formulation of policies in areas of major political concern ('high' politics).

References

Barkan JD, Mattes R, Mozaffar S, and Smiddy K (2010) *The African Legislatures Project: First Findings*. CSSR Working Paper No. 277. Cape Town: Democracy in Africa Research Unit, Centre for Social Science Research, University of Cape Town.

Commission on Macroeconomics and Health (2001) *Macroeconomics and Health: Investing in Health for Economic Development*. Report of the Commission on Macroeconomics and Health. Geneva: World Health Organization.

Evans PB, Rueschemeyer D and Skocpol T (eds) (1985) *Bringing the State Back In*. Cambridge: Cambridge University Press.

Hacker JS (2010) The road to somewhere: why health reform happened – or why political scientists who write about public policy shouldn't assume they know how to shape it. *Perspectives on Politics* 8: 861–76.

Healey J and Robinson M (1992) *Democracy, Governance and Economic Policy.* London: Overseas Development Institute.

Howlett M, Ramesh M and Perl A (2009) *Studying Public Policy: Policy Cycles and Policy Subsystems.* Don Mills, ON: Oxford University Press.

OECD (1997) *In Search Of Results: Performance Management Practices.* Paris: OECD.

Parkhurst JO (2001) The crisis of AIDS and the politics of response: the case of Uganda. *International Relations* 15: 69–87.

Schneider H (2002) On the fault-line: the politics of AIDS policy in contemporary South Africa. *African Studies* 61: 145–67.

Steinmo S and Watts J (1995) It's the institutions, stupid! Why comprehensive national health insurance always fails in America. *Journal of Health Politics, Policy and Law* 20: 329–72.

Tuohy CH (2004) Health care reform strategies in cross-national context: implications for primary care in Ontario. In Wilson R, Shortt SED and Dorland J (eds) *Implementing Primary Care Reform: Barriers and Facilitators.* Montreal: McGill-Queen's University Press, pp. 73–96.

Wanless D and the Health Trends Review Team (2002) *Securing Our Future Health: Taking a Long-Term View.* London: HM Treasury.

World Health Organization (2000) *World Health Report 2000: Health Systems, Improving Performance.* Geneva: WHO.

Interest groups and the policy process 6

Overview

The previous chapter focused on the formal institutions of government and how government policy makers are at the heart of the policy process. But neither politicians nor civil servants operate in a sealed system, especially not in well-functioning democracies, even if the government tends to be at the centre of collective decision making. To use the terminology of the 'policy triangle' in Chapter 1, there are many other *actors* in the policy process. Governments often consult external (non-governmental) groups to see what they think about issues and to obtain information. Governments may also fund non-governmental groups, or treat some preferentially. In turn, groups outside government attempt to influence ministers and civil servants. In most countries, there is a growing number of interest or pressure groups that want to influence government thinking on policy or the provision of services. They use a range of tactics to get their voices heard, including building relationships with those in power, lobbying them, mobilizing the media, setting up formal discussions or providing the political opposition with criticisms of government policy. Some interest groups are far more influential than others: in the health field, the medical profession and industries such as pharmaceuticals, insurance and food exert significant influence on governments in most countries. Increasingly, government operates in partnership with and through networks of these non-governmental actors. This is typically referred to as a shift from *government* to *governance* as governments are forced and choose to work with and through civil society and private sector organizations.

Learning objectives

After working through this chapter, you will be better able to:

- explain what an interest or pressure group is
- classify the different types of interest or pressure groups
- describe the tactics used by different interest groups to get their voices heard and exert pressure on governments
- appreciate the differential resources available to different sorts of interest groups
- identify how networks of interest groups and government actors form around particular fields of policy
- account for the increasing prominence of civil society groups and others in public policy making
- understand what is meant by the shift from 'government' to 'governance' in the way that fields of public policy are managed.

Key terms

Cause group. Interest or pressure group whose main goal is to promote a particular issue or cause.

Civil society. That part of society between the private sphere of the family or household and the sphere of government.

Civil society group. A group or organization which is outside government. It may or may not be involved in public policy (e.g. sports clubs are civil society organizations, but not primarily pressure groups). Private sector groups involved in the market (e.g. industry groups) are sometimes defined as in civil society, but are generally treated separately.

Governance. Denotes 'the rules of collective decision-making in settings where there are a plurality of actors or organisations and where no formal control system can dictate the terms of the relationship between these actors and organisations' (Chhotray and Stoker 2009: 3). Where once governments were perceived to be largely responsible for health governance, there has been a rearrangement of responsibilities, so that organizations outside government are also involved in health decision making.

Insider group. Interest groups that pursue a strategy designed to win themselves the status of legitimate participants in the policy process.

Interest (pressure) group. Any group outside the state including market and some civil society groups that attempts to influence policy to achieve specific goals.

Iron triangle. Small, stable and exclusive policy community usually involving executive agencies, legislative committees and interest groups (e.g. around defence procurement).

Issue network. Loose network comprising a large number of diverse members who usually come together to try to draw attention to an issue, address a specific problem or promote a particular solution.

Non-governmental organization (NGO). Any not for-profit organization outside government, often used to refer to structured organizations providing services.

Outsider group. Interest groups that have either failed to attain insider status or have deliberately chosen a path of confrontation.

Policy community (and sub-system). Relatively stable network of organizations and individuals involved in a recognizable field of wider public policy such as health policy. Within each of these fields, there will be identifiable sub-systems, such as for mental health policy, with their own policy communities.

Policy network. Generic term for inter-dependent organizations involved in an area of policy that exchange resources and bargain to varying degrees to attain their specific goals.

Sectional group. Interest group whose main goal is to protect and enhance the interests of its members and/or the section of society it represents.

Social movement. Loose grouping of individuals sharing certain views and attempting to influence others but without a formal organizational structure.

Introduction

In Chapter 2 you were introduced to the theory of pluralism, the view that power is widely dispersed throughout society such that no group holds absolute power. The pluralists were influential in drawing attention to the idea of the state arbitrating between competing interests as it develops policy. As a result, they focused on interest groups in order to explain how policy is shaped, arguing that, although there are elites, no elite dominates at all times. They contended that sources of power such as information, expertise and money, are distributed non-cumulatively. While this may be true for routine matters of policy ('low politics'), pluralism has been criticized for not giving sufficient weight to the fact that major economic decisions which are generally part of 'high politics' tend to be taken by a small elite in order to preserve the existing economic and political regime. In these circumstances, pluralism is clearly 'bounded' in that those interests wishing to replace a capitalist system of economic organization with a socialist one would not be invited to take part in the policy process.

Pluralists have also been criticized for focusing on Western liberal democracies, and failing to recognize differences between countries, not all of which have, until comparatively recently, national interest groups putting pressure on governments. Traditionally, in such countries, extra-governmental influences have tended to derive from personal and family connections in which ministers and officials are expected to use their position to enhance the situation of members of their families or tribes. However, in the 1980s and 1990s there was growing evidence of interest group activity in such settings. Related to this trend, there has been a proliferation of non-governmental organizations (NGOs), both national and international, in the health and development sectors in recent years. They are difficult to enumerate, but *The Economist* estimated that the number of international NGOs had risen from 6,000 in 1990 to 26,000 in 1996 and by 2002 the United Nations Development Programme (UNDP) Human Development Report estimated that there were 37,000 worldwide, a fifth of which had been formed in the 1990s (cited in McGann and Johnstone 2006). In part, this growth was due to waves of democratization leading to less authoritarian and elitist governments in a number of countries and, in part, to a concern to give greater opportunities to organizations outside government to make governments more accountable to their people.

Activity 6.1

Before reading any further, take a few minutes to think about your understanding of what is meant by 'interest groups'. Write your own definition and a list of the groups that could come under the heading of 'interest groups' in relation to health policy.

Feedback

At its simplest, an 'interest group' promotes or represents a particular part of society (e.g. people suffering from blindness or manufacturers of pharmaceuticals) or stands for a particular cause (e.g. environmentalism or free trade). Different types of interest group are discussed later in the chapter.

Your list of 'interest groups' involved in health policy is likely to have contained organizations and groups such as those representing:

*   staff, such as the medical, nursing and the allied health professions (e.g. physiotherapy, speech therapy)
*   providers, such as hospital associations
*   insurers such as sickness funds
*   payers such as employers' associations
*   different groups of patients
*   manufacturers/suppliers, such as pharmaceutical companies, medical equipment manufacturers and food corporations.

You may have wondered how different labels for organizations outside the formal system of government such as NGO, 'civic society group', 'interest group' and 'pressure group' related to one another. What follows now tries to clarify these different terms. Refer to the notes of your own definition as you go through this and modify them, if necessary.

Interest groups and civil society groups

'Pressure group' is another term for 'interest group' that you may hear used. While there are varying definitions of interest groups, most writers would agree on the following features:

*   they are voluntary – people or organizations choose to join them;
*   they aim to achieve some desired goals;
*   they generally do not attempt to infiltrate the process of decision making to the extent of becoming part of the formal government machinery.

Unlike political parties that are also voluntary and goal-oriented, pressure groups do not generally plan to take formal political power (e.g. by putting forward candidates for election). Sometimes they evolve into political parties and become involved in policy making from within government like the German Green Party which began life as an environmental pressure group. But most pressure groups exist outside government, even if some of them have very close relationships with government (as you will see in the discussion of 'insider' and 'outsider' groups, below).

It has been common to describe all interest groups, including industry interests as existing in *civil society*, meaning that they are located in the part of society that lies between the private space of the family or household and the public sphere of the government. Hence, the term *'civil society group'* is sometimes used synonymously with interest group, though public policy issues can be very peripheral to the identity of some civil society groups. For instance, sports clubs will only very occasionally take a position on an issue of public policy when it risks impinging on their sporting activities, whereas other groups are constantly in campaigning mode since this is central to their identity. Other groups such as organized religion sit somewhere in between. As a result, not all civil society groups should be seen as interest or pressure groups. Civil society organizations represent a wider range of organizations as Figure 6.1 tries to show.

If not all civil society groups are necessarily interest groups trying to influence policy, then it is logical to doubt whether it is helpful to see *all* interest groups as forming part of civil society. Some writers would exclude interest groups that are specifically related to market activities (i.e. trade and employer associations) from civil society, arguing that civil society is more specifically 'a sphere located between the state and market: a buffer zone strong enough to keep both state and market in check, thereby preventing each from becoming too powerful and dominating' (Giddens 2001). Certainly the altruistic motivations and goals of some civil society groups are very different from those of market-related interest groups that are self-interested. Figure 6.1 is drawn from this perspective. According to this scheme, civil society lies in the social space not occupied by the family/household, the state or the market.

NGOs form the most familiar part of civil society in the health and development sectors. The term NGO originally referred to any not-for-profit organization outside government but more recently has taken on the more specific meaning of a relatively structured organization with a headquarters and paid staff working in fields such as client advocacy or service delivery, in many cases providing a service that might have been provided directly by the state at an earlier stage. A good example is Médecins Sans Frontières (MSF) which began life by specializing in providing care in conflict and

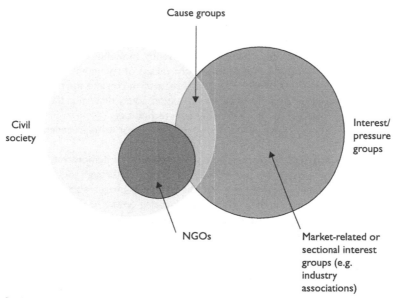

Figure 6.1 Civil society organizations, interest/pressure groups and NGOs

Note: not to scale

disaster zones, but has broadened in recent years to routine service delivery in under-served areas.

Many NGOs retain a desire to influence public policy and thus can act as pressure groups (hence the overlap shown in Figure 6.1 between NGOs and interest groups). MSF is no exception. Its *Campaign for Essential Medicines* challenged governments, inter-national organizations, the pharmaceutical industry and other NGOs to improve the rate of development of, and access to, life-saving medicines, diagnostic tests and vac-cines for patients in MSF programmes in low and middle income countries. The Campaign contributed to the reduced price of anti-retroviral drugs for HIV and encouraged a greater focus on neglected tropical diseases such as sleeping sickness, leishmaniasis and Chagas disease.

Usually, 'civil society group' has positive connotations, implying that such groups are a sign of a vigorous, healthy, non-authoritarian society. However, if a politician or public official calls an organization a 'pressure group', it may be a coded way of implying that it is narrowly focused, imbalanced in its point of view, illegitimate, or a nuisance. However, not all civil society groups are necessarily good for society. For example, organized criminal gangs are part of civil society.

Interest groups may start simply as a group of people concerned about a particular issue with little or no formal organization. When a large number of such groups get involved with the same issue, sociologists talk of them as forming a '*social movement*'. For example, the popular protests against authoritarian rule in countries like Tunisia and Egypt that formed the so called 'Arab Spring' of 2011 were social movements largely orchestrated through the elaborate use of social media, particularly by young people. As one expert commentator said of the demonstrations in an interview with the US think tank, The Council on Foreign Relations, in January 2011:

> What is also fascinating is that it is being facilitated by new technologies such as Facebook, YouTube, and Twitter, allowing people to communicate amongst them-selves in real time and in a very widespread way. The governments in the region are struggling to control it and to react to it. In Tunisia, they were unable to. In Egypt they've shut down Twitter intermittently, they shut down Facebook intermittently, they've tried to take control of the means of communication.
>
> In the past, when there were threats to the regime, the tanks would surround the television station and the radio station. Today that's not the case. If a regime feels threatened, it's going after this new technology.
> (http://www.cfr.org/egypt/arab-worlds-unprecedented-protests/p23908)

In Tunisia, video cameras in the mobile phones of demonstrators captured images of the first protests. These were widely transmitted through social media and contributed to spreading unrest elsewhere. The uploaded images also prompted Al Jazeera, the satellite television network, to begin focusing on the revolt, which toppled the Tunisian government and set the stage for the ensuing demonstrations in Egypt (Preston and Stelter 2011).

Different types of interest groups

Political scientists are fond of classifying the great diversity of interest groups into a number of analytical types. Perhaps the most important distinction is between:

- *Sectional* groups whose main goal is to protect and enhance the interests of their members and/or of the section of society they proclaim to stand for (the market-related interest groups in Figure 6.1 are sectional groups of this type).
- *Cause* groups whose main goal is to promote a particular issue or cause and whose membership is open to anyone who supports the cause without necessarily having anything to gain personally if the cause is successful (see Figure 6.1).

Examples of sectional interest groups include trade unions, employers' associations and bodies representing the professions. Examples of cause groups include campaigning groups such as those on abortion, free antenatal care, human rights, environment and conservation. Crudely, sectional groups tend to stand for producer interests (e.g. doctors, nurses, etc.) and cause groups tend to stand for consumer interests (e.g. organizations campaigning for people suffering from particular diseases, or for patients' rights in general) though this distinction should not be exaggerated (which is why Figure 6.1 can only be a guide).

Sectional groups

Sectional groups are usually able to bargain with governments because they typically provide a particular productive role in the economy. Their influence with government largely depends on how important government thinks this role is politically and economically. On occasions, they can challenge government policy, if they do not like what governments propose. For example, well-organized trade unions, particularly in the public sector, can persuade their members to withdraw their labour, thus harming both the economy and the reputation of the government, as well as withdrawing their financial support for political parties (mostly parties on the political left). Obviously the power of interest groups like trade unions depends on factors such as the structure of the economy (e.g. workers in a large number of small enterprises are far harder to organize than those in a small number of large firms), the structure of wage bargaining (in a more decentralized system, the power of unions is generally less than in more centralized systems), the number of unions, whether they are ideologically unified and how well funded they are. The media can be regarded as a special form of sectional interest with a particularly important role in agenda setting as well as in selling its services to maximize its profits (see Chapter 4).

In most sectors of policy, including health, producer interest groups tend to have the closest contacts with government and exercise the strongest influence, while consumer groups tend to have less influence, principally because their cooperation is less central to the implementation of policies. In health policy, the medical profession was traditionally regarded as occupying a dominant position not just in controlling the delivery of health care (particularly who is permitted to carry out which tasks), but also in shaping policy in relation to health care systems. In Western countries, physicians controlled and regulated their own training and day-to-day clinical work for much of the twentieth century. The scope of practice of other health workers such as nurses depended on the consent of doctors and their role was seen primarily as supporting doctors rather than acting independently. In the eyes of the public, the medical profession was seen as the most authoritative source of advice on health-related matters whether at the individual, community or national levels. Health care systems tended to be organized in deference to the preferences of medical interest groups (e.g. systems of reimbursement in public systems that mirrored the fee-for-service arrangements in private practice). However, from the 1980s there was a significant, multi-pronged challenge to the medical profession's privileged status.

Activity 6.2

What have been the major challenges to the dominant position of doctors in health care and policy over the past 40 years?

Feedback

Your answer probably included a number of different challenges coming from different sources. Here are some of the challenges you may have identified:

- Governments and insurers attempted to control doctors' use of resources by imposing budget caps, limiting the range of drugs that they can prescribe, or restricting patient referral to the least cost or most efficient providers.
- Governments and insurers brought in stronger management and encouraged competition (e.g. between public hospitals and between public and private providers) in order to make medical services more responsive and efficient.
- Governments developed systems for assessing the quality of clinical care and promoted evidence-based medicine rather than relying on precedent and individual clinical judgement.
- The so called 'medical model' of disease which explains ill-health in terms of biological factors and the appropriate response in individual, curative terms was challenged by the 'primary care approach' which emphasized inter-sectoral action beyond the confines of individual treatment and of the health care system, and community involvement and control of health care facilities to make them more responsive to local people's needs.
- There was a growing recognition that patients themselves had expertise in relation to their own ill-health, particularly where this was chronic, derived from their own experiences and from wider use of information sources such as the Internet, and that this could contribute to better outcomes, as long as it was recognized by doctors, and patients were permitted to share responsibility with professionals.
- Nurses and other health care workers became better educated and organized, and governments moved to widen the range of clinical tasks they were permitted to undertake, sometimes at the expense of doctors.

All of these challenges can be detected in government policies in the UK from the mid-1980s to the present. Governments not only introduced policies which were actively opposed by the medical establishment such as the 'internal market' in the NHS in 1991 and further market reforms in the 2000s, but they also contrived to split the profession, thereby weakening its ability to resist change. For example, in one strand of the internal market reforms of 1991, general practitioners were offered the opportunity of holding their own budgets for their patients' elective hospital care as well as for their pharmaceutical costs. A substantial minority were keen to do so, making it difficult for the doctors' trade union to sustain its opposition to the policy. Had the policy been imposed on all GPs, it would most likely have failed.

While it is undoubtedly true that medical interests have been challenged and have lost some influence in Western countries, the knowledge and authority with which medical organizations speak are still a key resource enabling them to influence health policy (Johnson 1995).

In many low income countries, professional associations have not played such an important role in health policy, although this may be changing. In part, this is because most publicly paid-for health care and preventive activity are undertaken not by doctors but by nurses and community health workers in these settings. The medical profession largely serves the small urban elites through private practice. Doctors are influential in public health policy in such countries, but often as civil servants in the ministry of health or as health ministers rather than through the medical associations.

Cause groups

Cause groups aim to promote an issue that is not necessarily specific to the members of the group themselves, although it can be. For example, disabled people or people living with AIDS may form a pressure group to shape policy directly related to them. On the other hand, people from all walks of life with a wide range of beliefs come together in organizations such as Greenpeace devoted to global conservation of species or Amnesty International which highlights human rights' abuses all over the world.

It is generally assumed, somewhat naively, that cause groups arise spontaneously through the actions of unconnected individuals based on their beliefs. However, some cause groups are actually 'front' groups which have been set up at arm's length from corporate interests as a way of getting their views into the civil society debate in a seemingly more persuasive way. The public relations arms of large corporations and trade associations reason that their messages are more likely to be listened to by the public if they are articulated by apparently independent interest groups. Thus the Global Climate Coalition campaigned against the 1997 Kyoto Protocol to the UN Framework Convention on Climate Change, which limits the emission of greenhouse gases on scientific and social grounds, without it being immediately apparent to the casual observer that the Coalition was funded by the oil and motor industries. Similarly, the tobacco industry supports libertarian organizations devoted to promoting the rights of smokers to smoke without hindrance from government regulation and the food industry has funded seemingly independent research bodies such as the World Sugar Research Organization.

In the past 35 years in Western countries, membership of cause groups has risen and membership of political parties has tended to fall. Political scientists argue that this is a result of a growing disillusionment, particularly among younger people, with conventional Left–Right party politics and with the seeming remoteness of representatives in a democratic system. It is also a function of people's concern about large single issues such as environmental conservation and climate change (both with major health implications) that had not been given high or consistent priority by conventional political parties, often because of pressure from business interests and threats that they would withdraw their funding of political parties.

Activity 6.3

What are the main resources that interest groups have to bring about the change that they desire? Think of a range of different interest groups that you are familiar with and list their attributes and resources.

Feedback

The resources that interest groups can mobilize vary widely. Some of the resources you may have listed include:

- Their members – the more members, all other things being equal, the more influence an interest group is likely to have, though in the case of patient groups, their personal experience may give them even greater legitimacy. Interest groups composed of other organizations, particularly where they are representative of these other associations (known as 'peak' or 'apex' associations), are particularly likely to have more influence and often draw on a wide range of skills, knowledge and contacts from within their constituent organizations.
- Their level of funding – funding affects all aspects of an interest group's activities such as its ability to hire professional staff to organize campaigns and work with the media, prepare critiques of government policy and develop alternatives, contribute to political parties, organize rallies and demonstrations, and so on. This explains, in large part, why health producer interest groups tend to be better organized than consumer groups since their members are often prepared to pay large subscriptions to ensure that their key economic and professional interests are well represented and defended.
- Their knowledge about their area of concern – some of this information and understanding may be unavailable from any other source. For example, a government may be dependent on a commercial interest group for access to confidential information about the likely financial impact of a proposed policy on its members that may be essential to justify the policy.
- Their persuasive skills in building public support for particular positions or policies by stimulating activity by others, such as the mass media.
- Their contacts and relationships with policy-makers, officials, ministers, opposition parties and the media.
- The sanctions, if any, at their disposal – these could range from embarrassing the government in international fora or the mass media to organizing consumer boycotts thereby harming the domestic economy or mounting protracted industrial action.

Strategies and relations to the state: 'insider' and 'outsider' groups

Interest groups can also be analysed in terms of how far they are recognized or legitimized by governments which, in turn, relates to their aims and their strategies. Grant (1984) identified two basic categories in this respect – *insider* and *outsider* groups. Insider groups are groups which are not officially part of the machinery of government but are regarded as legitimate by government policy makers, are consulted regularly and are expected to play by the 'rules of the game'. For example, if they accept an invitation to sit on a government committee, they can be relied upon to respect the confidentiality of the discussions that take place there until ministers are ready to make a statement about the agreed direction of policy. Insider groups thus become closely involved in testing policy ideas and in the development of their field. Typically, in health policy, producer groups such as medical and nursing associations expect to be consulted at an early stage or directly involved from the outset in policy developments and frequently are, even if they do not always get their own way.

In the UK, the Association of the British Pharmaceutical Industry (ABPI) has traditionally had insider status with the Department of Health on the grounds that the government is both concerned to promote the UK pharmaceutical industry and to ensure that safe and effective medicines are available at the earliest opportunity to patients. There are regular meetings between the industry, senior officials and ministers. Like so many sectional interests, the ABPI has also recruited retired civil servants to help it negotiate with government over drug regulation and prices, thereby improving its insider knowledge of the policy making process.

Outsider groups, by contrast, are either organizations that reject a close involvement in government processes on strategic grounds or have been unable to gain a reputation as legitimate participants in the policy process. Perhaps the most high profile outsider groups in the contemporary health field are anti-abortion and anti-vivisection organizations because of the vehemence of their views and their reputation for taking direct action against clinics, laboratories and sometimes those who work in them. One of the best-known public health direct action groups was BUGA UP (Billboard Utilising Graffitists Against Unhealthy Promotions). Founded in 1979 in Sydney, Australia, it was notorious (or celebrated, depending on your point of view) for illegally defacing outdoor advertising of unhealthy products, particularly tobacco and alcohol. Its tactic was to alter tobacco advertisements to provide a critical commentary on the industry's promotions. 'Anyhow, Have a Winfield' was changed to 'Anyhow, it's a Minefield' (Chapman 1996).

Interest groups may shift their strategies over time. For example, in its early life, Greenpeace favoured direct action as a way of drawing attention to conservation issues. Most notably it disrupted the activities of whaling vessels. More recently, Greenpeace has adopted a less flamboyant strategy through scientifically based advocacy though it does still use direct action from time to time. In the process, it has developed closer relations with governments, though is probably not regarded as a full insider group. Groups that shift their strategies or positions are known as *thresholder* groups.

The Treatment Action Campaign (TAC) in South Africa successfully used a wide range of insider and outsider strategies over time to advance a human rights approach to access to medicines for HIV, combining negotiation with government and outspoken criticism, constitutional litigation, alliance building with civil society organizations internationally, engagement with scientists and the media, and social mobilization including demonstrations, civil disobedience and campaigns (Heywood 2011; Robins 2004). Over time TAC's success in embarrassing and pressurizing the government led to close involvement in drafting the National Strategic Plan on HIV, AIDS and Sexually Transmitted Infections, 2007–11 which committed the government to a large increase in spending on anti-retrovirals.

Activity 6.4

Obtain information on a number of health-related interest groups (perhaps in a field of health that you are interested in) and try to work out what sorts of strategies they are using, their range of activities and whether they could be regarded as insider, outsider or thresholder groups.

Feedback

The stance of an organization will not always be apparent from its literature or website, but there are some clues you can look for. For example, the slogans of an organization give an indication of its stance towards government. If the organization is 'fighting' for animal rights, it is more likely to be an 'outsider' group than one that claims to be 'working' for animal rights. Similarly, an organization that lists its main activities as organizing demonstrations and mobilizing the media is likely to be pursuing an 'outsider' strategy, while an organization that describes its participation in government committees and consultations, or its links to elected representatives, is more likely to be following an 'insider' track.

Functions of interest groups

Taken together, the different types of interest groups indicate the range of functions that they can fulfil in society. Peterson (1999) argues that interest groups can potentially provide the following seven functions in society:

1 Participation – given that elections in democracies are both an infrequent and a highly indirect way for citizens to involve themselves in public issues, interest groups provide an alternative way for voters to get involved in politics and register their opinions to politicians.
2 Representation – where policy makers take into account the views of a range of interest groups, this normally widens the range of opinion under consideration.
3 Political education – provide a way for members to learn about the political process, for example, if they become office holders in an interest group.
4 Motivation – interest groups can draw new issues to the attention of governments, provide more information, change the way governments view issues and even develop new policy options through their scientific and political activities.
5 Mobilization – interest groups build pressure for action and support for new policies (e.g. by stimulating media interest in a topic).
6 Monitoring – increasingly, interest groups are assessing the performance and behaviour of governments, thereby contributing to the public accountability of leaders, for example, by seeing whether political promises are implemented. They are also increasingly involved in holding private corporations to account as national governments struggle to deal with the power of transnational businesses (see Chapter 8).
7 Provision – interest groups can use their knowledge of a particular patient group or area of policy to deliver services with or without government funding (e.g. missionary societies).

Interest groups are also increasingly involved in conducting or commissioning scientific research, providing technical advice and using legal action or the threat of legal action against governments and transnational corporations to promote their point of view and force change in policy. For example, national and international civil society organizations played an important part in the legal action against the South African government in the mid-2000s which forced the government to concede the principle that anti-retroviral drugs should be made available universally.

Activity 6.5

Taking the list of seven functions plus the ones mentioned in the paragraph immediately above, find examples of interest groups that carry out each of these activities. You may find that some organizations carry out many of these functions and others focus on just one. You can get this information from libraries, information centres, the ministry of health, newspapers, websites, annual reports and so on.

Feedback

Larger interest groups tend to have a wider range of functions and ways of operating. For example, Oxfam, the British-based international anti-poverty NGO describes itself as 'a development, advocacy and relief agency working to put an end to poverty world-wide'. Its activities cover 'motivation', 'mobilization', 'monitoring' and 'provision' according to Peterson's typology as well as 'representation' in some of the 70 or so countries it works in. Project HOPE (Health Opportunities for People Everywhere) is the largest US NGO devoted to international health. Its website describes its mission as: 'to achieve sustainable advances in health care around the world by implementing health education programs and providing humanitarian assistance in areas of need'. While its early work concentrated on emergency humanitarian health care relief work, its scope has broadened to include educating local health care professionals and lay health workers, and strengthening health care facilities. It currently works in 35 countries worldwide.

Some other international organizations are more politically focused. For example, Corporate Accountability International campaigns to protect the environment, public health and democracy from what it sees as abuses by transnational corporations. As a result, it played a significant role alongside many other groups in campaigns against the marketing of breast milk substitutes in developing countries in the 1970s and 1980s and in favour of the control of the promotion of tobacco products in the 1990s. Current campaigns focus on getting countries to ratify and implement the Framework Convention on Tobacco Control, and promoting and protecting public water supplies while discouraging the corporate promotion of bottled water.

Smaller NGOs tend to have more focused goals and activities. For example, the Fred Hollows Foundation is an NGO devoted to working with local blindness prevention agencies in around 20 countries to reduce unnecessary and avoidable blindness, with a primary focus on cataract. As with many NGOs, its main function is 'provision', including training local staff to deliver services and developing high quality, low cost technologies for eye care.

Relations between interest groups and government

Political scientists have observed that when it comes to policy formulation and implementation in health (as opposed to getting an issue onto the agenda in the first place), the participants (actors) are usually individuals and organizations with an enduring interest and knowledge of the field, even if, conceivably, a far wider range of actors could potentially be involved. Who is involved, for what reasons and how their relationships are structured have been the subjects of much research on what have been referred to at various times as 'policy networks', 'policy communities' and 'policy sub-systems'. The terminology and classifications can be confusing and even contradictory. They are all forms of network linking governments with 'insider' interest groups. By definition, 'outsider' groups are generally excluded fom these networks or very peripheral since they seek influence at a distance and through conflict.

A *network* in a policy area consists of organizations that have resources important to others in the policy area such as information, skills and influence, but which are dependent on others in the network for other resources (e.g. money, access to government decision makers). They thus have to exchange resources to achieve their goals (Rhodes 1997). Government becomes part of these networks depending on the degree to which it depends on interest groups to develop and implement its policies. Analyses of policy areas as networks of actors or interests are common (stakeholder analysis described in Chapter 10 is often used as part of a network analysis). However, network analysis is criticized for failing adequately to explain how policies change and how some interests gain or lose power. The advocacy coalition framework (ACF) is one approach to incorporate a theory of change into a network analysis and is described in Chapter 7.

Political scientists argue that the increasing significance of policy networks in public policy represents an important change in the process of governing, or making decisions. Policy networks reduce the ability of governments to act alone and require politicians and bureaucrats to learn new skills of working with and through interest groups in a less hierarchical and more negotiated, less controlling way. This trend is sometimes summed up as representing the transition from a world of *government* to one of *governance*. A key skill of governments in such a world is the ability to coordinate and hold to account a disparate set of actors, many of which are far from its direct control. One set of forces driving this transition relates to globalization which reduces, but by no means eliminates, the power of national governments as they become increasingly dependent on international agencies, agreements and business corporations (see Chapter 8).

One way of understanding the formal and informal network relationships between government and non-government (interest group) actors is to identify the various *policy sub-systems* in which they interact. At its simplest, a policy sub-system is a recognizable sub-division of public policy-making comprising the individuals and groups most often involved in decisions in that field. In health policy, for example, mental health policy formulation is distinctively different from policy on environmental health issues and involves different actors. Some sub-systems, known as *iron triangles*, are small, very stable and highly exclusive, three-way sets of relationships usually between politicians, bureaucrats and a commercial interest. In the case of food and agriculture policy in the US, the triangle is constituted by the Department of Agriculture, politicians from farming regions and the agribusiness (the food industry), and leads to the continuing subsidy of unhealthy food production. Other sub-systems are typically larger (i.e. involving more entities), more fluid and with less clear boundaries (e.g. family policy).

Marsh and Rhodes (1992) distinguish between 'policy communities' and 'issue networks' which can be regarded as the opposite ends of a continuum of different types of policy network. They see 'policy communities' as highly integrated networks involving a limited number of participants, each controlling some valued resources with some groups excluded, and marked by stable and frequent relationships, persistence over time in membership and consensus in terms of values and policy preferences. The main point about a policy community is that there is sustained interaction between the participants through a web of formal and informal relationships (Lewis 2005). By contrast 'issue networks' are loosely inter-dependent, unstable networks comprising a large number of members whose interaction fluctuates. There is a lack of consensus and may be conflict within the issue network. Its members have very different levels of resources and power inhibiting the level of bargaining within the network. Such networks usually draw attention to issues and help with agenda setting, whereas the predominant form of interaction in the policy community is one of bargaining over policy developments.

In health policy, organizations and individuals representing practitioners (health professionals), users, the public, researchers (from laboratory sciences to the social sciences), commentators (journalists and policy analysts), businesses (drug companies, medical equipment manufacturers), hospitals and clinics, insurers, government officials, politicians and international organizations are involved with government to differing degrees depending on their resources and the issue at stake. Some sets of relationships are closer to the integrated policy community end of the spectrum and others are closer to the fluid issue network end.

Activity 6.6

Think of a tight 'policy community' or loose 'issue network' around a specific health policy issue in your own country. It could be focused on any public health issue such as whether or not condom use should be promoted to prevent HIV infection. List those interest groups known to be or likely to be critical of the current policies in your country and those likely to be supportive.

Feedback

Obviously your answer will depend on the policy network and issue you considered. For example, if you chose the issue of condom use and HIV, your answer will reflect the precise arrangements for HIV prevention in your country and the groups involved in trying to influence policy in this field. The list might include the following:

- In support of policies to increase condom use: ministry of health, national HIV/AIDS commission or programme, interest groups of people living with HIV/AIDS and their supporters, sexual and reproductive health NGOs, family planning associations, employers (those aware of the economic costs of AIDS).
- Against policies to increase condom use: some religious groups, some international donors (i.e. those promoting abstinence), sections of the media (others may be supportive), certain professional associations.

Which sorts of interest groups are most influential?

Among interest groups, business interests are generally the most powerful in most areas of public policy, followed by interest groups representing workers. This is because both capital and labour are vital to the economic production process. In capitalist societies, ownership of the means of production is concentrated in the hands of business corporations rather than the state. As a result, business has huge power vis-à-vis government, particularly in the current globally interconnected environment in which corporations can potentially shift their capital and production relatively easily between countries if their interests are being harmed by government policies (see Chapter 8).

As Chapter 3 showed, there is a wide range of industrial and commercial interests involved in health policy. Even in health care systems where most services are provided in publicly owned and managed institutions, there will be extensive links with private sector actors who bring new ideas and practices into the public sector (e.g. improving safety procedures in operating theatres by learning from the aviation industry) as well as providing essential services (e.g. construction firms building hospitals and IT companies providing information systems). However, provider professionals and workers as well as governments have an important influence on policy in addition to business interests. In the case of governments, this is because of the large contribution of public finance and provision in most (particularly high income) countries. In the case of the doctors, this is because of the medical monopoly over a body of knowledge allied to the control that they are able to exert over the market for their services. Consumer (user) and public interests are also increasingly heard and responded to.

Through a study of successive hospital reforms in New York in the 1960s and 1970s, the sociologist Robert Alford (1975) argued that beneath the surface interplay of a wide range of interests in the health care arena in high income countries, lay three *structural* or fundamental interests that defined how health care politics operated and whose inter-relationships determined how the system was governed:

1 the *professional monopolists* – the doctors and to a lesser extent the other health professionals whose dominant interests are served by the existing economic, social and political structures of government and the health system;
2 the *corporate rationalizers* – who challenge the professional monopolists by attempting to implement strategies such as rational planning of facilities, efficient methods of health care delivery and modern management methods over medical judgement. These can be private insurers, governments as payers, health planners, employers wanting to curb the cost of insuring their workers, commercial hospital chains, etc.;
3 the *equal health advocates* and *community health advocates* – the wide range of relatively repressed cause and sectional interest groups lobbying for patients' rights, fairer access to health care for poor and marginalized groups and more attention to be given to the views of patients and populations in health care decision making.

In the 1970s, when Alford published his theory of structural interests, consumers and the public had relatively little voice in shaping health care policies but managers and planners were increasingly trying to assert greater control over how systems were financed and organized. In the past 35 years, corporate rationalizers (both public and private) and patient and community health advocates have been seen as increasing their influence in health care policy making in high income countries (Evetts 2006). However, trends in professional autonomy are not all pointing in the same direction or moving at the same speed. For example, in Russia, there are signs of a revival of traditional medical professionalism after the Soviet era when the professions were subordinated to the Communist Party (Yurchenko and Saks 2006). While the *structuralist* approach is a useful way of understanding the broad contours of policy and who is likely to have the greatest influence, in order to understand the dynamics of particular policy trajectories, it is necessary to analyse the interactions within the formal and informal networks of groups that grow up around specific issues and their relationship to the wider socio-political context.

What impact do interest groups have?

It is increasingly apparent that interest groups are playing a more influential role in health policy including in low and middle income countries where they have traditionally been weak or absent. Of course, the extent of influence on policy from outside government varies from place to place and from issue to issue. This changing relationship between government and interest groups can be seen as part of the wider shift in the way that governments operate, discussed above, from a hierarchical, directive and controlling mode towards operating through networks of government, civil society and private sector organizations.

The history of the global response to AIDS is noteworthy for the very high level of involvement and influence of civil society organizations acting as interest groups. 'Nothing for us; without us' was a common rallying cry leading to the institutionalization of the GIPA principle (greater involvement of people living with AIDS). As a consequence,

> Never before have civil society organizations – here defined as any group of individuals that is separate from government and business – done so much to contribute to the fight against a global health crisis, or been so included in the decisions made by policy-makers.
>
> (Zuniga 2005)

The AIDS history is also notable for the diversity of interest group activities, the large number of national AIDS organizations involved in policy making (over 3,000 in 150 countries in the mid-2000s) and the shift of activism from the high to low and middle income countries as Case Study 7 shows.

Case Study 7: the history of the role of civil society groups in global policy to combat HIV

Phase of activism	Main activities	Main demands	Impact
Early 1980s in US and Western countries: civil rights activism	Protest, lobbying and activism modelled on US black civil rights movement of 1960s	Protection of human and civil rights; PLWA are not to blame; inclusion of PLWA in policy process – inclusion and partnership	Traditional STI approach of isolation, surveillance, mandatory testing and strict contact notification replaced by rights based model promoted by WHO from 1987

(Continued overleaf)

Case Study 7 Continued.

Phase of activism	Main activities	Main demands	Impact
Mid-/late-1980s in US and Western countries: aggressive, scientific activism	New more aggressive organizations such as ACTUP and TAG lobbying politicians; simultaneous street protests and scientific debates with government; AIDS pressure groups winning places on government committees	Government funding for treatment and price reductions for early ART	Access to effective treatment for PLWA; showed that new drugs did confer benefits and that early trials did not warrant denying treatment to PLWA; ensured that trials included women, minorities, etc.
1990s in US and Western countries: institutionalized and internalized activism	US/Western activist groups shrinking because of success; activists increasingly accepted and working within health policy system; established CSO role in provision	Ensuring that HIV remains a policy and resource allocation priority in the West; attention should be given to HIV in poorer countries	Increased awareness of distribution of HIV and AIDS globally
Later 1990s in low and middle income countries: growing activism	Overseas funding to raise awareness and educate people, and support CSOs; explosion of CSOs; North-South cooperation between CSOs	Franker public discussion of HIV and AIDS, better leadership, concerted government responses, provision of AZT and treatment of co-infections	Notable impact in pioneer countries such as Brazil and Uganda; latter showed that ART could be provided in a middle income setting with good results and that comprehensive response could save health care costs
Late 1990s/early 2000s: global movement for treatment access	Period of advocacy sparked by successful CSO protest and resistance to attempt by US/SA pharmas to prevent SA government from offering low cost, generic ART; growing international coalition of NGOs pushing for low cost ART by promoting production of generic drugs and pressurizing pharmas to reduce their prices in low income settings	Universal access to affordable treatment as a human right; HIV to be seen as a security and development issue with major negative economic consequences	CSOs contributed to recognition that public health considerations had some weight alongside trade and intellectual property considerations in WTO; new funding initiatives (Global Fund to Fight AIDS, TB and Malaria, and US President's Plan for AIDS Relief – PEPFAR); gradual roll-out of ART helped by lower drug prices in developing world

Case Study 7 Continued.

Phase of activism	Main activities	Main demands	Impact
2000s	Advocacy continues but is complemented by an increasing role in service delivery – particularly with funds from Global Fund and PEPFAR	Universal access to HIV prevention, treatment and care; PEPFAR and Global Fund should finance generic ARVs; Recognition of men who have sex with men, sex workers and people who inject drugs as higher risk groups	Mobilization of resources – from 1.6b in 2001 to 15.9b in 2010; Unprecedented roll out of treatment coverage in low and middle income countries from 300,000 in 2001 to 6.6m in 2010 (22-fold increase); Drop in new infections from 3.1m in 1999 to 2.6m in 2010 (20% reduction); High risk populations named for first time in a UN General Assembly Declaration in 2011

Note: ACTUP, AIDS Coalition to Unleash Power; ART, anti-retroviral treatment; AZT, Azidothymidine; CSO, civil society organization; PLWA, people living with AIDS; STI, sexually transmitted infection; TAG, Treatment Action Group; SA, South Africa.

Sources: Seckinelgin (2002), Zuniga (2005), UNAIDS (2011)

Activity 6.7

Why has the AIDS policy arena attracted such a high level of civil society group involvement as shown in Case Study 7?

Feedback

A number of factors help to explain the high level of interest group activism, particularly in the early stages of the pandemic in high income countries which provided models for later activism in low and middle income countries:

1 The demographic profile of the early affected population and most subsequent infections – HIV tends to infect young adults and in countries like the UK, it initially affected a relatively affluent male homosexual population in cities.
2 HIV and even AIDS before therapy was available is not an immediate killer, allowing an opportunity for activism, unlike some other diseases.
3 Spillover from other social movements – in the US and Western Europe, the most affected population group was homosexual men who had recent experience of the gay rights movement of the 1970s. They used some of the same civil rights strategies and refused to play the role of 'patients'. In low and middle income

countries subsequently, AIDS activism was inspired by and allied itself to wider social justice movements such as those for debt relief.

4 The slowness of the official response in high income countries – it took between two and four years, and sometimes longer, between the first diagnosis and the development of official awareness campaigns.

Activity 6.8

Why do you think AIDS activism was less prominent in low and middle income countries in the 1980s and early 1990s?

Feedback

There are a number of inter-related reasons for this phenomenon. You may have written down some or all of the following:

1 A lack of data and, therefore, lack of awareness of the pandemic.
2 Unresponsiveness of political leaderships, especially in undemocratic countries in Africa (which were more common in the 1980s).
3 Denial by governments of the prevalence of the disease in countries and popular views that AIDS was a Western, alien problem only affecting homosexuals.
4 The fact that AIDS in low and middle income countries did not affect a cohesive, well-off group such as the male homosexual population in the US but poor people who could easily be silenced and ignored.
5 Other priorities competing for the attention of interest groups and health systems such as more immediately lethal diseases and malnutrition.
6 Lack of donor interest and funding to NGOs in the area of AIDS.

Is interest group participation a good thing in policy terms?

Up to now, the involvement of interest groups and the evolution of networks have been analysed without attempting to draw attention to their positive and negative consequences for policy making. Generally, in democratic societies, the involvement of organizations outside the government in policy processes is seen as a good thing. However, there are potential drawbacks.

Activity 6.9

List the possible positive and negative consequences of having a wide range of interest groups involved in the shaping of health policy.

Feedback

Your lists will probably have included some of the following possible advantages and drawbacks shown in Table 6.1

Table 6.1 Possible advantages and drawbacks of interest group involvement in shaping health policy

Potential advantages of 'open' policy processes	Potential negative consequences of 'open' policy processes
Wide range of views is brought to bear on a problem including a better appreciation of the possible impacts of policy on different groups	Difficult to reconcile conflicting and competing claims for attention and resources of different interest groups
Policy making process includes information that is not accessible to governments	Adds to complexity and time taken to reach decisions and to implement policies
Consultation and/or involvement of a range of interests gives policy greater legitimacy and support so that policy decisions may be more likely to be implemented and more sustainable	Concern to identify who different interest groups 'truly' represent and how accountable they are to their members or funders Activities of interest groups may not be transparent. Proliferation of 'front' groups enables corporate interests to develop multiple, covert channels of influence
New or emerging issues may be brought to governments' attention more rapidly than if process is very 'closed', allowing rapid response	Less well-resourced, less well-connected interests may still be disadvantaged by being overlooked or marginalized
	Interest groups may not be capable of providing the information or taking the responsibility allocated to them
	Interest groups can be bigoted, self-interested, badly informed, abusive and intimidatory – being in civil society does not confer automatic virtue

Summary

There are many groups outside government which try to influence public policy on particular issues at various stages of the policy process. In some countries, there are many of these groups and they are strong; in other countries there are few nongovernmental actors and their influence on policy makers is relatively limited. Until the 1990s, policy in many low and middle income countries was dominated by elites closely affiliated with the government of the day (including representatives of donor agencies). However, since the 1990s, in many low and middle income countries the number of different groups and alliances of groups trying to influence government policies has grown and governments have increasingly come to recognize that they should listen. NGOs that had previously confined themselves to delivering services have become more involved in policy advocacy. Most recently, alliances between interest groups in different countries, most notably between NGOs in high, middle and low income settings, have become more prominent in their efforts to influence governments' policies in the health field.

Interest groups differ in the way they are treated by governments. Some are given high legitimacy, 'insider' status and are regularly involved in policy development. Sectional groups often fall into this category because they are powerful and can employ sanctions if they do not approve of a government's policy. In contrast, cause groups may be highly regarded and consulted but have less recourse to sanctions. They may be perceived as 'outsider' groups or even deliberately pursue an 'outsider' strategy organizing demonstrations and ensuring a high level of media coverage in a bid to embarrass or put pressure on government.

The increasing significance of interest groups organized within policy networks around particular areas of public policy represents a challenge to the assumption that governments can act alone, and requires politicians and bureaucrats to learn new skills of working in a less hierarchical and more negotiated way. This trend has been referred to as a shift from 'government' to 'governance'. A key skill of governments in such a world is the ability to coordinate and hold to account a diverse set of actors, many of which are far from its direct control.

References

Alford RR (1975) *Health Care Politics*. Chicago: University of Chicago Press.

Chapman S (1996) Civil disobedience and tobacco control: the case of BUGA UP. Billboard Utilising Graffitists Against Unhealthy Promotions. *Tobacco Control* 5(3): 179–85.

Chhotray V and Stoker G (2009) *Governance Theory and Practice: A Cross-Disciplinary Approach*. Basingstoke: Palgrave Macmillan.

Evetts J (2006) Short note: the sociology of professional groups. *Current Sociology* 54: 133–43.

Giddens A (2001) Foreword. In Anheier H, Glasius M and Kaldor M (eds) *Global Civil Society*. Oxford: Oxford University Press. Available at: http://www.lse.ac.uk/Depts/global/Yearbook/PDF/forward.pdf.

Grant W (1984) The role of pressure groups. In Borthwick R and Spence J (eds) *British Politics in Perspective*. Leicester: Leicester University Press.

Heywood M (2011) South Africa's Treatment Action Campaign: combining law and social mobilization to realize the right to health. *Journal of Human Rights Practice* 1: 14–36.

Johnson T (1995) Governmentality and the institutionalisation of expertise. In Johnson T, Larkin G and Saks M (eds) *Health Professions and the State in Europe*. London: Routledge, pp. 7–24.

Lewis J (2005) *Health Policy and Politics: Networks, Ideas and Power*. Melbourne: IP Communications.

Marsh D and Rhodes RAW (1992) Policy communities and issue networks: beyond typology. In Marsh D and Rhodes RAW (eds) *Policy Networks in British Government*. Oxford: Oxford University Press.

McGann J and Johnstone M (2006) The power shift and the NGO Credibility Crisis. *The International Journal of Not-for-Profit Law* 8(2), January.

Peterson MA (1999) Motivation, mobilisation and monitoring: the role of interest groups in health policy. *Journal of Health Politics, Policy and Law* 24: 416–20.

Preston J and Stelter B (2011) Cellphones become the world's eyes and ears on protests. *New York Times*, 18 February. Available at: http://www.nytimes.com/2011/02/19/world/middleeast/19video.html?_r=1&ref=tunisia (accessed 24 August 2011).

Rhodes RAW (1997) *Understanding Governance*. Buckingham: Open University Press.

Robins S. (2004) 'Long live Zackie, Long Live': AIDS activism, science and citizenship after Apartheid. *Journal of Southern African Studies* 30: 651–72.

Seckinelgin H (2002) Time to stop and think: HIV/AIDS, global civil society, and the people's politics. In Glasius M (ed.) *Global Civil Society Year Book, 2002*. London: London School of Economics and Political Science. Available at: http://www.lse.ac.uk/Depts/global.Yearbook/index.htm.

UNAIDS (2011) *AIDS at 30: Nations at the Crossroads.* Geneva: UNAIDS.

Yurchenko O and Saks M (2006) The social integration of complementary and alternative medicine in official health care in Russia. *Knowledge, Work and Society* 4: 105–27.

Zuniga J (2005) Civil society and the global battle against HIV/AIDS. In Beck E, Mays N, Whiteside A and Zuniga J (eds) *Dealing with the HIV Pandemic in the 21st Century: Health Systems' Responses, Past, Present and Future.* Oxford: Oxford University Press, pp. 706–19.

7 | Policy implementation

Overview

It will now be apparent that the policy process is complex and interactive: many groups and organizations at national and international levels try to influence what gets onto the policy agenda and how policies are formulated. Yet policy making does not come to an end once a course of action has been determined. It cannot be assumed that a policy will be implemented as intended since decision makers typically depend on others to see their policies turned into action. This chapter describes and analyses this process.

Learning objectives

After working through this chapter, you will be better able to:

- contrast 'top-down' and 'bottom-up' theories of policy implementation
- understand other approaches to analysing policy implementation including those that attempt to synthesize insights from both 'top-down' and 'bottom-up' perspectives
- identify some of the tensions affecting implementation between international bodies and national governments, and between central and local authorities within countries
- describe some of the factors that facilitate or impede the implementation of policies.

Key terms

Advocacy coalition. Group within a policy sub-system distinguished by a shared set of norms, beliefs and resources. Can include politicians, civil servants, members of interest groups, journalists and academics who share ideas about policy goals and to a lesser extent about solutions.

Bottom-up approach to understanding implementation. Approach to analysing and explaining policy implementation that focuses on how local-level actors and contextual factors influence policy implementation. Recognizes the strong likelihood that implementing actors at subordinate levels have discretion and play an active part in the process of implementation producing policy results which may be different from those envisaged.

Implementation. Process of turning a policy into practice or action.

Implementation gap. Difference between what the policy architect intended and the end-result of a policy.

Policy instrument. One of the range of options at the disposal of the policy maker in order to give effect to a policy goal (e.g. privatization, regulation, subsidy, etc.).

Principal–agent theory. Theory of organizational and government behaviour that focuses on the relationship between principals (e.g. purchasers) and their agents (e.g. providers), together with the contracts or agreements that enable the purchaser to specify what is to be provided and check that this has been accomplished.

Street-level bureaucrats. Front-line staff involved in delivering public services to members of the public who have some discretion in how they apply the objectives and principles of policies handed down to them.

Top-down approach to understanding implementation. Approach to analysing and explaining policy implementation structured according to a largely linear, rational perspective on the policy process which follows policy initiated at higher levels of the policy system (e.g. national government) through its subsequent execution at subordinate levels. This perspective recognizes a relatively clear division between policy formulation and implementation and focuses on how aspects of policy design at higher levels affect local implementation.

Introduction

Implementation has been defined as 'what happens between policy expectations and (perceived) policy results' (DeLeon 1999). Until the 1970s, policy scientists had tended to focus their attention on the agenda setting, policy formulation and decision making 'stages' of the policy process (see Chapter 1 for an overview of the 'stages', and Chapters 4, 5 and 6 for an account of agenda setting, and policy formulation within and outside government). While the notion of there being formal 'stages' is far from the messy reality of most policy processes, it remains a useful device for drawing attention to different activities and actors, and for organizing the collection of data about policy. The changes that followed policy decisions had been relatively neglected. However, it became increasingly apparent that many public policies had not worked out in practice as well as their proponents had hoped. A series of studies in the late 1960s of anti-poverty programmes, initially in the US, led to an increasing focus by practitioners and analysts on showing the effects of policies (see Chapter 9) and explaining why their consequences were often not as planned (Pressman and Wildavsky 1984).

Today, it is commonplace to observe an '*implementation gap*' between what was planned and what occurred as a result of a policy. For example, there are numerous case studies of the impact of health policies 'imposed' by international donors on poor countries in the 1980s and 1990s, showing that they had less than positive results for a range of reasons. For example, El Salvador received loans from the Inter-American Development Bank (IDB) to improve its health infrastructure. However, there was no concomitant closing of old facilities or improvement of existing, dilapidated facilities. As a result, the ministry of health's maintenance and repair budget could not cope with maintaining the larger capital stock and facilities fell further into disrepair. In the late 1990s, the Nicaraguan Ministry of Health was funded to donate cement to rural house-holders to build latrines, but they chose not to follow the technical building recom-mendations or sold the cement.

Much government reform is currently focused on trying to devise systems that increase the likelihood that governments' policies will be implemented in the way that government ministers intended and that provide information on the impact of policies. For example, the Labour government in the UK in the 2000s emphasized what it called 'delivery', by which it meant the imperative that policies should verifiably make a difference to people's lives. It set a series of quantitative targets with explicit achievement dates and held individual ministries and agencies accountable for their delivery. Similarly, the UN set its Millennium Development Goals in 2000 in order to focus the efforts of its own agencies and world governments on quantitative, timed targets to reduce poverty, malaria and AIDS, and increase access to education by 2015. Unfortunately, progress has been patchy. While it seems likely that the number of people living in extreme poverty will be halved by 2015, progress is much slower in relation to health-related goals such as reducing child and maternal mortality, though maternal mortality has fallen significantly in some countries. It is unlikely that all the goals will be met (http://www.undp.org/mdg/progress.shtml). The variable results indicate the value of studying the detail of implementation processes in different con-texts.

Activity 7.1

Why do you think that some programmes driven by overseas donors in low and middle income countries been less successful than expected? What sorts of obsta-cles face ministries of health in implementing such programmes?

Feedback

The range of reasons has at various times included the following: limited systems in recipient countries to absorb the new resources, lack of government capacity in recipient countries to make good use of resources, the pressure to achieve quick and highly visible results driven by short funding cycles, the importation of alien policy models based on theories tested in other contexts (e.g. in Afghanistan, the World Bank reformed the health system by using its successful experience in Cambodia to introduce a purchaser–provider separation linked to performance-based contracting for services, regardless of the differences between the two coun-tries), differences of view and operating procedures between donors and recipient countries, high costs imposed on recipients by donors' administrative requirements (e.g. the costs of having repeatedly to prepare proposals for fixed term funding) and a failure to identify opposing interests and/or find ways of changing their positions. In general, in the health sector, there has been too much emphasis on increasing the number of trained staff and facilities (e.g. clinics) and not enough attention given to the decision making, managerial and supervisory systems that enable health care to be properly delivered, but which are harder to put in place and take longer to build (Potter and Brough 2004).

Early approaches to explaining policy implementation

'Top-down' approaches

'Top-down' approaches to understanding and thereby, it is hoped, improving policy implementation are closely allied with the rational model of the entire policy process which sees it as a linear sequence of activities in which there is a clear division between policy formulation and policy execution (implementation). The former is seen as explicitly political and the latter as a largely technical, administrative or managerial activity. Policies set at a national or international level have to be communicated to subordinate levels (e.g. health authorities, hospitals, clinics) which are then charged with putting them into practice. The 'top-down' approach was developed by policy analysts from early studies in the 1960s and 1970s of the 'implementation deficit' or 'gap' to provide policy makers with a better understanding of which systems they needed to put in place to minimize the 'gap' between aspiration and reality (that is, to make the process approximate more closely to the rational ideal). These studies were empirical but then led to recommendations for change. Thus, according to Pressman and Wildavsky (1984), the key to effective implementation lay in the ability to devise a system in which the causal links between setting goals and the successive actions designed to achieve them were clear and robust. Goals had to be clearly defined and widely understood, the necessary political, administrative, technical and financial resources had to be available, a chain of command had to be established from the centre to the periphery, and a communication and control system had to be in place to keep the whole system on course. Failure was caused by adopting the wrong strategy and using the wrong machinery.

Later 'top-down' theorists devised a list of six necessary and sufficient conditions for effective policy implementation (Sabatier and Mazmanian 1979), indicating that if these conditions were realized, then policy should be implemented largely as intended:

1 clear and logically consistent objectives;
2 adequate causal theory (i.e. a valid theory as to how particular actions would lead to the desired outcomes);
3 an implementation process structured to enhance compliance by implementers (e.g. appropriate incentives and sanctions to influence subordinates in the required way);
4 committed, skilful implementing officials;
5 support from interest groups and legislature;
6 no changes in socioeconomic conditions that undermine political support or the causal theory underlying the policy.

Proponents of this approach argued that it could distinguish empirically between failed and successful implementation processes, and thereby provided useful guidance to policy makers in the future. Its most obvious weakness was that the first condition was rarely fulfilled in that most public policies were found to have fuzzy, potentially inconsistent objectives.

Activity 7.2

Given what you know already about policy in the health field, what criticisms would you level at the 'top-down' perspective to understanding implementation? How good an explanation of policy implementation does it offer, in your opinion?

The main criticisms of the 'top-down' approach to the analysis of implementation are that:

- It gives too much weight to the perspective of central decision makers (those at the top of any hierarchy or directly involved in initial policy formulation) and not enough to the role and perspectives of other actors (e.g. NGOs, professional bodies, the private sector) and factors shaping the behaviour of people at other levels in the implementation process (e.g. regional health authorities and front-line staff) when designing implementation plans.
- As an analytical approach, it risks over-estimating the impact of government action on a problem compared with other social and economic factors.
- It is difficult to apply in situations where there is no single, dominant policy or lead agency involved – in many fields, there are multiple policies in play and a complex array of agencies implementing them.
- Its distinction between policy decisions and subsequent implementation can be analytically misleading since it ignores the possibility that policies might be changed as they are being implemented.
- It does not explicitly take into account the impact on implementation of the extent of change required by a policy.

In essence, the critics argued that the reality of policy implementation was messier and more complex than even the most sophisticated 'top-down' approach could cope with and that the practical advice it generated on reducing the 'gap' between expectation and reality was, therefore, largely irrelevant. To reinforce these points, Hogwood and Gunn (1984) drew up an even more demanding list of ten pre-conditions for what they termed 'perfect implementation' in order to show that guidance on implementation derived from the 'top-down' approach to the analysis of processes of implementation was unrealistic in most situations:

1 The circumstances external to the agency do not impose crippling constraints.
2 Adequate time and sufficient resources are available.
3 The required combination of resources is available.
4 The policy is based on a valid theory of cause and effect.
5 The relationship between cause and effect is direct.
6 Dependency relationships are minimal – in other words, the policy makers are not reliant on groups or organizations which are themselves inter-dependent.
7 There is an understanding of, and agreement on, objectives.
8 Tasks are fully specified and in the correct sequence.
9 Communication and coordination are perfect.
10 Those in authority can demand and obtain perfect compliance.

Since it was very unlikely that all ten pre-conditions would be present at the same time, critics of the 'top-down' approach argued that the approach was neither a good description of what happened in practice nor a helpful guide to improving implementation.

'Bottom-up' approaches

The 'bottom-up' approach to understanding the implementation process is rooted in an awareness that implementers often play an important function in implementation, not just as managers of policy handed down from above, but as active participants in a complex process that informs those higher up in the system, and that policy should be made with this insight in mind. Even in highly centralized systems, studies show that some power is usually granted to subordinate agencies and their staff. The subordinate implementers often change the way a policy is implemented and in the process may even end up redefining the objectives of the policy.

One of the most influential studies in the development of the 'bottom-up' analytical perspective on implementation was by Lipsky (1980) who studied the behaviour of what he termed 'street level bureaucrats' in relation to their clients in the 1970s. 'Street level bureaucrats' included front-line staff administering social welfare benefits, social workers, teachers, local government officials, doctors and nurses. He showed that even those working in the most rule-bound environments had some discretion in how they dealt with their clients, and that staff such as doctors, social workers and teachers had high levels of discretion which enabled them to get round the dictates of central policy and reshape policy for their own ends.

Lipsky's work helped re-conceptualize the implementation process, particularly in the delivery of health and social services which is dependent on the actions of large numbers of professional staff, viewing it as a much more interactive, political process characterized by largely inescapable negotiation and conflict between interests and levels within policy systems. As a result, researchers began to focus their attention on the actors in the implementation process, their ideas, their goals, their strategies, their activities and their links to one another. Interestingly, 'bottom-up' studies showed that even in the rare situations where the conditions specified as necessary by the 'top-down', rational model were in place (e.g. a good chain of command, well-defined objectives, ample resources, and a communication and monitoring system), policies could still be implemented in ways that policy makers had not intended. Indeed, well-meaning policies could make things worse, for example, by increasing staff workload so that they had to develop undesirable coping strategies (Wetherley and Lipsky 1977).

Such studies of 'street level bureaucrats' still have relevance. For example, Walker and Gilson (2004) studied how nurses in a busy urban primary health care clinic in South Africa experienced and responded to the implementation of the 1996 national policy of free care (removal of user fees). They showed that while the nurses approved of the policy of improving access, in principle, they were negative towards it in practice because of the way it exacerbated existing problems in their working environment and increased their workload, without increasing staffing levels or the availability of drugs. They were also dissatisfied because they felt that they had not been included in the process of policy formulation.

This finding has been reinforced by more recent research showing that poor relationships and a lack of trust between mid-level managers and health workers can generate resistance to policies even when health workers stand to gain from a policy (Scott et al. 2011). The nurses in Walker and Gilson's (2004) study also believed that many patients abused the free system and some patients did not deserve free care because they were personally responsible for their own health problems. Such views were presumably at odds with the principles underlying the policy of free care and made nurses slow to grant free access to services to certain groups of patients.

Insights from the 'bottom-up' perspective on policy implementation have guided a range of studies in health care systems of the way in which the relationships between central, regional and local agencies influence policy. The ability of the centre to control lower levels of the system varies widely and depends on the institutional arrangements, comprising factors such as where the funds come from and who controls them (e.g. the balance between central and local, and national and international sources of funding), legislation (e.g. setting out which level of authority is responsible for which tasks), operating rules and the ability of the government to enforce these (e.g. through performance assessment, audit, incentives, etc.). However, implementation also depends on understanding and working with the cultures, learning styles and networks of local actors. Blaauw and colleagues (2003) argue that insufficient attention has been given in practical implementation strategies to what they call the 'software' of health systems, meaning their everyday organizational reality and, in particular, to developing the tools for building networks, persuasion, information and changing cultures.

Relationships between centre and periphery in health systems influence the fate of many policies. Sometimes, as the South African example above showed, policies are diverted to some degree during their implementation. At other times, they are entirely rejected. In New Zealand in the early 1990s, the government introduced user charges for public hospital outpatients and inpatients in order, among other things, to remove the perceived incentive for patients to go to hospital rather than use primary care where they already faced user charges. Whatever its intellectual merits, the policy was extremely unpopular among the public, patients, and the hospital managers and staff who had to collect the fees. The user charges were progressively withdrawn until they disappeared about two years after their introduction.

Activity 7.3

Write down in two columns the main differences between the 'top-down' and 'bottom-up' analytical approaches to understanding policy implementation. You might contrast the following aspects of the two approaches: where the analysis starts; how the main actors are identified; how the policy process is viewed; how the implementation process is evaluated; and the overall focus of the analysis.

Feedback

Your answer should have included some of the differences shown in Table 7.1.

Table 7.1 'Top-down' and 'bottom-up' approaches to analysing policy implementation

	Top-down approaches	Bottom-up approaches
Analytical starting point	Central government decision	Local implementation actors and networks of relationships
Process for identification of major actors	From top-down and starting with government	From bottom-up, including both government and non-government actors

	Top-down approaches	Bottom-up approaches
View of the policy process	Largely rational process, proceeding from problem identification to policy formulation at higher levels to implementation at lower levels	Interactive process involving policy makers and implementers from various parts and levels of government and outside, in which policy may change during implementation.
		Implementers are active participants in making policy, not just transmitters of policies made elsewhere
Evaluative criteria	Extent of attainment of formal objectives rather than recognition of unintended consequences	Extent to which implementation processes are designed to take into account local participants' views and influences on how policy unfolds
Overall analytical focus	Designing the system to achieve what central/top policy makers intend – tends to focus on 'structure' and management (i.e. how systems and organizations can drive the implementation process using regulations, sanctions and incentives)	Recognition of strategic interaction among multiple actors in a policy network – focus on the culture and relationships between actors and their ability to shape their environment and thus how policy unfolds

Source: Sabatier (1986), adapted and expanded

While the insights derived from the 'bottom-up' approach are likely to appeal to health care workers and middle-ranking officials because they bring their views and the constraints on their actions into view, the approach raises as many questions as the 'top-down' perspective, both as an explanation of how policies are implemented and as a guide to action. One obvious question both analytical approaches and their findings raise is whether or not the approach chosen by government to its policy making and particularly to implementation should be shaped predominantly by insights from the top-down or bottom-up perspective. Another question is how the divergence of views and goals between actors at different levels identified by 'bottom-up' analysis can or should be reconciled in practice. Specifically, in a democracy, how much influence should unelected professionals have in shaping the eventual consequences of policies determined by elected governments? Should plans for policy implementation be equally informed by the perspectives and needs of, say, national policy makers and local implementers?

Activity 7.4

Write down any other analytical drawbacks of the 'bottom-up' approach that you can think of.

Feedback

In addition to the value (normative) questions mentioned in the paragraph above, you could have listed:

- If there is no distinction analytically or in reality between 'policy formulation' and 'implementation', then it is difficult to separate the influence of different levels of government and of elected politicians and subordinate staff on policy decisions and consequences. This is important for democratic and bureaucratic accountability.
- If there are no separate decision points in the policy process, it becomes very difficult to undertake any evaluation of a particular policy's effects (as you will see in Chapter 9).
- The approach risks under-emphasizing the indirect influence of higher levels of government in shaping the institutions within which lower level actors operate and in distributing the political resources they possess, including permitting them to be involved in shaping implementation.

The list of drawbacks in the feedback above is a reminder that it pays to be cautious if judging one theory superior to another in such a complex field as policy. Most theory in policy science inevitably simplifies the complexity of any particular set of circumstances in order to bring greater understanding.

Other ways of understanding policy implementation: beyond 'top-down' and 'bottom-up' perspectives

The approaches debated thus far have largely been developed by political scientists and sociologists. However, management scientists and economists have also been drawn to trying to explain why there are frequently gaps between policy intention and eventual outcomes, and how to reduce their scale and likelihood.

Principal–agent theory

From the principal–agent perspective, sub-optimal policy implementation is an inevitable result of the structure of the institutions of modern government in which decision makers ('principals') have to delegate responsibility for the implementation of their policies to their officials (e.g. civil servants in the ministry of health) and other 'agents' (e.g. managers, doctors and nurses in the health sector or private contractors) whom they only indirectly and incompletely control, and who are difficult to monitor. These 'agents' have discretion in how they operate on behalf of political 'principals' and may not even see themselves as primarily engaged in making a reality of the wishes of these 'principals'. For example, even publicly employed doctors tend to see themselves as members of the medical profession first and foremost rather than as civil servants. Discretion opens up the potential for ineffective or inefficient translation of government intent into reality since 'agents' have their own views, ambitions, loyalties and resources which can hinder policy implementation. The inherent problem for politicians is to get the compliance of their officials and others who are contracted to deliver services at all levels. The more levels of hierarchy there are, the more principal–agent relations there are, as each level is dependent on the next level below or beside it, and the more complex is the task of controlling the process of implementation.

The amount of discretion and the complexity of the principal–agent relationships are, in turn, affected by:

1 *the nature of the policy problem* – this can be, for example, macro versus sectoral or micro (affecting the scale of change required and size of the affected group), simple versus complex, ill-defined versus clear, have many causes versus a single cause, be highly politically sensitive versus neutral politically, requiring a short or long period before impacts will become apparent, costly versus inexpensive, and so on. In general, long-term, ill-defined, interdependent (goals affected by other policies), high profile problems affecting large numbers of people are far more difficult to deal with than short-term, specific issues with a single cause and a large technical component. Most public policy debate focuses on the former which are known, understandably, as 'wicked problems' or problems to which there is never likely to be an easy solution. A typical example would be how to simultaneously balance the public desire to punish and deter criminals by giving them prison sentences with the evidence that prison does not help rehabilitate criminals and may even increase their odds of reoffending.

2 *the context or circumstances surrounding the problem* – for example, the political situation, whether the economy is growing or not, the availability of resources and pace of technological change.

3 *the organization of the machinery required to implement the policy* – most obviously this includes the number of formal agencies and informal relationships involved in making the desired change, and the skills and resources that have to be brought to bear.

Activity 7.5

The three sets of factors listed above help explain why some policies are easier to implement than others. Take a health policy with which you are familiar and describe the nature of the problem, the context and the machinery required to implement the policy. Under each of the three headings listed above, try to assess whether the factors you have listed are likely to make implementation of the policy easier or more difficult.

Feedback

Your answer will clearly depend on the policy you chose to analyse. For example, if your chosen policy had simple technical features (e.g. introduction of a new drug), involved a marginal behavioural change (e.g. a minor change in dosage), could be implemented by one or a few actors (e.g. pharmacists acting alone), had clear, non-conflicting objectives (e.g. better symptom control with no cost implications) and could be executed in a short period of time (e.g. drugs were easy to source and distribute), you would be lucky and you would be able to conclude that implementation would be relatively straightforward. Unfortunately, the majority of health policy issues and policies are more complex. Policy analysts are fond of contrasting the challenge of goals such as putting a man on the moon with the stock-in-trade of public policy such as reducing poverty. The former was carried out in a tightly organized, influential, well-resourced organization focused on a single goal with a clear end point. The latter is driven by a large number of causes, involves a wide range of agencies and actors and has inherently fuzzy objectives (Howlett et al. 2009).

New Public Management: markets and performance payment

The insights of principal–agent and related theories led to a greater appreciation of the importance of the design of institutions and the choice of policy instruments for implementation, so that the 'top' had the information to monitor activities and hold to account the staff at 'street level' at reasonable cost. One aspect of this was a growing focus on the actual and implied *contracts* defining the relationships between principals and their agents in order to ensure that the principal's objectives were followed by agents. So, from the 1980s, in a number of high, middle and low income countries, the civil service was reformed to make more explicit what officials were expected to deliver to ministers in return for their salaries. Multi-purpose ministries were restructured and agencies with a small number of policy objectives were set up with clear performance targets incorporated in contracts with the parent ministry. Performance indicators were used to assess whether their performance in meeting government objectives was improving or not.

In public services, the conventional role of government as direct provider of services was also critically reviewed in many countries, with a view to improving the efficiency and responsiveness of services both to the objectives of ministers and the needs of citizens as consumers. The catch phrase of the reformers was that government should be 'steering not rowing' the ship of state (Osborne and Gaebler 1992), confining itself to what only it could do best. As a result, some services that had been directly provided in the public sector (e.g. by publicly owned hospitals) were contracted out to private for-profit or not-for-profit providers on the grounds that they would be better able to focus on delivering government policy objectives.

From the early 1980s, policy makers were encouraged to consider the potential of the whole range of policy instruments available to governments to ensure the efficient delivery of goods and services, each entailing differing scope of government involvement and of compulsion. There are a number of different ways of describing the policy instruments or tools at the disposal of governments to implement their policies, but most identify the following basic types:

* *information and persuasion* – these encourage changes in behaviour by providing information such as health education programmes, clinical guidelines, training, research and evaluation, but without associated compulsion to act in a particular way;
* *regulation* – these require changes in behaviour by providing sanctions for those who do not comply with the regulations. Legislation is the most obvious form of regulation. Typical forms of regulation include licensing (e.g. of clinics and health professionals) and minimum standards (e.g. of nurse staffing levels), but others include redistribution such as through taxation, subsidy and reallocation of resources such as the clinical workforce between geographic areas.
* *public provision* – the government provides key public services itself or through publicly owned and directly managed agencies. This is particularly likely when the service has the features of a 'public good' (i.e. the benefits of the service accrue to

everyone and they depend on high population participation such as defence and immunization).

* *markets and market-like incentives* – these encourage behaviour change through using the incentives associated with markets, such as introducing competition between a wider range of different suppliers of public services into previously monopoly situations and/or allowing users greater choice of provider. Other market instruments involve governments developing markets where previously none existed (e.g. carbon emission trading and carbon offsetting to prevent health-damaging climate change).

The New Public Management (NPM), as it became known, reflected the preference in mainstream economics for markets over other approaches to producing goods and services and the fashionable theory that the self-interested behaviour of voters, politicians and bureaucrats tends to lead to an increase in taxation, public spending and government activity, often unnecessarily and inefficiently compared with the private sector (see fuller discussion of NPM in Chapter 3). NPM was driven by economic critiques of policy implementation and the importation into the public sector of policy instruments and management techniques used in large private enterprises. It remains the dominant approach to public sector management worldwide.

Broadly, by the end of the 1990s, market or market-like systems (e.g. the separation of purchaser and providers within a publicly owned and financed health system or paying hospitals for the treatments they delivered), and voluntary instruments of persuasion (e.g. voluntary codes of behaviour) had become more prominent in many countries, leading to a more mixed set of policy instruments in sectors such as health. These included ways of giving patients more information and more choice over where and from whom they received their care. The assumption of reformers was that such arrangements would improve the implementation of policy designed to improve the efficiency and effectiveness of public services.

As well as changes to instruments, there were also changes to the processes by which decisions were made. One such change was the trend towards decentralization of parts of the decision making function, from central to local levels, while reducing the number of tiers in the management hierarchy. In many jurisdictions, subordinate agents were given greater control over their own affairs on a day-to-day basis but remained accountable for the attainment of the government's key goals. The theory was that this would free agents to pursue the objectives of their principals unfettered by unnecessary interference and allow principals to judge the performance of their agents objectively, and would remove from agents the excuse that their poor performance was the result of inappropriate interventions by principals. These more autonomous entities are referred to as 'public firms' or 'public enterprises'. Since 1991, NHS hospitals in the UK have operated in this way as 'self-governing' bodies with some, limited freedom from direct ministerial control. From 2004, in England, better performing NHS hospitals were encouraged to apply for 'foundation status' which, in principle, gave them even greater freedom to operate more entrepreneurially and to keep the rewards of their good performance by retaining any savings they made. Similar reforms have been pursued in middle income countries such as Zambia where performance improvements by service providers have been rewarded with greater freedom from government control (Bossert et al. 2003).

Another related, increasingly popular policy instrument for service improvement derived from NPM thinking is performance-based funding, also known as payment for performance. In this approach, a percentage of the revenue of a service provider is dependent on the achievement of pre-specified standards and/or targets. For example, around a quarter of the income of general medical practices in the UK NHS comes from their performance in relation to a wide range of performance criteria such as the proportion of their patients with normal blood pressure.

Performance-based funding is used by a number of large development organizations, both public and philanthropic. For example, the Global Fund to Fight AIDS, Tuberculosis and Malaria supports bids initially on the basis of the quality of the proposals received, but subsequent funding is dependent on recipient countries demonstrating results against performance targets the countries themselves have proposed.

Activity 7.6

What are the arguments in favour of payment for performance systems as a way of improving policy implementation? Can you think of any potential disadvantages of such systems of paying for services?

Feedback

The main advantages put forward in support of payment for performance systems are that: (1) they focus service providers on improving the outcomes of services and on delivering value for money rather than client throughput; (2) the financial risk for poor performance lies to varying degrees with the provider not the payer; and (3) they improve accountability for public services.

The main disadvantages suggested are that: (1) they encourage 'cherry picking' of those clients most likely to benefit rather than those in greatest need; (2) they encourage an excessive focus on meeting the specified standards and targets rather than providing a balanced high quality service; (3) they lead to clients being coerced so that targets can be met; (4) outcomes can be difficult to attribute to providers; and (5) small-scale providers are deterred from entering the market because they find it harder to manage the financial risks involved.

Activity 7.7

Identify the main elements of the 'New Public Management' from what you have just read about principal–agent theory and related ideas.

Feedback

NPM is a hybrid of different intellectual influences and practical experience, and emphasizes different things in different countries, but the following elements are commonly seen as distinctive in NPM:

1 Clarification of roles and responsibilities for effective policy implementation by separating strategic (i.e. advising ministers on policy direction) from operational (i.e. service delivery) functions within the government machinery. For example, this

has led to governments setting up agencies to run public services at arm's length from central government (e.g. courts, prisons and health services) with greater operational freedom and attempting to slim down central government ministries providing policy advice.

2 Separation of 'purchase' from 'provision' within public services in order to allow the contracting out of services to the private or voluntary sector if this is regarded as superior to in-house, public provision.

3 The establishment of more independent public providers (e.g. turning English NHS hospitals into Foundation Trusts at arm's length from direct government control).

4 Greater competition between providers driven by giving users more choice.

5 Focus on performance assessment and incentives to improve 'value for money' and to ensure that services deliver what policy makers intended (e.g. including payment for performance).

6 Setting standards of service which citizens as consumers can expect to be delivered.

Towards a synthesis of 'top-down' and 'bottom-up' perspectives

While economists tended to see the choice of the best policy instrument to implement a policy as a technical exercise and were keen to recommend approaches based on markets and competition in the 1990s and 2000s, political scientists studied how governments behaved and with what consequences. For example, Linder and Peters (1989) identified the following factors as playing a critical role in shaping the policy implementation choices of governments:

1 *Features of policy instruments* – some instruments are intrinsically more demanding technically and politically to use. They vary on at least four dimensions: resource intensiveness; targeting; political risk; and degree of coerciveness. Ripley and Franklin (1982) suggested that distributive policies (i.e. allocating public funds to different groups, for instance, when directly providing publicly financed services) tend to be relatively easy to implement, regulatory policies (e.g. allowing nurses to prescribe drugs previously restricted to doctors) were moderately difficult, and redistributive policies (i.e. policies involving the re-allocation of income or opportunities between socio-economic groups) were very difficult to implement since there were obvious losers from the last category of policy whereas the costs of the first category were spread across the population less visibly.

2 *Policy style and political culture* – in different countries and different policy fields, participants and the public were accustomed to, for instance, different degrees of government control and/or provision. Policies departing from these traditions were more difficult to implement.

3 *Organizational culture* – the past operating experience and ways of doing things of the implementing organizations, linked to point 2.

4 *Context of the problem* – the timing (e.g. in relation to how well the economy was performing), the range of actors involved, the likely public reaction, etc.

5 *Administrative decision makers' subjective preferences* – based on their background, professional affiliations, training, cognitive style, and so on.

These factors highlight two general sets of variables affecting policy implementation, namely, the *extent of government capacity* and, therefore, its ability to intervene, and the *complexity of the particular policy field* it is attempting to influence. Attempts to reconcile the 'top-down' and 'bottom-up' approaches have focused on the interplay between these two sets of variables. Crudely, 'top-down' theory provides the focus on government capacity, whereas 'bottom-up' theory offers the focus on sub-system complexity since the former emphasizes how institutional design and socio-economic conditions (context) constrain and shape the process of implementation and the latter emphasizes how the beliefs of participants, their relationships and networks, and inter-organizational dynamics shape and constrain implementation. One attempt to bring together these different strands of theory and research was developed by Paul Sabatier and various colleagues (Sabatier and Jenkins-Smith 1993).

The policy sub-system or advocacy coalition framework (ACF)

Sabatier's framework is a general approach to understanding the policy process and policy change since it rejects the idea of separating 'implementation' from other stages as unrealistic and misleading. Instead, policy change is seen as a continuous process that takes place within policy sub-systems bounded by relatively stable limits and shaped by major external events. Within the sub-system (e.g. mental health policy), 'communities' or networks of actors interact over considerable periods of time. The actors include all those who play a part in the generation, dissemination and evaluation of policy ideas. Sabatier does not include the public in any policy sub-system on the grounds that ordinary people as individuals rather than as members of organizations do not generally have the time or inclination to be direct participants.

The large number of actors and networks within each sub-system are organized into a smaller number of *advocacy coalitions*, in conflict with one another. Each competes for influence over government institutions by advocating its solutions to policy problems. An 'advocacy coalition' is a group distinguished by a distinct set of norms, beliefs and resources, and can include politicians, civil servants, members of civil society organizations, researchers, journalists and others. Advocacy coalitions are defined by their *ideas* rather than by the exercise of self-interested power (see Chapter 9 for more on their role in bringing ideas from research to bear on policy). Within advocacy coalitions there is a high level of agreement on fundamental policy positions and objectives, though there may be more debate about the precise means to achieve these objectives. Sabatier argues that the fundamental (or 'core') norms and beliefs of an advocacy coalition change relatively infrequently and in response to major changes in the external environment such as shifts in macro-economic conditions or the replacement of one political regime by another. Otherwise, less fundamental, 'normal' changes in policy beliefs occur as a result of policy-oriented learning in which a coalition tests and refines its beliefs either in order to achieve its goals or in response to challenges. The changes take place through the interaction between advocacy coalitions within the policy sub-system.

The final element in Sabatier's model is to identify the existence of so called '*policy brokers*', that is, actors concerned with finding feasible compromises between the positions advocated by the coalitions (a role similar to that of Kingdon's 'policy entrepreneurs' in Chapter 4). 'Brokers' may be civil servants experienced in a particular sub-system or bodies designed to produce agreement, such as committees of inquiry.

Subsequent empirical work has shown that the advocacy coalition model works fairly well in explaining policy change over a decade in relatively open, decentralized, federal, pluralistic political systems such as the US, but works less well in political systems such as the UK which are more closed and where there is less interplay between advocacy coalitions. It has also been little used in the context of low or middle income countries where policy making has been traditionally even more closed and elitist. Looking at its utility in specific policy sub-systems, it appears to fit well with sub-systems such as AIDS policy and other aspects of public health where government typically has to try to reach agreement among conflicting advocacy coalitions. It is less applicable to the policy sub-systems of 'high politics' such as defence and foreign policy (e.g. decisions to go to war) where policy decisions are normally made within a small and tightly defined elite since the national interest as a whole may be perceived to be at stake.

A good example of the application of the ACF is the analysis of the changes in government policy towards the use of illicit drugs in Switzerland in the 1980s and 1990s by Kübler (1999). Over this period, policy shifted from a predominantly prohibitionist position in the early 1980s to a harm reduction position with some moves to decriminalizing the use of drugs. How and why did this change occur? Until the mid-1980s, drug policy was dominated by an 'abstinence coalition' of prosecutors, judges, police and public health specialists. As a result, access to needles and syringes for drug use was made as difficult as possible despite the risk of needle sharing and associated infection. The arrival of AIDS in the mid-1980s – a major change in the external environment – changed the debate; unlike hepatitis, there was no vaccination or cure for AIDS and there was the risk of the spread of HIV to the general population through drug-related sex work. As a result, some health experts who had supported the abstinence coalition began to advocate a change in policy on the grounds that an abstinence-oriented policy was ineffective in preventing HIV. The idea that controlling HIV was more important than abstinence rapidly led to the concept of harm reduction and a coalition of public health and infectious disease specialists, plus social workers. This coalition was soon supported by leftist local politicians, and began to press for harm reduction facilities. In the late 1980s and early 1990s, needle exchanges and safe injection rooms were set up in the large cities with local funding, but the federal (national) government also began to be interested in testing harm reduction approaches scientifically, thereby allowing it to contribute resources.

The harm reduction coalition's political strategy was two-pronged: on the one hand, to lobby local and national governments for a change in their policies; and, on the other, to produce change without waiting for the active support of local government by mobilizing finance and expertise that allowed the establishment of harm reduction facilities by NGOs. The goal of the latter was to demonstrate that harm reduction was the correct policy and thereby attract additional support. By the early 1990s, the harm reduction coalition was driving drug policy decision making in most parts of Switzerland, but faced a further challenge as a result of the emergence of a third advocacy coalition concerned with quality of life in cities. Plans for new harm reduction facilities usually led to protests from local residents and businesses fearing that facilities would not only attract drug users but also disorder, crime and debris (e.g. used needles). Neighbourhood quality of life advocates frequently allied with the abstinence coalition so as to be able to claim that their opposition to harm reduction facilities was more than simple self-interest.

The harm reduction coalition was forced to confront the public order implications of its position and some members began to advocate an approach that gave equal weight to public order and drug users' health so as to rescue the harm reduction approach. The idea of *Stadtverträglichkeit* ('city compatibility'), or the search for the equilibrium between repression and harm reduction interventions, became a substantial secondary element in the harm reduction coalition's belief system. The re-balancing of the objectives of local drug facilities proved a practical success. As a result, neighbourhood quality of life advocates no longer supported the abstinence coalition and withdrew from drug policy, and the harm reduction coalition was able to consolidate its dominant position.

Activity 7.8

Which external event fundamentally altered the debate and actors involved in the above case study of drug policy in Switzerland in the 1990s? Describe the advocacy coalitions involved and their policy core beliefs. Which part of Sabatier's advocacy coalition framework did not appear to be present in the Swiss case study?

Feedback

The AIDS epidemic fundamentally altered the range of policy ideas at play in the drug field and mobilized a new set of actors – the harm reduction coalition. This coalition began to press local and national governments to change direction away from abstinence and prohibition towards a policy focused on the health of drug users.

There were two major advocacy coalitions competing in the drug policy sub-system: the abstinence coalition which believed in repression of drug use and making drug use as unattractive as possible, and the harm reduction coalition which believed in improving the health and social situation of drug users and reducing the harm associated with drug use as a way of motivating users to come off drugs. A third minor coalition, the urban quality of life coalition, entered the policy sub-system for a time. It believed in policies to improve the experience of living in cities and to enhance the economy of cities.

There were no obvious 'policy brokers' at work in the Swiss case study trying to produce a deal between the abstinence and harm reduction coalitions, perhaps because their belief systems were so incompatible. Only when the public order issue arose did some members of the harm reduction coalition try to identify a consensus between their own beliefs and those of the quality of life advocates, though only at the level of secondary aspects of the respective belief systems.

Activity 7.9

Although the advocacy coalition framework is not specifically a theory of policy implementation, what can be learned about policy implementation from the Swiss case study, above?

Feedback

The main observation concerning implementation is the fact that policy is and needs to be adapted as it is being implemented. In this case, the harm reduction coalition had to respond to the concerns of city dwellers about the disruption to neighbourhoods caused by the concentration of people with drug habits around the facilities it had championed. The operational policies of the facilities had to be altered to take account of concerns wider than the health of drug users so that the harm reduction strategy could be sustained in the face of opposition.

There are a number of different approaches to understanding implementation which transcend the contrast between 'top-down' and 'bottom-up' perspectives. Through the concept of 'advocacy coalitions', Sabatier's framework has the virtue of highlighting the possibility that many of the most important conflicts in policy cut across the simple divide between policy makers and those formally charged with putting policy into practice.

What help to policy makers are the different approaches to understanding policy implementation?

Most of the research discussed in this chapter was not directly devoted to providing practical advice for policy makers, though some fairly simple messages emerge. For example, there is little doubt that policies which are designed to be incremental (with small behavioural change), can be delivered through a simple structure involving few actors and have the support of front-line staff are more likely to succeed than those that are not. However, this is no great help to those charged with bringing about radical policy change in complex systems where conflicts of fact and opinion abound.

Grindle and Thomas (1991) encourage policy makers to analyse carefully their political, financial, managerial and technical resources and work out how they may be mobilized as well as those of their likely opponents before making decisions about how to bring about change. The key message from their approach is a reminder that the political aspects of the policy sub-system are just as important as aspects of government capacity such as the quality of the technical advice available. Where governments lack capacity and the sub-system is complex, involving a large number of interdependent actors, the advice from this perspective might be to use subsidies to encourage particular forms of behaviour rather than attempt direct provision. For example, rather than attempting to employ primary care doctors, the government might subsidize the cost of patients' visits to private doctors.

This chapter demonstrates a range of frameworks for analysing policy implementation, each of which has something valuable to offer. Elmore (1985) argues that thoughtful policy makers should use a variety of approaches to analysing their situation simultaneously, inspired by both 'bottom-up' and 'top-down' understandings of how implementation is brought about. A key skill is the ability to map the participants ('stakeholders' in modern jargon), their situations, their perspectives, their values, their strategies, their desired outcomes and their ability to delay, obstruct, overturn or help policy implementation (see Chapter 10 for more on this).

As a broad generalization, in the various health policy sub-systems, most governments are ambitious (they want to make a significant impact), but the sub-systems are complex, and governments have relatively modest levels of direct control over many of the key actors; for example, they are highly dependent on a range of influential professional groups. This suggests that persuasion and bargaining will often be important parts of any strategy of implementation.

Drawing these threads of advice together, Walt (1998) sets out a strategy for planning and managing the implementation of change in the health sector which is summarized in Table 7.2.

Table 7.2 Strategy for planning and managing the implementation of change

Area or aspect of implementation	Type of action or analysis
Macro-analysis of the ease with which policy change can be implemented	Analyse conditions for facilitating change and, where possible, make adjustments to simplify; i.e. one agency, clear goals, single objective, simple technical features, marginal change, short duration, visible benefits, clear costs
Making the values underlying the policy explicit	Identify values underlying policy decisions. If values of key interests conflict with policy, wide coalition of support will have to be built and costs to key interests minimized
Stakeholder analysis	Review interest groups (and individuals) likely to resist or promote change in policy at national and institutional levels; plan how to mobilize support by consensus building or rallying coalitions of support
Analysis of financial, technical and managerial resources available and required	Consider the distribution of costs and benefits; assess likely self-interested behaviour within the system; review incentives and sanctions to change behaviour; review need for training, new information systems or other supports to policy change
Building strategic implementation process	Involve planners and managers in analysis of how to execute policy; identify networks of supporters of policy change including 'champions'; manage uncertainty; promote public awareness; institute mechanisms for consultation, monitoring and 'fine tuning' of policy

Source: Walt (1998), adapted

Summary

Implementation cannot be seen as a separate part of a sequential policy process in which political debate and decisions take place among politicians and civil servants, and then managers and administrators at a lower level implement these decisions. It is best viewed as a mostly complex, interactive process in which a wide range of actors influence both the direction of travel as well as the way that given policies are executed, within the constraints of existing institutions, prevailing ideas and competing interests. Implementation is a political process shaped by government capacity and system complexity. Experience suggests that this basic insight from the social sciences of the interplay of actors (agency) and institutions (structure) is still imperfectly built into plans for putting policy into practice.

To avoid the gap between policy expectation and reality, policy makers should develop a strategy for implementation that explicitly takes account of financial, managerial and technical aspects of the policy (capacity) as well as the anticipated resistance and support from all the actors in the sub-system within and outside government.

References

Blaauw D, Gilson L, Penn-Kekana L, and Schneider H (2003) *Organisational Relationships and the 'Software' of Health Sector Reform*. Background Paper. Disease Control Priorities Project (DCPP). Johannesburg: Centre for Health Policy, School of Public Health, University of the Witwatersrand.

Bossert T, Bona Chita M, and Bowser D (2003) Decentralization in Zambia: resource allocation and district performance. *Health Policy and Planning* 18: 35769.

DeLeon P (1999) The missing link revisited: contemporary implementation research. *Policy Studies Review* 16: 311–338.

Elmore R (1985) Forward and backward mapping. In Hanf K and Toonen T (eds) *Policy Implementation in Federal and Unitary Systems*. Dordrecht: Martinus Nijhoff.

Grindle M and Thomas J (1991) *Public Choices and Policy Change*. Baltimore, MD: Johns Hopkins University Press.

Hogwood B and Gunn L (1984) *Policy Analysis for the Real World*. Oxford: Oxford University Press.

Howlett M, Ramesh M and Perl A (2009) *Studying Public Policy: Policy Cycles and Policy Subsystems*. Don Mills, ON: Oxford University Press.

Kübler D (1999) Ideas as catalytic elements for policy change: advocacy coalitions and drug policy in Switzerland. In Braun D and Busch A (eds) *Public Policy and Political Ideas*. Cheltenham: Edward Elgar, pp. 116–21.

Linder SH and Peters BG (1989) Instruments of government: perceptions and contexts. *Journal of Public Policy* 9: 35–58.

Lipsky M (1980) *Street Level Bureaucracy: Dilemmas of the Individual in Public Services*. New York: Russell Sage Foundation.

Osborne DE and Gaebler TA (1992) *Reinventing Government: How the Entrepreneurial Spirit Is Transforming the Public Sector*. Reading, MA: Addison-Wesley.

Potter C and Brough R (2004) Systemic capacity building: a hierarchy of needs. *Health Policy and Planning* 19: 336–45.

Pressman JL and Wildavsky A (1984) *Implementation*, 3rd edn. Berkeley, CA: University of California Press.

Ripley R and Franklin G (1982) *Bureaucracy and Policy Implementation*. Homewood, IL: Dorsey.

Sabatier PA (1986) Top-down and bottom-up approaches to implementation research: a critical analysis and suggested synthesis. *Journal of Public Policy* 6: 21–48.

Sabatier PA and Jenkins-Smith HC (eds) (1993) *Policy Change and Learning: An Advocacy Coalition Approach*. Boulder, CO: Westview Press.

Sabatier PA and Mazmanian DA (1979) The conditions of effective implementations: a guide to accomplishing policy objectives. *Policy Analysis*: 5: 481–504.

Scott V, Mathews V and Gilson L (2011) Constraints on implementing an equity-promoting staff allocation policy: understanding mid-level managers' and nurses' perspectives affecting implementation in South Africa. *Health Policy and Planning*, advance access, published March 30 2011 doi: 10.1093/heapol/czr020.

Walker L and Gilson L (2004) 'We are bitter but we are satisfied': nurses as street-level bureaucrats in South Africa. *Social Science and Medicine* 59: 1251–61.

Walt G (1998) Implementing health care reform: a framework for discussion. In Saltman RB, Figueras J and Sakellarides C (eds) *Critical Challenges for Health Care Reform in Europe*. Buckingham: Open University Press, pp. 365–84.

Wetherley R and Lipsky M (1977) Street-level bureaucrats and institutional innovation: implementing special education reform. *Harvard Educational Review* 47: 171–7.

8 Globalizing the policy process

Overview

In this chapter you will learn about the global dimensions of the health policy process. First, you will consider why globalization has intensified the need for states and other national level policy actors to cooperate internationally, then identify actors who seek to develop health policies at the global level and those who operate internationally to influence health policy at the national level, and finally consider policy transfer between the global and national levels.

Learning objectives

After working through this chapter, you will be better able to:

- explain what is meant by globalization
- appreciate how globalization impacts on health policy
- understand why states cooperate to address health problems and why they increasingly do so with private and civil society actors
- identify the range of actors who operate globally in the area of health policy making.

Key terms

Global civil society. Civil society groups which are global in their aims, communication or organization.

Global public goods. Goods which are undersupplied by markets, inefficiently produced by individual states, and which have benefits which are strongly universal.

Globalization. Complex set of processes which increases interconnectedness and interdependencies between countries and peoples.

Introduction

Most of this book has addressed policy making in the national context, apart from the set of contextual factors highlighted in Chapter 1 that were described as 'international' or 'global'. These factors were treated as external ('exogenous') to domestic policy making. With the intensification of global integration, these global factors are playing an increasingly prominent role in national policy making.

Few countries or health policies are immune from global influences. You have seen in Chapter 3 that health policies, even in high income countries, are subject to pressures from transnational corporations. For example, how tobacco firms resist putting warnings on cigarette packs. National policies are also subject to international trade rules, for example, the challenge by the Canadian government to the French ban on the importation of Canadian asbestos on alleged health grounds. High income countries also voluntarily adopt policies so as to coordinate action to address global health threats, for example, harmonizing border controls to combat infectious diseases, such as Severe Acute Respiratory Syndrome (SARS).

Similarly, and arguably to a much greater extent, health policies in low and middle income countries are subject to these external forces. Policy conditions may be set by donor organizations on ministries of health in return for access to loans or grants. Policies may also be established in response to pressure from global social movements, for example, South Africa's decision to provide treatment for people living with HIV. Moreover, implementation of policies, such as childhood immunization programmes, may be dependent on external support from global public–private partnerships such as the Global Alliance for Vaccines and Immunizations (GAVI Alliance). Reflecting shifts in the global geo-political realm, the health ministers of the so-called BRICS nations (Brazil, Russia, India, China and South Africa) met for the first time in Beijing in July 2011 to coordinate policy and, as an emerging economic and political bloc, to influence the global health agenda. While national policies have always been subject to external influences, globalization has amplified and multiplied them.

For health policy analysts, a key concern relates to how globalization affects policy making. This can be broken down into three questions. First, how do global interactions facilitate the transfer of policies among countries and organizations? Second, who influences the transfer of policies? Third, how has globalization shaped the content of health policy? This chapter addresses these questions – but doing so requires that you first have some background knowledge of globalization and an overview of how governments have traditionally cooperated in health.

Globalization

The term globalization is ubiquitous and used in many different ways. Views are polarized on whether or not globalization is a good thing or not, and, because the term is used in different ways, some dispute the very existence of the phenomenon. You can distinguish at least five ways in which the term globalization is used. First, globalization is associated with the increasing volume, intensity and extent of cross-border movement of goods, people, ideas, finances, or infectious pathogens (internationalization). Second, globalization sometimes refers to the removal of barriers to trade which have made greater movement possible (liberalization). Third, some associate globalization with the trend towards a homogenization of cultures (universalization) or fourth of a convergence around Western, modern and particularly US values and policies (McDonaldization).

Jan Scholte (2000) argues that what is novel about the contemporary world is the reconfiguration of 'social space' and specifically the emergence of 'supraterritorial' or 'transworld' geography. This is the fifth form of globalization. While 'territorial' space (villages and countries) remains important to people and policy makers, what has changed is that people and organizations have increasing connections to others in ways that transcend territorial boundaries. For example, people can have loyalties, identities and interests that go beyond an allegiance to the nation–state, linked to values, religion, ethnicity or sexual identity. Moreover, technologies seemingly compress both time and space. Not only do people and things travel much further, much faster and much more frequently, at times they do so in ways that defy territorial boundaries. Problems can occur everywhere and nowhere. For example, a virus can almost simultaneously infect millions of computers irrespective of their physical location. On any one day, millions of people will connect on the social networking site, Facebook. Hundreds of millions of currency transactions take place in 'cyberspace' on a daily basis. These examples illustrate the fifth dimension of globalization – one that is fundamentally new.

While some might rightly question whether or not all these trends are really new or unprecedented, most agree that they are taking place on a greater scale and with greater intensity than ever before. As a result, there is increasing inter-dependence between countries.

It is argued that globalization has spatial, temporal and cognitive dimensions (Lee et al. 2002). The spatial dimensions have already been alluded to (we are increasingly 'overcoming' distance) as have the temporal ones (through telecommunications and transport activity, the world has speeded up). The cognitive element concerns the thought processes that shape perceptions of events and phenomena. The spread of communication technologies conditions how ideas, values, beliefs, identities and even interests are produced and reproduced. For some, globalization is producing a global village in which all villagers share aspirations and interests, whereas others see Western-inspired values, particularly consumerism and individualism, coming to dominate. Yet others perceive an increasingly polarized world between those who benefit from globalization and those who merely serve it.

Activity 8.1

Provide an example of each of the five meanings of globalization.

Feedback

- internationalization – more people flying around the world; the ability to buy 'seasonal' fruits all year around
- liberalization – removal of protection for domestic production of cigarettes
- universalization – same shops and same brands found around the world or the same words used on signs (the internet, STOP)
- McDonaldization – Starbucks in Beijing and Burma
- superterritoriality – buying airline tickets over the Internet from a third country

To fully appreciate the health policy implications of globalization, it is necessary to understand some of the ways that globalization impacts on health.

Globalization and health

The impact of globalization on health is most evident in the area of infectious diseases. Microbes can now find their way to multiple destinations across the world in less than

24 hours. The SARS outbreak in 2003 spread rapidly from China to neighbouring countries and on to places as geographically distant as Canada. Not only did the virus cause illness and death, it was estimated to have cost Asian economies US$30 billion and the economy of Toronto US$30 million per day at its peak. In 1990, a ship pumping its bilge in a Peruvian harbour spread cholera throughout Latin America causing 4,000 deaths and 400,000 infections in the first year and considerable costs in terms of lost trade and travel. This was part of the seventh cholera epidemic which spread more quickly than the preceding six. In 2003 and 2004, polio spread from Nigeria to 12 polio-free countries in Central, West and Southern Africa. These outbreaks demonstrate that if an epidemic is not detected or contained by a national health system, it can rapidly become a health threat in other parts of the world because of globalization.

It is not only infectious diseases that benefit from globalization. The global production, distribution and marketing of foods, for example, carry with them health risks linked to unhealthy diets. Behaviours may also be prone to globalization in relation to smoking, use of alcohol, the sex trade, and so on. Globalization can also affect the ability of the health care system to respond to health threats. One pressing example relates to health workers. The World Health Organization estimated in 2010 that an additional 4.2 million health care workers were required globally to provide services. High income countries which cannot meet the demand for health workers domestically tend to recruit workers from poorer countries. India and the Philippines have responded to this global demand by training workers for export. Other countries, such as Nigeria and South Africa, have been losing health workers by default rather than design as they are unable to retain staff due to poor working conditions. As a result of insufficient training and migration, Africa alone is estimated to face a shortfall of 1.5 million health workers. The shortage of health workers is recognized as one of the most fundamental constraints to achieving health and development goals.

Activity 8.2

Most health issues and problems are affected in one way or another, often both positively and negatively, by forces associated with globalization. Select a health issue or problem with which you are familiar and attempt to identify the transnational dimensions of the determinants of the problem.

Feedback

You will have first identified the determinants of the health issue. Subsequently, you would need to think about how globalization (in its many guises) may have affected the determinants of the health issue you have identified. Take, for example, the incidence of sexually transmitted infections (STIs) in Bangladesh. Arguably, the most important determinants are the position of women, access to treatment for infected people, and human mobility. Globalization has likely affected each of these determinants in different ways. For example, trade liberalization and other factors, such as entry permit relaxation, have resulted in large movements of workers to and from the Gulf States as well as busy overland trucking routes between India, Bangladesh, Nepal and Burma. This has facilitated a booming sex industry with attendant consequences for STI rates. Trade liberalization and increased foreign investment have resulted in the rapid development of an urban clothing industry which now accounts for one of the country's largest industrial sectors. The industry employs largely young women – an estimated 3 million of them. This has improved the bargaining position of women in general and perhaps in relation to sexual relationships, and has also delayed sexual debut, both of which may help slow the spread of STIs.

It is important to consider that countries, peoples and problems are differentially integrated. Some countries in sub-Saharan Africa are not as well integrated into the global economy, as are, for example, China and India. Nonetheless, as a result of globalization, countries will not be able to directly control all the determinants of ill-health of their populations and will therefore have to cooperate with other actors outside their borders to protect the health of those within them.

Traditional inter-state cooperation for health

States have always been concerned about the spread of disease over their borders. For example, as early as the fourteenth century, the city–state of Venice forcibly quarantined ships which were suspected of carrying plague-infected rats. The practice spread to other ports. These early initiatives paved the way for more formal international agreements in the nineteenth century which aimed to control the spread of infectious disease through restrictions on trade. These, in turn, resulted in the International Health Regulations (IHR), which were accepted by all members of WHO in 1969. The regulations provide norms, standards and best practice to prevent the international spread of disease, but equally importantly require states to report on six diseases. The regulations provide a useful illustration of how states have cooperated to address common problems. The IHR also, however, illustrate the limits of such cooperation. In particular, many states failed to report to WHO, and there was nothing that WHO could do about the lack of compliance. After consideration of the effects of globalization on the spread of disease and the emergence or re-emergence of a wider range of communicable diseases and public health threats, the regulations were revised and re-negotiated over a ten-year period leading up to 2005. The revised regulations require member states to report to WHO on 'events that constitute a public health emergency of international concern' and provide the Organization, for the first time, with authorization to take into consideration 'unofficial reports'. This provides WHO with the power to better monitor outbreaks and marks an evolution in international cooperation to broader forms of public–private interaction that we will return to later in the chapter.

States may cooperate in many ways, both formally and informally. You will now learn about the other formal arrangements that have been established to facilitate cooperation, focusing particularly on multilateral organizations.

The United Nations

The United Nations (UN) system was established at the end of the Second World War to maintain peace and security and to save further generations from the scourge of war. At the heart of the system was the sovereign nation–state which could take up membership in the various UN organizations (such as WHO or UNICEF). These organizations were established to promote exchange and contact among member states and to provide a platform to cooperate to resolve common problems. Member states dictated the policies of the organizations with little interaction with non-governmental bodies. Thus, through the UN system, as you will see later in this chapter, governments, particularly those of high income countries, were able to influence international health policy. At the same time, UN organizations themselves were also, to varying degrees, able to influence national policy.

The World Health Organization (WHO) was founded in 1948 as the UN's specialized health agency with a mandate to lead and coordinate international health activities. Currently, most nation–states (193) belong to WHO and non-voting 'associate membership' allows 189 NGOs in 'official relations' to participate in the governance of the organization. WHO is governed through the World Health Assembly (WHA). Composed of representatives of member states, typically their ministers of health, the WHA meets annually to approve the Organization's programme and budget, and to make international health policy decisions. WHO's Constitution grants the WHA the authority 'to adopt conventions or agreements with respect to any matter within the competence of the Organization'. Decisions are made on the basis of one vote per member and are binding on all members unless they opt out in writing. The Constitution does not, however, provide for sanctions for failure to comply with resolutions. In practice, most of the decisions are expressed as non-binding recommendations, in particular, as technical guidelines, which states may adopt, adapt or dismiss depending on their perceived relevance and national politics.

The WHA is advised by an Executive Board which facilitates the work of the Assembly and gives effect to its decisions and policies. The WHO Secretariat is led by an elected Director-General, who is supported by over 8,000 experts and support staff working at headquarters in Geneva, in six regional offices and in over 150 country offices. Collectively, they attempt to fulfil the following functions:

- articulating consistent, ethical and evidence-based policy and advocacy positions;
- managing information by assessing trends and comparing performance; setting the agenda for, and stimulating research and development;
- catalysing change through technical and policy support, in ways that stimulate cooperation and action and help to build sustainable national and inter-country capacity;
- setting, validating, monitoring and pursuing the proper implementation of norms and standards. For example, in response to the health workforce crisis discussed above, in 2010, WHO used its constitutional authority to develop a code – the WHO Global Code of Practice on the International Recruitment of Health Personnel;
- stimulating the development and testing of new technologies, tools and guidelines for disease control, risk reduction, health care management, and service delivery;
- negotiating and sustaining national and global partnerships.

Of these functions, WHO is best respected for the technical norms and standards developed by its extensive networks of experts and its technical advice to member states. However, while WHO may provide the technical basis for health policies around the world, it has virtually no power to 'impose' these policies on sovereign states – its influence rests on its technical authority.

Like other UN organizations, WHO has been the subject of much criticism. Concerns have been raised over weak leadership, poor management and performance and a lack of accountability. In relation to the Organization's ability to develop normative standards to support national health policy making, criticism has focused on its failure to prioritize, and to fully use the tools at its disposal. Concerns have also been expressed about inadequate conflict of interest management. In 2011, WHO's Director-General conceded that the Organization was over-extended and unable to respond quickly to global health challenges, and met criticisms by embarking on reform to increase focus on core business, enhance financing and management and strengthen WHO's role in global health governance.

Other organizations within the UN system also have some responsibility for health. These include the World Bank, the United Nations Children's Fund (UNICEF), the United Nations Fund for Population (UNFPA), the United Nations Joint Programme on HIV/AIDS (UNAIDS), the United Nations Development Programme (UNDP), the Food and Agricultural Organization of the United Nations (FAO), the World Food Programme (WFP) and the UN Office on Drugs and Crime (UNODC).

Unsurprisingly, as these organizations matured and grew in size, they began not only to serve their members' needs (i.e. to provide a platform for information sharing and collaboration), but to pursue their own organizational interests in policy debates at both the national and international levels. In this process, UN organizations became actors in their own right; often competing with each other and pursuing different health policy alternatives. For example, the 1980s were marked by a major conflict between WHO and UNICEF over the interpretation of primary health care policy. WHO took the position that a multi-sectoral and preventive approach that improved water and sanitation, literacy, nutrition and was based on mass participation was required to improve health in poor countries. In contrast, UNICEF advocated focusing on a few narrow health care interventions that had proved cost-effective and implementing them through vertical programmes (e.g. childhood immunization). Although this public quarrel was short-lived, it points to differences between UN organizations over policies which they promote to member states.

In part, as a response to the challenge of somewhat overlapping mandates and the need for improved coordination among UN agencies, UNAIDS was established in 1996. Fifteen years on, it remains an innovative partnership that aspires to lead the world to achieve universal access to HIV prevention, treatment, care and support – not only coordinating the ten co-sponsoring UN agencies but also setting the agenda for bilateral organizations and member states. Yet, as another UN body, it adds to the complexity of the global health landscape and the scope for international disagreement.

One UN organization with significant influence on health policy is the World Bank. The World Bank has a mandate to provide financial capital to assist in the reconstruction and development of member states. Unlike other UN organizations which make decisions on the basis of one country–one vote, voting rights in the World Bank are linked to capital subscriptions of its members. As a result, the World Bank has often been perceived as a tool of high income countries. The World Bank entered the health field through lending for population programmes in the 1960s, began lending for health services in the 1980s and led international health policy on financing reforms. In 2000, it was the largest external financier of health development in low and middle income countries. Its influence derived not just from the loans it disbursed but also from the perceived objectivity and authority of its economic analysis (at least by elite institutions and donors if not others), and its relationships with powerful finance ministries in borrowing countries. In effect, acceptance of policy conditions associated with health sector loans could be linked to World Bank support for projects in energy or industrial sectors which other ministries cared deeply about. Although the World Bank's policies have been contested, most donors, industry and governments have supported them in general. By the late 2000s, however, the World Bank was no longer the largest external financier of health development – that distinction was held by The Global Fund to Fight AIDS, TB and Malaria – although the World Bank's influence remained significant.

The World Trade Organization (WTO)

A significant addition to the international architecture since the establishment of the UN emerged in 1995 with the founding of the World Trade Organization (WTO). The WTO administers and enforces a series of international trade agreements with the goal of facilitating trade. These global ground rules for trade can impact on health directly through access to medicines, trade in health services or flows of health workers, and indirectly through exposure to consumption and environmental risks that arise from trade. Domestic policies dealing with these issues have become more constrained as a result of the WTO agreements because, by joining the organization, states commit themselves (with no reservations allowed) to alter their policies and statutes to conform with the principles and procedures established in all the WTO agreements. For example, in September 2011, the WTO released the report of a panel which had considered a complaint brought by Indonesia concerning a ban which the US had imposed on importations of Indonesia's clove-flavoured tobacco products. The panel found that the US ban discriminated against Indonesian clove cigarettes in favour of menthol cigarettes of US origin. As a result of the decision, the US will have to choose between appealing the outcome, or implementing the decision by prohibiting menthol cigarettes or permitting clove cigarettes.

The WTO Trade Policy Review Body also conducts periodic surveys of member government's policies to ensure that they are WTO-consistent. Alleged violations can also be notified to the WTO by other member states. Panels of experts review the alleged violations and their decisions, including the need to amend laws to make them WTO-compliant, are binding on member states.

A number of the WTO agreements have implications for health policy. TRIPS, or the Agreement on Trade Related Intellectual Property Rights, has had the highest profile because of its impact on policies concerned with generic drug production and trade – and thus the costs of medicines. The Agreement on Technical Barriers to Trade, the Agreement on the Application of Sanitary and Phytosanitary Measures and the General Agreement on Trade in Services have all been invoked to challenge the health policies of member states when other governments fear that they serve to protect domestic industries instead of protecting health.

Bilateral cooperation

Bilateral relationships (that is, government to government) including cooperation and assistance, are as old as the notion of nation–states. Currently, there are several bilateral organizations, including the United States Agency for International Development (USAID), the UK Department for International Development (DfID) and the Swedish International Development Agency (SIDA), that play roles at the international, regional and national levels. They are often major financiers of health programmes in low and middle income countries and of health programmes of UN organizations. Bilateral cooperation often involves a political dimension and these organizations may use their support to pursue a variety of objectives (diplomatic, commercial, strategic) within the UN system and recipient countries. For example, UK bilateral support often favours Britain's ex-colonies, while a large proportion of US bilateral assistance is earmarked for Egypt and Israel, and that of Japan for South-East Asian countries.

While most bilateral donors profess to adhere to the principle of national sovereignty and 'ownership' over the health policy agenda and pledge to align their support with countries' priorities, in practice, 'external partners' are often intimately involved in setting the health policy agenda (through, for example, influencing priorities by their engagement in policy coordination forums or by stipulating which programmes and services they will fund) and in policy formulation – through, for example, the technical support they provide to ministries of health.

In 2000, the bulk of all aid was provided by 15 or so rich countries. That is changing as Western donors are increasingly joined by new donors from the Gulf States and emerging economies such as China. For example, India, which had over its history been the largest recipient of aid, became a significant donor. China has also moved from being a net recipient to donor, complementing the medical teams that it has been sending to African countries since the 1960s, with significant loans and grants for the construction of hospitals and roads. China also supports anti-malarial programmes across the continent through, for example, the donation of anti-malarial drugs in what has been described as a 'tie of Sino-African friendship'. China's first White Paper on development stresses the principle of equality and mutual benefit through South–South cooperation, although questions have been raised about the extent to which Chinese aid activities are commercial ventures rather than traditional development assistance. Whatever the truth of the case, in 2011, Brazil, India and Russia were at various stages in the planning of aid agencies which will provide new models of cooperation and introduce more competition in the aid industry.

Health as a foreign policy instrument

Overall, reported development assistance for health roughly quadrupled from approximately US $5.6 billion in 1990 to around US$21.8 billion in 2007 (although there are many difficulties in defining and measuring it). The proportion channelled through the United Nations and development banks has declined as the proportion channelled through Global Health Partnerships and NGOs has increased. What is striking, however, is the explicitness with which support for global health has come to be seen as a foreign policy instrument by governments. This can in part be explained by the tendency to frame health as a 'security issue' – particularly following the 9/11 and supposed anthrax attacks on the US in 2001. Health as a foreign policy issue was given a further political boost by the SARS threat in 2003 and later by avian influenza. For a period, international public health enjoyed the 'high politics' status of defence and the economy, and the term 'health diplomacy' was coined. One visible manifestation was the Oslo Declaration in 2007 – issued by the Ministers of Foreign Affairs of Brazil, France, Indonesia, Norway, Senegal, South Africa, and Thailand – which proclaimed global health as a pressing, neglected foreign policy issue.

Activity 8.3

List five to seven examples of multilateral and bilateral organizations that operate in a country with which you are familiar.

You have learned that states have a long history of collaboration in relation to health and that they have established a variety of institutions to this end. The impetus for such collaboration has been varied. Some states have clubbed together so as to create global public goods; goods which markets will not produce and governments cannot efficiently produce on their own but have benefits which are universal (e.g. eradicating polio, developing an AIDS vaccine). At times, cooperation has been predominantly altruistic – perhaps because of shortcomings or lack of resources in other states (e.g. through humanitarian or development cooperation arrangements). But cooperation has also arisen for reasons of enlightened or naked self-interest (e.g. shore up disease surveillance in low income countries to reduce the threat of bio-terrorism in high income ones). At times, 'cooperation' resulting in policy change has been achieved through threats or coercion, e.g. during 'mopping up' campaigns to achieve universal immunization or as a result of trade sanctions imposed through the WTO regime. Whatever the impetus for interaction, domestic policy processes are not hermetically sealed from international processes; international actors are often actively engaged in national policy making.

Modern cooperation in global health

So far, collaboration has been discussed in the context of formal interaction among states and between states and the international system. Yet two of the features of the contemporary global health landscape are the emergence of many non-state actors and the emergence of policy making through informal mechanisms. Both of these developments will now be considered. Particular emphasis is placed on the activities of global civil society, transnational corporations and global public–private partnerships. The aim is to demonstrate that these actors actively participate in international and national health policy processes.

Global civil society

There has been a spectacular proliferation of global civil society groups over the past 50 years; from 1,117 international associations registered with the Union of International Associations in 1956 to over 16,500 in 1998, with 34,995 active by 2011 – while 64,587 were registered (UIA 2011). As early as 1994, Lester Salamon argued that a global 'associational revolution' was under way that would be as 'significant to the latter 20th century as the rise of the nation–state was to the latter 19th'.

Global civil society encompasses a diverse set of actors targeting a diverse set of issues. For example, there are global civil society organizations active in:

* reproductive health – such as the International Women's Health Coalition;
* trade agreements – such as Health Action International (a coalition of 150 NGOs from 70 countries);

- rights of people living with HIV – for example, the 15,000 members of the International Community of Women Living with HIV/AIDS who live in 120 countries representing 17 million women living with HIV;
- ethical standards in humanitarian relief – for example, the Sphere Project, launched by a group of humanitarian NGOs, the Red Cross and Red Crescent movement, which defines and upholds standards of response to the plight of people affected by disasters;
- banning landmines – for example, the International Campaign to Ban Landmines is coordinated by a committee of 13 organizations bringing together over 1,300 groups from over 90 countries.

Global civil society is heterogeneous, comprising everything from a group of people linked together via the Internet to communicate a shared vision across national frontiers to organizations which have vast amounts of political assets. For example, the People's Health Movement offers an alternative global health agenda as well as an alternative to the World Health Assembly by way of its Assembly, while its publication *Global Health Watch* provides an alternative to the WHO's annual *World Health Report.*

One civil society organization has in some important respects eclipsed UN agencies as the epicentre of global health. The Bill and Melinda Gates Foundation was established in 2000 and is now a central actor in international health. The Foundation, with an endowment of over US$36 billion (in 2011), has made over US$14 billion in grant commitments for health in developing countries. Its annual disbursements for global health are larger than the annual budget of the World Health Organization.

The Foundation is led by Bill and Melinda Gates as well as Bill Gates Sr., and run by a relatively small executive staff. The Foundation wields considerable influence over health policy and priority setting in international health as a result of the magnitude of resources at its disposal.

The Foundation has played a catalytic role in changing the organizational landscape in international health. Whereas the other major financier of health development, the World Bank, largely provides loans to governments, the Foundation has mainly supported non-governmental organizations, particularly public–private partnerships with grants. Indeed, one of the most striking features of the Foundation is the number of global public–private partnerships and alliances that it has engineered, incubated and supported financially as well as providing staff to sit on many of their governing bodies. For example, the Foundation played a central role in conceiving the GAVI Alliance, the Foundation for Innovative New Diagnostics, and the Global Alliance for Improved Nutrition, among others. While the Foundation's support has been critical in financing research (for example, trebling the amount spent on malaria research during the 2000s), development and product access for a range of neglected conditions, equally important has been its success in getting public and private sector actors to collaborate on policy projects.

The Foundation has been involved in health policy in other ways as well. Through its grant making, it has supported evidence-informed policy making (see Chapter 9). Universities, think tanks and policy research institutes, academies of science as well as public awareness and advocacy organizations have all been major recipients of Gates Foundation grants. For example, it supported the establishment of a Global Health Policy Research Network whose working groups produce influential analytical reports.

Funding provided by the Foundation acts to set public priorities in a wide range of countries as well as national and international health organizations by default as governments, non-governmental organizations and international organizations gravitate to where the resources are found. Moreover, as a result of large investments in international health activities and the standing of Bill Gates, the Foundation has easy access to influential decision makers at all levels.

Like their national counterparts, international or global civil society organizations play a range of roles in the policy process – either influencing formal international organizations (such as the Global Fund to Fight AIDS, TB and Malaria) or influencing debates at the national level. They adopt different strategies: some as 'insider' groups, through accreditation to the United Nations, for example, or through global policy communities and issue networks as in the case of the work of Médecins Sans Frontières (MSF) on principles for humanitarian interventions in conflict zones; some as 'outsider' groups which use confrontational tactics such as the Occupy groups in various cities of the world protesting against the huge inequalities produced by the global financial system in 2011; and some act as 'thresholder groups' which shift between the two positions. For example, MSF was part of a wider issue network working with WHO, UNAIDS and other groups to increase access to AIDS drugs, but was also a member of a network of activist groups using confrontational tactics to lower AIDS drug prices, among other demands.

In Chapter 6 you learned that civil society often performs critical roles in the policy process, including participation, representation and political education, and that individual civil society organizations can motivate (draw attention to new issues), mobilize (build pressure and support), and monitor (assess the behaviour of states and corporations and ensure implementation) in respect of particular issues and policies. Partially as a result of improved global communications, global civil society plays the same roles at the sub-national, national and international levels.

Activity 8.4

As you read the following account by Jeff Collin and colleagues (2002) of the role of global civil society in a high profile health policy process, make notes and draw a two- or three-sentence conclusion on the functions it performs at different political levels.

Case Study 8: global civil society and the Framework Convention on Tobacco Control

In May 2003, the text of the Framework Convention on Tobacco Control (FCTC) was agreed after almost four years of negotiation by the member states of the WHO. The process was highly contested and often polarized with industry pitted against public health activists and scientists, and both sides seeking to influence the negotiating positions of member states. While the text provides the basis for national legislation among ratifying countries, the process highlights the important role that global civil society can play in international health forums and its limits as well. First, interested NGOs with 'consultative status' at WHO participated formally, but in a circumscribed manner (i.e. not voting), in the negotiation process – but were able to use this status to lobby official delegations. Moreover, many NGOs pressed WHO to accelerate the process by which international NGOs enter into official relations with the Organization – and a decision was made to provide official relations for the purposes of the FCTC process. Second, WHO hosted public hearings in relation to the Convention at which many civil society organizations provided testimony and written statements. Third, civil society groups, such as

Campaign for Tobacco Free Kids and Action on Smoking and Health (ASH), pro-vided an educative function – organizing seminars, preparing briefings for delegates on diverse technical aspects of the Convention, publishing reports on technical issues and issuing a daily news bulletin on the proceedings. A fourth, and perhaps unique, role involved acting as the public health conscience during the negotiations. For example, some NGOs drew attention to the obstructionist positions of some member states and industry tactics – often in a colourful manner such as issuing an Orchid Award to the delegation that they deemed had made the most positive contribution on the previous day and the Dirty Ashtray award to the most destruc-tive. Fifth, individuals working for civil society organizations were, on some occa-sions, able to participate directly in the negotiations through their inclusion in national delegations. Over the course of the negotiations, global civil society organ-izations became a more powerful lobbying force through the formation of a Framework Convention Alliance which sought to improve communication between groups directly involved in systematically building alliances with smaller groups in developing countries. By the end of the negotiations, over 180 NGOs from over 70 countries were members. The Alliance thus provided a bridge to national level actions which involved lobbying, letter writing, policy discussions, advocacy cam-paigns and press conferences before and after meetings.

Feedback

There is general agreement that civil society provided critical inputs to the FCTC process which influenced the content of the Agreement in a variety of ways. Yet there were limits to its influence. For example, the final negotiations were restricted to member states – thus, effectively restricting the direct contribution of civil society. Perhaps more importantly, the transnational tobacco companies have greater politi-cal resources that they can deploy to block the implementation of the Convention.

Keck and Sikkink (1998) have drawn attention to the advocacy role that global civil society networks and coalitions play in world politics in diverse areas such as policies on breast milk substitutes and female genital mutilation. Such coalitions aim to change the procedures, policies and behaviour of states and international organizations through persuasion and socialization – by engaging with and becoming members of a larger policy community on specific issues. Keck and Sikkink argue that the power of such networks and coalitions stems from their information, ideas and strategies to 'alter the information and value contexts within which states make policies'. In Chapter 6 you learned about the role of cause groups in altering perceptions of interests through discursive and other tactics in relation to HIV. Groups such as the Treatment Action Campaign (largely national) and ACTUP (global) have redefined the agenda and altered the perspectives of corporations (e.g. persuading them to lower the cost of drugs, drop lawsuits against governments wanting to implement TRIPS flexibilities, etc.) and successfully invoked policy responses at the national and international levels (Seckinelgin 2003).

Unsurprisingly, civil society has turned to the internet as a tactic for organizing sup-port to influence policy. In Chapter 4 you read about Avaaz, a global web movement which empowers people to influence decision making everywhere. One of its projects was to petition Pope Benedict XVI to stop condemning HIV prevention programmes with his public comments on the use of condoms.

The growth and growing influence of global civil society have been welcomed by many diverse groups. For some, it is welcomed due to the declining capacity of some states to manage policy domains, such as health. For others, it is a means to improve the policy process by bringing new ideas and expertise into the process, by reducing conflict, improving communication or transparency. For others, civil society involvement provides the means to democratize the international system – to give voice to those affected by policy decisions, thereby making these policies more responsive. Civil society is also thought to engage people as global citizens and to 'globalize from below'. Others equate civil society with pursuing humane forms of governance; providing a counterweight to the influence of the commercial sector. Despite these promises, there are others who are less sanguine about it.

Activity 8.5

You have read some of the positive reasons for welcoming the growth of global civil society. What criticisms do you think have been made of global groups?

Feedback

Your list may include:

- *The legitimacy of 'global' groups* may be questioned as a result of Global Northern domination – most funds and members come from the Global North and the agenda is set accordingly. Only approximately one-third of the NGOs accredited to the UN Economic and Social Council (ECOSOC) are based in the Global South (the much more populous part of the globe).
- *Concerns about elitism.* While global civil society is often thought to represent the grass roots, in practice, some organizations are described as 'astroturf' in that they draw their membership from, or are funded by, Southern elites.
- *Lack of democratic credentials.* Many organizations have not considered the extent to which they involve and truly represent the individuals and groups that they claim to advocate for, and how to do so better.
- *Lack of transparency.* Many groups fail to identify clearly who they are, what their objectives are, where their funds originate and how they make decisions. Some are fronts for industry and would be better described as being market actors.
- *'Uncivil' civil society.* Global civil society is a catch-all phrase for a diverse group of entities. Transborder criminal syndicates and pro-racist groups both have a place in this sector.

Transnational corporations

In Chapter 3 you learned about the heterogeneous character of the commercial sector and the ways that the sector wields influence in domestic health policy debates. The commercial sector, particularly transnational corporations (TNCs), commercial associations and peak associations, also pursue their interests through the international system. In 1998, the Secretary General of the International Chamber of Commerce (ICC) wrote that 'Business believes that the rules of the game for the market economy, previously laid down almost exclusively by national governments, must be applied globally if they are to be effective. For that global framework of rules, business looks to the United Nations and its agencies' (Cattaui 1998). The ICC was particularly interested in the WTO fostering rules for business 'with the proviso that they must pay closer attention to the contribution of business'. The then ICC President made clear that 'We want neither to be the secret girlfriend of the WTO nor should the ICC have to enter the World Trade Organization through the servants' entrance' (Maucher 1998). As a result, the ICC embarked on a systematic dialogue with the UN and a multi-pronged strategy to influence UN decision making – including an overt attempt to agree a framework for such input. The activities resulted in a joint UN–ICC statement on common interests as well as a 'Global Compact' of shared values and principles which linked large TNCs with the UN without the shackles of formal pre-scriptive rules or a binding legal framework.

While the Global Compact is a highly visible, tangible and controversial expression of the interaction of the commercial sector with the international system, other avenues have also been utilized. The following illustrative list of the ways that the commercial sector exercises its influence in relation to inter-governmental organiza-tions and their work should alert you to the need to include this group of actors in health policy analysis:

• influencing agendas and proceedings of inter-governmental organizations such as WHO, for example, through industry roundtables with the Director General, involvement in expert advisory and working groups, staff from industry assuming temporary positions and covert infiltration;
• delaying the introduction of international legal instruments;
• blocking the adoption of an international instrument, for example, the sugar industry mobilized significant opposition to the international dietary guidelines proposed by FAO/WHO in 2003 (Waxman 2004a);
• influencing the content of international agreements, for example, Philip Morris suc-cessfully lobbied the US administration to adopt a pro-tobacco position on the text of the FCTC (Waxman 2004b);
• challenging the competence and mandate of an international organization to develop norms in a particular policy area; for example, the food industry opposed and attempted to circumscribe the extent to which WHO could address the obesity epidemic (Waxman 2004a).

This list reveals that the commercial sector is actively involved in international organi-zations – organizations which started life as tools to facilitate inter-country coopera-tion. The following case study provides an in-depth look at industry involvement in the development of global trade rules.

Activity 8.6

As you read through the case study on intellectual property rights (IPR) consider the following questions, making notes as you go.

1 Why does industry want binding as opposed to voluntary rules governing IPR?

2 Why does industry seek global rules?

3 Why did the American administration support the Intellectual Property Committee?

4 Why are these trade rules important for public health?

Case Study 9: the globalization of intellectual property

Sell (2003) provides a fascinating account of industry influence on the development of an inter-governmental agreement on IPRs that is virtually global in scope. The impetus for global rules arose from the concern among certain industries that weak intellectual property protection outside the US was 'piracy' and represented a huge loss and threat to further investment in knowledge creation. As a result, the Chief Executive Officers of 12 US-based TNCs (in chemicals, information, entertainment and pharmaceuticals) established the Intellectual Property Committee (IPC) to pursue stronger and world-wide protection of IPR. The Committee was formed in 1986, just before the launch of the Uruguay Round of trade negotiations which culminated in the establishment of the WTO.

The Committee worked as an informal network. Its goals were to protect IPR through trade law. The Committee began by framing the issue – linking inadequate protection to the US balance of payments deficit. Based on these economic arguments, its considerable technical expertise and links to administration officials, it was able to win the support of the US administration. The IPC then set about convincing its industry counterparts in Canada, Europe and Japan of the logic of its strategy (linking IPR to trade law) and gained their support to put the issue on the agenda of the Uruguay Round negotiations. The IPC commissioned a trade lawyer to draft a treaty which would protect industry interests. This draft was adopted by the US administration as 'reflecting its views' and came to serve as the negotiating document in Uruguay. The IPC was able to position one of its members, the chief executive of Pfizer, as an adviser to the US delegation. Although India and Brazil attempted to stall negotiations and to drop IPR from the round, economic sanctions brought them into line. As a result, the Agreement on Trade Related Intellectual Property Rights (TRIPS) emerged and, according to industry, 'The IPC got 95% of what it wanted.'

As a WTO agreement, TRIPS has a particularly powerful enforcement mechanism and is likely to have profound implications for public health. The Agreement obliged countries that had hitherto not protected product or process patents to make provisions for doing so and in particular to set the patent period at 20 years. Industry argues that monopoly protection is required to encourage investment in research and development. Critics are concerned that this will place unnecessary restrictions on the use of generic products, inevitably increase drug costs and erect barriers to scientific innovation.

Feedback

1 Industry wanted binding rules so that all firms would have to comply. Voluntary schemes often result in piecemeal compliance.

2 Industry wanted global rules as they did not want countries to be allowed to opt out.

3 The US administration is thought to have supported the IPC for a number of reasons. First, the administration accepted the framing of the problem and the magnitude of the problem as estimated by industry. Second, industry provided unique expertise in the area which the US government did not have. Third, these industries provided a great deal of campaign finance and invest heavily in lobbying.
4 The public health impact might be positive and negative. There will likely be more private investment in health research and development. Yet, the availability of these advances might be limited to those able to pay.

As you learned in Chapter 3, the commercial sector influences domestic health policy in a variety of ways and can be a force for positive or negative change. You will recall that the commercial sector also develops private health policy initiatives without the involvement of the public sector. For example, it has developed numerous codes of conduct that are global in scope.

Global public–private health partnerships

One of the features of the globalizing world is the tendency of actors from distinct sectors and levels to work collectively as policy communities and issue networks on policy projects, as described in Chapter 6. One of the most visible forms of collaborative efforts (albeit at the formalized end of the spectrum) in the health sector is the multitude of global public–private health partnerships (GHPs) which have been launched since the mid-1990s. While the GHP label has been applied to a wide range of cooperative endeavours, most bring together disparate actors from public, commercial and civil society organizations who agree on shared goals and objectives and commit their organizations (sometimes numbering in the hundreds as is the case with the Global Partnership to Stop TB) to working together to achieve them. Some partnerships develop independent legal identities, such as the International AIDS Vaccine Alliance or the GAVI Alliance, whereas others are housed in existing multilateral or nongovernmental organizations, such as Roll Back Malaria and Health Metrics Network in WHO.

GHPs assume a range of functions. Some undertake research and development for health products, for example, the Medicines for Malaria Venture raises funds from the public sector and foundations which it uses to involve pharmaceutical and biotechnology companies to focus on producing malaria vaccines for use in low and middle income countries. Others aim to increase access to existing products among populations that could otherwise not afford them. The International Trachoma Initiative, for example, channels an antibiotic donated by Pfizer to countries which use it as part of a public health approach to controlling trachoma. A small number of GHPs mobilize and channel funds for specific diseases or interventions. The most prominent is the Global Fund to Fight AIDS, TB and Malaria which, since its launch in 2002, has approved funding of over US$21 billion in 150 countries. Some GHPs operate primarily in advocacy mode, such as the International Partnership for Microbicides. In the course of their work, many GHPs develop policies, norms and standards that might have been developed by governments or inter-governmental organizations in a previous period, and most actively seek to set agendas, influence the priority given to health issues and become involved in policy formulation or implementation by national governments and international organizations.

From a policy perspective, what makes GHPs noteworthy is the fact that they have come to represent important actors in global and national health policy arena. Even partnerships hosted by other organizations (e.g. Stop TB) assume distinct identities and pursue specific objectives in the health policy arena. Their influence often stems from the range of political resources at their disposal which gives them an edge over organizations working independently. Resources range from political access and savvy, multiple sources of knowledge and perspectives relating to many facets of a policy process, as well as breadth and depth of skills in research capacity, product distribution or marketing techniques. Their power is also a function of their ability to unite a number of important policy actors behind a particular position; actors who may have pursued competing policy alternatives or who may have not been mobilized at all. Consequently, GHPs have become powerful advocates for particular health issues and policy responses (Buse and Tanaka 2011).

Activity 8.7

Closer relationships between public and private sectors, including through partnerships, while welcomed by most, have drawn criticism from some quarters. Write down four or five reasons which may explain critics' misgivings of GHPs as they relate to health policy making.

Feedback

Your response may have included any of the following points, most of which are more or less valid at least some of the time:

- GHPs may further fragment the international health architecture and make policy coordination among organizations even more difficult.
- GHPs increase the influence of the private sector in public policy making processes which may result in policies which are beneficial to private interests at the expense of public interests.
- Following on from the previous point, there are concerns that decision making in GHPs may be subject to conflicts of interest. Although many GHPs develop technical norms and standards, few have mechanisms for managing real, apparent or potential conflicts of this nature.
- Through association with public sector actors, GHPs may enhance the legitimacy of socially irresponsible companies (what critics term 'blue wash').
- Private involvement may skew priority setting in international health towards issues and interventions which may, from a public health perspective, be questionable. GHPs have tended to be product-focused (often curative) and deal with communicable as opposed to non-communicable diseases. Addressing non-communicable diseases is both more difficult and may directly affect the interests of commercial lobbies (e.g. food, beverage and alcohol).
- GHPs may distort policy agendas at the national level. They behave as other international actors in that they pursue particular policy objectives – they are just another actor.
- Decision making in GHPs is dominated by a Northern elite which stands in contrast to decision making in many UN organizations (i.e. one country; one vote). Moreover, representatives from the South tend also to be members of elites.

Although critics have raised valid concerns about public–private partnerships, in an increasingly integrated world it is natural that policy is increasingly made through policy communities and issue networks. These open up new sites for actors to pursue policy goals and in so doing add further complexity to the health policy arena.

Globalizing the policy process

In Chapter 6, the concept of an 'iron triangle' was introduced – the idea that three broad sets of actors are active in the policy process at the national level (i.e. elected officials, bureaucrats and non-governmental interest groups – particularly the commercial sector). The changes described in this chapter suggest that policy making has an increasing global dimension and specifically that global and international actors often play important roles. Cerny coined the term 'golden pentangles' to reflect these changes to the policy process (2001). While domestic bureaucrats, elected officials and interest groups remain influential, they have been joined on the one hand by formal and institutionalized activities of international organizations (e.g. the World Bank, the World Trade Organization, the G20, etc.) – the fourth side of the pentangle – and less formal, often networked, entities (e.g. public–private partnerships) and transnational civil society and market activities on the other – the fifth side. Depending on the issue, any or all five categories of actors may be involved and one or more sets may dominate. The image of the pentangle is useful to policy analysts in that it draws attention to the range of interests that may be active and the complexity of any policy process. For governments, particularly those in low and middle income countries, managing this cacophony of inputs in the political system is a difficult business.

Ministries of health in low and middle income countries face an increasing number of actors in the policy process in addition to managing numerous bilateral relationships with diverse donor organizations – often in the context of discrete projects. One minister has been quoted as follows:

> When I was appointed minister, I thought I was the minister of health and responsible for the health of the country. Instead, I found I was the minister for health projects … run by foreigners.

By the early 1990s, it was increasingly clear that the demands placed on many ministries by donors who pursued different priorities and demanded separate and parallel project accounting mechanisms were overwhelming, undermining limited capacity and making it a challenge to formulate coherent and consistent policy in the sector. As a result, a broad consensus emerged on the need for improved coordination and efforts were placed on establishing 'sector-wide approaches' (SWAPs). These involved articulating an agreed policy framework and medium-term expenditure plan. All external donors were expected to operate within the framework, only to finance activities contained in the plan (preferably through a common pool and ideally intermingled with domestic funds) and to accept consolidated government reports.

Given the politics of development cooperation, success with SWAPs was mixed; many donors continued to fund off-plan externally designed projects which were poorly harmonized and subject to burdensome and complex reporting and accounting practices – often for purposes of attribution. In countries where progress was made, these gains were often threatened by the arrival of new global public–private partnerships. By 2010, many countries hosted over 25 health GHPs which often operated as vertical programmes with parallel systems – thus pulling the ministry of health in differing directions as they competed for attention and priority. As a result, there were renewed and high profile pleas for coherence at the country level. Similarly, it was recognized that country-level coordination needed to be supported by global-level coordination. The most prominent manifestation of this is the Millennium Development Goals (MDGs) agreed in 2000 by 189 countries, with the support of the International Monetary Fund (IMF) and the World Bank, the Organization for Economic Cooperation and Development (OECD), and the G8 and G20 countries. The eight MDGs have specific targets and include verifiable indicators against which progress is measured by 2015, and reported to the UN General Assembly. The goals galvanized the global community and lent a large degree of coherence to global health.

Activity 8.8

Why has it been so challenging to coordinate efforts to support government health policies at the country level? Give two or three reasons.

Feedback

Your answer should have discussed the fact that different actors pursue different interests. Often these interests are difficult to reconcile. Bilateral donor organizations may pursue diplomatic or commercial interests in addition to health and humanitarian objectives through development cooperation. These may be at odds with priorities established through a consultative process within the recipient country. As you learned above, international organizations can pursue distinct and multiple objectives as well. All organizations, including global health partnerships, will compete to get their issues onto the policy agenda and to see that they receive attention. External agencies may, for example, prefer the use of their own countries' commodities and equipment, may advocate for transparency, value for money, decentralization or resource re-allocation which may significantly affect domestic interests. Hence, there will always be a political as well as a technical dimension to coordination, with external agencies attempting to set agendas and get national counterparts to implement their preferred policy alternatives.

The pentangle model raises questions of whether or not the addition of new categories of actors leads to greater pluralism and whether or not increased interaction leads to the consideration of a wider range of policy alternatives. There is no one answer to these questions as they depend on the policy and context. The few empirical studies of health sector policy making suggest that although some areas have included a greater range of groups, decisions tend to be dominated by members of policy elites, often representing a narrow range of organizations, albeit from public, civil society and for-profit sectors (i.e. elite pluralism).

As for the question of whether or not globalization increases the range of policy options under consideration, it would appear that policy agenda setting and formulation are marked by increasing convergence – particularly in relation to the health sector reforms outlined in Chapter 3. Yet the transfer of policies from country to country – often through international intermediaries (such as global partnerships or international organizations) – which results in convergence is not a straightforward process. Explicit cross-border and cross-sector lesson learning (e.g. through study tours) or the provisions of incentives (e.g. loans, grants) does not automatically lead to policy transfer and change. Often the processes are drawn-out, and involve different organizations and networks at various stages.

Summary

In this chapter you have learned that globalization is a multifaceted set of processes that increases integration and interdependence among countries. Integration and inter-dependence have given rise to the need for multi-layered and multi-sector policy making (above and below the state as well as between public and private sectors). State sovereignty over health has generally, albeit differentially, diminished. Yet the state retains a central regulatory role even if it has to pursue policy through conflict and collaboration with an increasing number of other actors at various levels in policy communities.

References

Buse K and Tanaka S (2011) Global public-private health partnerships: lessons learned from ten years of experience. *International Dental Journal* 61(suppl. 2): 2–10.

Cattaui MS (1998) Business partnership forged on a global economy. ICC Press Release. 6 February. Paris: International Chambers of Commerce.

Cerny P (2001) From 'iron triangles' to 'golden pentangles'? Globalizing the policy process. *Global Governance* 7(4): 397–410.

Collin J, Lee K and Bissell K (2002) The Framework Convention on Tobacco Control: the politics of global health governance. *Third World Quarterly* 23(2): 265–82.

Keck ME and Sikkink KI (1998) *Activists Beyond Borders*. Ithaca, NY: Cornell University Press.

Lee K, Fustukian S and Buse K (2002) An introduction to global health policy. In Lee K, Buse K and Fustukian S (eds) *Health Policy in a Globalizing World*. Cambridge: Cambridge University Press, pp. 3–17.

Maucher HO (1998) *The Geneva Business Declaration*. Geneva: ICC.

Salamon LM (1994) The rise of the non-profit sector. *Foreign Affairs* 73(4): 109–22.

Scholte JA (2000) *Globalisation: A Critical Introduction*. Houndsmill: Palgrave.

Seckinelgin H (2003) Time to stop and think: HIV/AIDS, global civil society and peoples' politics. In Kaldor M, Anheier HK and Glasius M (eds) *Global Civil Society Yearbook 2003*. Oxford: Oxford University Press, pp. 114–27.

Sell S (2003) *Private Power, Public Law: The Globalisation of Intellectual Property*. Cambridge: Cambridge University Press.

UIA (2011) *Yearbook of International Associations*. Vol. 1 *Organisational Descriptions*. London: Union of International Associations.

Waxman HA (2004a) The WHO global strategy on diet, physical activity and health: the controversy on sugar. *Development* 47(2): 75–82.

Waxman HA (2004b) Politics of international health in the Bush administration. *Development* 47(2): 24–8.

Research, evaluation and policy 9

Overview

This chapter looks at how and in what circumstances the findings from research, evaluation and other forms of evidence are used in the policy process. In terms of the now familiar device of seeing the policy process as a 'policy cycle', evaluation is commonly portrayed as the fourth and final phase (e.g. is the policy effective?), but it is also, in principle, the beginning of another cycle (if the policy is not delivering what was intended, what needs to change or should it be abandoned?). Research can contribute to policy in other ways and at other stages in the policy cycle (e.g. helping define the nature and severity of problems in the first place and thereby helping get issues on the policy agenda or providing the basis to choose among policy alternatives in the formulation stage). This chapter explores different models of the nature of the relationship between researchers and decision makers, and some of the steps that both are encouraged to take to improve the 'fit' between research and policy decisions. Although the idea that researchers and policy makers inhabit different cultural and occupational worlds explains a great deal of the difficulties of communication between the two, studies of the policy process reveal that the principal divide is often between different 'advocacy coalitions' which may involve both researchers, policy makers and other interest groups, competing for the ascendancy in particular policy contexts on the basis of their ideas about policy problems and solutions.

Learning objectives

After working through this chapter you will be better able to:

- define 'evidence', 'research' and 'evaluation', and the different ways 'evidence' of different types may be used in the policy process
- contrast different models of the relationship between research and policy, and their links to general perspectives on the policy process
- identify some of the barriers to research uptake by policy makers and reasons why the relationship between research findings and policy decisions is rarely, if ever, direct and linear
- identify some of the factors that facilitate the uptake of research findings by policy makers
- set out some of the strategies that researchers and policy makers are increasingly using in an attempt to close the 'gap' between research findings and policy decisions, and assess their likelihood of success
- critique the 'two communities' conceptualization of researchers and policy makers, and use other approaches such as the Advocacy Coalition Framework.

Key terms

Audit. Examination of the extent to which an activity corresponds with pre-determined standards or criteria.

Dissemination. Process by which research findings are made known to key audiences, including policy makers.

Evaluation. Research designed specifically to assess the operation and/or impact of a programme or policy in order to determine whether the programme or policy is worth pursuing further.

Evidence. Any form of knowledge, including, but not confined to research, of sufficient quality to be used to inform decisions.

Evidence-based medicine. Movement within medicine and related professions to base clinical practice on the most rigorous scientific basis, principally informed by the results of randomized controlled trials of effectiveness of interventions.

Evidence-based (or evidence-informed) policy. Movement within public policy to give evidence greater weight in shaping policy decisions, better described as 'evidence-informed' policy than 'evidence-based' since it is obvious in public policy that evidence is only one factor influencing decision making.

Formative evaluation. Evaluation designed to assess how a programme or policy is being implemented with a view to modifying or developing the programme or policy in order to improve its implementation.

Knowledge transfer. Strategy usually incorporating a variety of 'linkage' and 'exchange' activities designed to reduce the social, cultural and technical 'gap' between researchers and policy makers.

Monitoring. Routine collection of data on an activity usually against a plan or contract.

Research. Systematic activity designed to generate rigorous new knowledge and relate it to existing knowledge in order to improve understanding of the physical or social world.

Summative evaluation. Evaluation designed to produce an overall verdict on a policy or programme in terms of the balance of costs and benefits.

Introduction

This chapter focuses on how research, evaluation and other types of evidence may affect policy through introducing new ways of seeing the world, new techniques for improving health, or reasons for changing existing policies. *Research* is a systematic process for generating new knowledge and relating it to existing knowledge in order to improve understanding about the natural and social world. Research uses a wide variety of methods, theories and assumptions about what counts as valid knowledge. 'Applied' research takes new knowledge from 'basic' research and tries to apply it to solving practical problems.

For some people, *evaluation* is distinct from research, but since evaluations use research methods, it makes sense to see them as one type of research, defined as: 'any scientifically based activity undertaken to assess the operation and impact of [public] policies and the action programmes introduced to implement those policies' (Rossi and Wright 1979).

It is common to make a distinction between *formative* and *summative* evaluation. The former is best thought of as an evaluation designed to contribute directly to assisting those responsible for a programme to shape the programme while it is being designed or implemented. Formative evaluations generally take place during the early stages of a programme and focus on activities and processes with a view to providing advice directly to the policy makers that can be used to modify and develop the programme. By contrast, summative evaluations are designed to try to provide a verdict on a policy or programme. In other words, they focus on measuring the impact or outcome and costs as well as, the extent to which a programme has met its objectives. They tend to produce their findings later and to use quantitative methods. Formative evaluations tend to use qualitative methods such as observation and semi-structured interviews.

Evaluations are seen as particularly policy relevant forms of research since they are normally commissioned by decision makers or funders to assess whether or not policies or programmes are going well and to what effect. Within the conventional device of the 'policy cycle', evaluation is portrayed as an important fourth and final stage to see if a policy has been effective. However, since policy is a continuous process, evaluation can contribute at any stage. For example, an evaluation could show that a policy intervention was not working as intended and was generating unanticipated problems thereby contributing to the first stage of problem identification in another policy cycle.

Policy makers have access to, and use, forms of *evidence* other than scientific research. For example, research is usually distinguished from *audit* which examines the extent to which a process or activity corresponds with predetermined standards or criteria of performance (e.g. checking that the facilities and staffing at a clinic are adequate to deliver babies safely). It is also distinguished from *monitoring* which constitutes the continuous, routine collection of data on an activity (such as treatments delivered) to ensure that everything is going according to plan. For a government, regular surveys, focus groups and/or stakeholder analysis (which you will learn about in Chapter 10) can be seen as a form of monitoring. Both audit and monitoring may be used to inform policy as well as information from other sources such as opinion polls and community consultations. As a result, *evidence*, from the point of view of a policy maker, is likely to include a broader range of knowledge than that derived exclusively from research.

A movement which started in the early 1990s – *evidence-based medicine* – advocated the greater and more direct use of research evidence in clinical practice decisions, in particular promoting the application of the findings of systematic reviews of randomized controlled trials. In the latter part of the 1990s, the movement broadened into a call for *evidence-based policy*. Proponents wish to give research evidence greater weight than other considerations in shaping policy not just clinical decisions. Others have a more modest goal, advocating *evidence-informed* policy making, defined as 'the integration of experience, judgement and expertise with the best available external evidence from systematic research' (Davies 1999). Both formulations of evidence-based policy can be seen as a reaction to policies driven entirely by conviction.

How do research and evaluation influence policy?

Slogans such as 'evidence-based policy' and the related catch-phrase coined in government in the UK of 'what counts is what works' assume that ideally there should be a direct, sequential and relatively rapid relationship between research findings and policy decisions. This is known as the *engineering* model in which either a problem is identified by policy makers and 'solved' by researchers or new knowledge (e.g. of a previously unidentified health risk) leads to policy change. It is another formulation of the rational, linear approach to policy development outlined in Chapter 2 which argues that policy choices should be made in the light of what works best. Just as there have been many criticisms of the rational model of policy making, the engineering model of the links between research and policy has also been extensively critiqued. One problem is that there are relatively few empirical examples of a direct link between a particular set of research results and a specific policy change. Harrison (2001) identifies at least seven conditions that would have to be met for the 'perfect implementation' (see Chapter 7, for more on this notion) of research:

1 the existence of comprehensive, authoritative statements based on systematic reviews of research evidence;
2 the ability of such statements to provide a direct guide to decision-making in specific circumstances;
3 knowledge of such statements by all relevant actors;
4 adequate resources (e.g. time) to act upon the authoritative statements of evidence;
5 sufficient incentive to apply the evidence;
6 absence of substantial disincentives (material or non-material) to apply the evidence;
7 an implementation chain sufficiently short to ensure a good likelihood of compliance with the implications of the evidence.

Another difficulty with the model is the way it assumes that research precedes the policy solution to a pre-defined problem, when there are plenty of examples of policy solutions being promoted and implemented without it being clear which policy problem they are supposed to be a response to. For example, many people argue that the vogue for privatization and contracting out of public services in low and middle income countries was a solution in search of a problem, ill-suited to circumstances in many such settings.

Despite this, the rational, linear model of the relation between research and policy still tends to inform the day-to-day working assumptions of many researchers and policy makers. As Lomas (2000a) puts it, tongue in cheek, 'The research-policy arena is assumed to be a retail store in which researchers are busy filling shelves of a shop front with a comprehensive set of all possible relevant studies that a decision-maker might some day drop by to purchase.'

Studies of the complex way in which policy is made in practice led to a different more indirect conceptualization of the relationship between research (and other forms of evidence) and policy, and to the recognition that research conclusions can be 'used' in a wide variety of different ways by policy makers. Researchers observed that new knowledge and insights appeared to percolate through the political environment like water falling on limestone: the water is absorbed, disappears into multiple channels and then emerges unexpectedly some time later elsewhere. Weiss (1979) suggested that it was more accurate to term this process one of *enlightenment*. Concepts and ideas derived from research filtered into the policy networks that shaped the policy process in a particular field and had a cumulative, indirect effect rather than an immediate, direct effect on policy (for instance, it took seven years from the publication of the crucial research on smoking and lung cancer before the UK Ministry of Health began to take its implications seriously and many more years before the first restrictions on advertising of cigarettes were introduced). Under this model, the primary impact of research and researchers is at the level of ideas and ways of thinking about problems which are then taken up by others rather than in providing specific answers to specific policy puzzles. 'Research is considered less as problem solving than as a process of argument or debate to create concern and set the agenda' (Black 2001).

Activity 9.1

Compare and contrast the engineering (or problem-solving) model of how research may influence policy with the enlightenment model. Think of some of the limitations of each approach as a guide to how to ensure that research evidence is used for policy making.

Feedback

Your answer is likely to have included the points given in Table 9.1.

Table 9.1 Differences between the 'engineering' and 'enlightenment' models of how research influences policy

Engineering or problem-solving model	Enlightenment model
Sees the relationship between research and policy as rational and sequential	Sees the relationship as indirect and not necessarily logical, predictable or neat
A problem exists because basic research has identified it	Problems are not always recognized, or at least not immediately
Applied research is undertaken to help solve the problem	There may be a considerable period of time between research and its impact on policy. Much research develops new ways of thinking rather than solutions to specific problems
Research is then applied to helping solve the policy problem. Research produces a preferred policy solution	The way in which research influences policy is complex and hidden. Policy makers may not want to act on results or may use findings in ways that researchers do not approve of
Rarely or never describes how the relationship between research and policy works in practice. Assumes that this happens in a straightforward, uncontroversial manner	Research influences policy generally indirectly and the process is frequently obscure and hard to explain

Other researchers showed that research could be used in entirely political ways by governments and powerful interest groups as an instrument to advance their interests. This *strategic* model views research as ammunition to support predetermined positions or to delay or obstruct politically uncomfortable decisions (Weiss 1979). There is certainly empirical support for this somewhat cynical view of the nature of politics and the use of research. A classic recurring example of the strategic use of research is for a government to argue that no decision can be made on a contentious issue without further research and analysis, and then to appoint a commission of enquiry taking several years to do the necessary work. The effect of this action is to take the issue off the policy agenda. With any luck, a different government will be in office when the awkward report arrives from the commission.

An example of the interpretation and use of research findings in public health that can be interpreted in 'strategic' terms relates to the presentation and use of evidence of a decline in HIV prevalence in Uganda in the 1990s. While the totality of the epidemiological evidence indicated some improvement in the situation, commentary and discussion were dominated by the 'headline' figures of a huge reduction from 30 per cent to 10 per cent in prevalence between 1992 and 1996. Parkhurst (2002) argues that this selective, perhaps deliberately uncritical, interpretation of part of the evidence was the product of pressure on international donors from the international political community to show the success of the global anti-AIDS effort and a desire on the part of the Ugandan government to present its AIDS programme in the best possible light. Another attraction of the Ugandan good news story was that it provided an international role model of a government that had taken AIDS seriously with very positive results.

A less cynical model of the relation between research and policy, drawing on some of the same political insights, is the *elective affinity* model. This theory holds that policy makers are more likely to react positively to research findings and insights if they have participated in the research process in some way, if the findings are disseminated at the right time in relation to the decision making process and, most importantly, if the implications of the findings coincide with the values and beliefs of the policy audience (Short 1997). Essentially, this approach emphasizes the importance of ideological compatibility between the researchers and the policy makers at a particular point in time (see the discussion of Advocacy Coalitions, below) as well as the extent of contact between researchers and policy makers (see the development of 'linkage', below, as a way of increasing the likelihood that research will be used for policy). It indicates that research that introduces new thinking and challenges the status quo will be ignored unless it fits with dominant policy makers' ideology. If it does not fit, the research may play an 'enlightenment' role over a much longer period of time with much more uncertain consequences.

While all these models, apart from the engineering model, rightly see research and evaluation as only one input to a complex policy process, they implicitly tend to support the view that researchers and policy makers are each relatively homogeneous groups with similar views and distinctly different from one another. In fact, a notion of *two communities* of research and policy underlies not only many theories of the relationship, but also much of the practical thinking about how the relationship can and should be improved. The 'two communities' model emphasizes the idea that researchers and policy makers live in different cultures based on different assumptions about what is important and how the world works.

Activity 9.2

As a demonstration of the 'two communities' hypothesis, tabulate the main differences you can think of between, say, university researchers and government officials in terms of the type of activities they engage in, their attitudes to research, who they are accountable to, their priorities, how they build their careers and obtain their rewards, their training and knowledge base, the organizational constraints they face, and so on.

Feedback

Your analysis might look something like Table 9.2.

Table 9.2 The 'two communities' model of researchers and policy makers

	University researchers	*Government policy makers*
Work	Discrete, planned research projects using explicit, scientific methods designed to produce unambiguous, generalizable results (knowledge focused); usually highly specialized in research areas and knowledge; report findings using technical language	Continuous, unplanned flow of tasks involving negotiation and compromise between interests and goals; assessment of practical feasibility of policies and advice on specific decisions (decision focused). Often required to work on a range of different issues simultaneously
Attitudes to research	Justified by its contribution to valid knowledge; research findings lead to need for further investigations since there is always some uncertainty in findings	Only one of many inputs to their work; justified by its relevance and practical utility (e.g. in decision making); some scepticism about the value of research findings versus their own experience; value research which supports their policy decisions and reinforces their world view
Accountability	To scientific peers primarily, but also to funders	To politicians primarily, but also the public, indirectly
Priorities	Expansion of research opportunities and influence of experts in the world	Maintaining a system of 'good governance' and satisfying politicians; may wish to protect or expand the role of their agency;
Careers/ rewards	Built largely on publication in peer reviewed scientific journals and peer recognition rather than practical impact though this varies by discipline	Built on successful management of complex political processes (as well as relationships) and involvement with 'successful' policy initiatives rather than use of research findings for policy
Training and knowledge base	High level of training, usually specialized within a single discipline; little knowledge about policy making processes	Often, though not always, generalists expected to be flexible; often little or no scientific training
Organizational constraints	Relatively few (except resources); high level of discretion, e.g. in choice of research focus	Embedded in large, inter-dependent bureaucracies and working within political limits, often to short timescales; such organizations likely to be highly risk-averse
Values/ orientation	Place high value on independence of thought and action; belief in unbiased search for generalizable knowledge	Oriented to providing high quality advice, but attuned to a particular political and economic context and to informing specific decisions

Barriers to the use of research

As you were completing your table, you probably began to think about the various factors that are likely to intervene in the process of translating research into policy or act as barriers in that process. The 'two communities' perspective focuses attention on barriers relating to the different questions that researchers and policy makers may be interested in answering, as well as problems associated with the translation, dissemination and communication of research findings. However, there are more fundamental obstacles that relate more directly to the nature of public policy and politics.

Political and ideological factors

You should by now be familiar with the notion that 'policy' is a process that takes place in a particular context influenced by the values and interests of the participants. As a result, politics and ideology inevitably affect the way that research is used. For example, who initiates, undertakes, participates in and oversees an evaluation, and why it is wanted, are likely to influence how far it is used by policy makers. In low and middle income countries, evaluations of public health programmes are mostly a requirement of external donors, ostensibly as the basis for decisions about whether funding should be continued or not. They tend to be undertaken by foreign experts commissioned by the donors. As a result, the evaluations are less likely to be taken seriously by national governments or those working in the programmes, irrespective of the technical quality of the analysis they contain, even if they do influence the decisions of donors. In general, it is safe to assume that the validity and reliability of a piece of research may be necessary for it to have any chance of influencing policy but these characteristics alone are not sufficient to guarantee its influence.

Political and ideological context matters in the interpretation and use of research evidence. In the late 1990s, the president of South Africa, Thabo Mbeki controversially rejected the orthodox scientific view that the HIV virus caused AIDS and espoused the position of a small minority of dissident scientists. Thereby, he called into question the view that AIDS is a viral infection spread mainly by sexual contact (Schneider 2002).

Activity 9.3

Why do you think President Mbeki was attracted to the dissident scientific position on the link between HIV and AIDS?

Feedback

You may have suggested one or more of the following reasons:

1 It enabled him to play down what he took to be a racist insinuation that the high prevalence of AIDS in South Africa was the result of the sexual behaviour of black South Africans and black Africans in general.
2 It enabled him to assert the right of the elected government to decide not only who had the right to speak about AIDS and determine the appropriate response, but even who had the right to define what the AIDS problem was.

3 It enabled him to support indigenous science against a Western orthodoxy based largely, but not exclusively, on research from outside Africa.
4 It enabled the new post-apartheid state and African National Congress government to identify themselves as leaders in Africa in the resistance to the dominance of biomedical research by former colonial and other wealthy countries.

Policy on the non-pharmacological use of drugs is another notoriously contested area where research findings and scientific advice based on that evidence are frequently controversial. The UK Advisory Council on the Misuse of Drugs (ACMD) advises the responsible minister on government policy towards the misuse of drugs and, in particular, which of three categories, A to C, based on harm, should apply to individual drugs, with A the most harmful and C the least. Periodically, the ACMD has advised the government against a reclassification only to be ignored. For example, in May 2008, the government decided to reclassify cannabis from C to B against the advice of the Council. The chair of the ACMD, Professor David Nutt, argued publicly against the reclassification of cannabis. Despite his disagreement with the minister responsible, he remained as chair of ACMD. However, in October 2009, he was reported in the media as having given a lecture in which he attacked, 'the artificial separation [in UK policy] of alcohol and tobacco from illegal drugs'. He argued that alcohol and tobacco were more harmful than many illegal drugs and that politicians had 'distorted' and 'devalued' the evidence of harm. His argument was that a more balanced assessment would tend towards more restrictions on alcohol and tobacco, and fewer on some illicit drugs. This was seen by the minister as damaging efforts to give the public a clear message about the dangers of illegal drugs as well as straying beyond the field of illegal drug policy and he was dismissed (http://news.bbc.co.uk/1/hi/uk/8334774.stm, accessed 30 October 2011). This led to a vigorous media debate about the role of scientific evidence and scientific advice in UK policy making. Nutt's critics accused him of deliberately straying beyond the boundaries of scientific advice into political advocacy and ignoring the other factors that the minister had to take into account. His supporters lamented the intimidatory tactics of ministers and the low priority given to scientific evidence versus populist policy making.

Of course, it is not just politicians whose approach to, and use of, research can be shaped by ideology. Research requires resources and researchers have to apply to public and private sources of funds to support their projects. In turn, public and private funding bodies influence what kind of research will be undertaken and which researchers will be selected to do the research. Globally, the share of total health research funding from governments has been falling even though total spending has been rising in real terms. By 2001, 44 per cent of the total (as against 47 per cent in 1998) came from governments; and, of the remainder, 48 per cent came from the for-profit private sector and 8 per cent from the private not-for-profit sector (Global Forum on Health Research 2004a).

In the early 1990s around 75% of pharmaceutical companies' research funds went to university researchers who are, by and large, interested in disseminating the findings of their research widely. By 2000, this proportion had fallen to 34% with the rest accounted for by in-house research or research in private institutes linked to the industry or to advertisers (Petersen 2002). Even if there is no direct interference in privately funded research undertaken outside universities, it is clear that the incentive on such researchers is to produce findings that maintain a flow of funds from their sponsors. For example, while the data collected are likely to be used by the sponsoring companies, they are less likely to be made publicly available. The results are also likely to be interpreted in ways that are broadly supportive of the pharmaceutical industry or suppressed if they are unpalatable.

For example, Boots, a leading British pharmaceutical company, funded research on the effectiveness of its drug, Syntharoid, after small-scale tests had suggested it might be better than alternative drugs. Although more definitive research showed no benefits, Boots was able to prevent publication of the findings for a further seven years during which time it was able to sell the drug successfully (Rampton and Stauber 2001).

The impact of research on policy in the health field is also shaped by the interests of different countries with very different economic resources in supporting research on health problems relevant to their settings. In general, health research applied to the needs of people in low and middle income countries is still under-resourced, given the potential for such research to help reduce the large burden of preventable death and ill-health in those countries. About US$106 billion was spent globally on health research in 2004, of which roughly 10 per cent was spent on the problems facing low income countries which account for 90 per cent of the global burden of disease (measured in terms of disability-adjusted life years) (Global Forum for Health Research 2004a). This was described in 1998 as the '10/90 gap' by those pressing for a more equal distribution of global research effort. Thus one reason why poorer countries make less use of research is related simply to the fact that there is so little basic and applied research on many of the health problems they face. For example, of the 1,233 drugs that reached the global market between 1975 and 1997, only 13 (1 per cent) were for use in combating tropical infections which primarily affect the poor (Global Forum for Health Research 2004b). Although more funders of research in low and middle income countries have come onto the scene since the late 1990s, there is a continuing mismatch between the needs of such countries and the level of research investment.

Policy and scientific uncertainty

Particularly in the case of policy or programme evaluations, interpreting and using the findings can be difficult for two reasons: (1) the goals of the original programme are often deliberately broad and open to interpretation; and (2) the effects are likely to be small in relation to all the other influences on the outcome(s) of interest. Indeed, it is now generally accepted that the better designed the evaluation, the smaller the effect it is likely to demonstrate. It can be difficult for policy makers to know whether the fact that an evaluation fails to show a programme achieving the results intended is due to the intrinsic methodological difficulty of disentangling the specific contribution of the programme from other factors, or whether the programme has genuinely failed to meet its objectives. This is particularly likely in relation to policies designed to tackle long-standing, complex, multi-causal problems such as child poverty or poor health in early life and their subsequent effects. These tend to be the most important programmes attracting a high degree of public interest and debate.

All research findings carry a degree of uncertainty, but sometimes there is a particularly high level of uncertainty affecting the way in which the research can be used for policy. Mathematical modelling of the future trajectory and severity of an epidemic is important in planning an appropriate government response, but is intrinsically uncertain since it is dependent on current knowledge and assumptions about the future. For example, a large amount of scientific effort went into modelling the probable spread and impact of the swine 'flu epidemic of 2009–10 in order to find ways of reducing harm. In the event, the outbreak was far less severe than predicted and the modellers and public health authorities were criticized, among other things, for being insufficiently critical of evidence from the pharmaceutical industry seen as biased in favour of selling more vaccine and therapeutic drugs. Cynics argued that predictions were also used self-interestedly to bolster the budgets of public health agencies.

If there is little agreement as to what the main goals of a programme are and how progress towards them should be measured, then an evaluation is open to a variety of interpretations in policy terms. For example, a programme may improve equity but harm efficiency, yet unless the precise weight which should be given to each of these objectives has been set down in advance by policy makers, it is difficult to know how to use the results of an evaluation looking at both.

Another point of contention surrounding the interpretation and use of research relates to its generalizability and relevance to a particular policy context. Faced with research from elsewhere that does not support their policy line, policy makers tend to play down the relevance of the research. By contrast, scientists tend to emphasize the generalizability of their findings to a wider range of settings, sometimes inappropriately.

Different conceptions of risk

Individual conceptions of risk also shape the way that evidence influences health policies. People's perceptions of the likelihood of harm from environmental hazards generally exceeds their perception of the risks of harm caused by alcohol, tobacco or poor diets in spite of the fact that far more people are at risk of disease from the latter group than the former.

The mass media reinforce these perceptions by tending to focus on the dramatic, the rare and the new, thereby highlighting some pieces of research ahead of others and potentially putting politicians under pressure to act in the absence of good evidence. For example, in the UK in 2002–03, media coverage of one small study of the potential risk of autism associated with receiving the combined measles, mumps and rubella (MMR) vaccination was huge. Unfortunately, many parents chose not to have their children vaccinated, thereby exposing them to other greater health risks. Media coverage led to high levels of public anxiety and pressure on government to act to reduce risks to health. This was before a systematic review of the evidence had shown that the link between autism and MMR was almost certainly non-existent. The government resisted the pressure to change its childhood immunization policy even though this was unpopular at the time, but immunization rates were reduced for several years leading to an increase in cases, including avoidable deaths.

Perceived utility of research

Today, researchers of all kinds, but particularly social scientists, are far more willing than in the past to try to make their research potentially useful. Their ability to do so partly depends on the kinds of information generated by their research. Weiss (1991) identified three basic forms of output from research, generated to differing degrees by different research styles:

- data and findings;
- ideas and criticism – these spring from the findings and typify the enlightenment model of how research influences policy;

- arguments for action – these derive from the findings and the ideas generated by the research but extend the role of the researcher into advocacy.

Each is likely to be perceived as useful in different circumstances. Weiss argues that apparently objective data and findings are likely to be most useful when a clear problem has been recognized by all actors and there is already a consensus about the range of feasible policy responses. The role of research is then to help decide which option to choose.

Ideas and criticism appear to be most useful in an open, pluralistic policy system distinguished by a number of different policy groupings in stable communication with one another when there is uncertainty about the nature of the policy problem (or, indeed, whether one exists worthy of attention) and where there is a wide range of possible responses.

Research as argument may be used when there is a high degree of conflict over an issue. It has to be promoted in an explicitly political way if it is to have an impact. Its use depends on the lobbying skills of the researchers and whether the key policy audiences agree with the values and goals inherent in the research. If they do not, the research will be ignored. Thus this is a high risk strategy for researchers since, unlike simply letting the research percolate into policy and practice (following the 'enlightenment' model), it requires researchers to abandon their customary status as disinterested experts and enter the rough-and-tumble of political argument which could be career-threatening.

Timing

Another factor affecting whether or not research is used in policy making is timing. As Chapter 4 showed, the insight that new issues get onto the government's policy agenda when 'windows of opportunity' open shows that researchers can do all they like to establish the nature of a problem and develop suitable responses, but their recommendations will not be taken up unless the political context is conducive. Frequently, a change of government has this effect. For example, researchers in South Africa had tried to place the issue of maternal health on the government's agenda to little effect until the first fully democratically elected government in 1994 changed the political climate (Daniels et al. 2008). New officials were appointed with strong links to networks of 'policy entrepreneurs' and researchers in the field of maternal health. The government became more open, the idea that maternal mortality was a problem took root and a national policy response was formulated. In this case, the network of researchers and advocates took advantage of, and benefited from, a context they could not have created.

Decision makers often criticize researchers for taking too long when they are facing pressure to act. Sometimes, researchers have an influence because their findings happen to appear at just the right time in a policy development process, but it is difficult to predict this and build it into the plan of a research project. There may be a trade-off between the timeliness and the quality of research which is particularly apparent to the researchers. However, high quality is no guarantee that policy makers will take notice of research and vice versa when it suits them. The first reasonably rigorous estimate of the number of deaths associated with the 2003 invasion of Iraq by the US, the UK and their allies published in The Lancet (Roberts et al. 2004) was treated sceptically by government on both sides of the Atlantic principally because its central estimate differed so much from previous much lower estimates of casualties, despite its superior methods.

Communication and reputation

The above study of deaths in Iraq shows clearly that the ease with which a piece of research can be communicated has a bearing on its use for policy purposes. The more complex, opaque and indeterminate the results and presentation of findings, the less likely, all other things being equal, they are to be taken notice of and accepted. Yet, no matter how well research is communicated, if it proposes radical structural change to institutions and society, it is much more likely to be ignored. The perceived quality of the research, together with the reputation of the journal, the researchers and the institution where they are based also affect the attention that research will receive from policy makers.

The political and media reaction to the Iraq mortality study demonstrated all of these considerations. The fact that the researchers appropriately presented their results as a range of estimates with differing probabilities of being correct confused some and enabled others conveniently to portray the estimates as 'soft' compared with the previous estimates. Yet, the researchers were highly reputed scientists from the prestigious Johns Hopkins School of Public Health in the US, among other institutions, so their findings were difficult to ignore. Finally, the timing of the publication played its part in how the research was received. The paper appeared just before the US Presidential elections of 2004 in which the Iraq War was a central issue between the Democratic challenger and the Republican incumbent. *The Lancet* and the researchers were criticized by Republicans for fast-tracking the research to publication for political reasons. They judged that the sooner their much higher estimate was in the public domain, the better this would be for informed decisions about the future prosecution of the war.

Activity 9.4

List the main obstacles or barriers to research being accepted and used by policy makers discussed above.

Feedback

The main obstacles identified, particularly in low and middle income countries (Trostle et al. 1999; Court et al. 2005; Hyder et al. 2011) include:

- technical research reports written for other researchers, not for policy makers that are difficult to understand, and lack effective summaries and analysis of policy implications;
- lack of research on important policy issues or research which is not perceived as relevant to the country (e.g. undertaken on behalf of donors not national governments) or decision context (e.g. does not offer any solutions to a problem);
- limited access to research findings in policy agencies (e.g. lack of information services);
- lack of funds to pay for relevant research;
- political context, including the extent of civil and political freedom, political conflict, the role of vested interests and autonomy of policy officials;
- low priority in policy agencies to the use of research versus experience, political imperatives, etc.;
- lack of communication channels between researchers and policy makers;

- politically and ideologically controversial policy issues in which values come into conflict with the evidence which may then be used selectively;
- findings that would require a major change in policy, organizations or professional practice;
- low credibility of the researchers or the research (e.g. from outside the country or from institutes without a strong reputation or risk of bias from source of funding);
- poor quality research;
- high level of uncertainty associated with the research findings, and/or difficulties and differences in the interpretation of findings;
- decisions that need to be taken before research can be completed so that research lacks timeliness.

Activity 9.5

For each of the potential obstacles to research being accepted and used by policy makers, identify one or two possible ways of overcoming each of them.

Feedback

Many of the enabling or facilitating factors are the converse of the obstacles. The following are widely regarded as helpful for getting research used for policy (Innvaer et al. 2002; Lavis et al. 2005):

- timely, context-specific evidence that includes aspects relevant to decision making such as cost (not just effectiveness), acceptability to users and feasibility of implementation;
- systems for assuring the quality and integrity of research, including international support to local researchers;
- non-technical summaries of research that are widely accessible at low or no cost and written differently for different policy audiences;
- policy staff and intermediaries such as journalists who understand the principles and methods of research, and are open to discussing the implications of research for policy change;
- getting research into the hands of influential third parties such as policy advocates, respected experts, NGOs, etc.;
- development of formal and informal channels of communication and fora for interaction between researchers and policy makers to share knowledge and build trust (e.g. policy dialogues in which senior government officials, opposition parties, NGO representatives, academics and others are briefed and then meet to discuss policy options);
- attention to the design of policy organizations so that they have systems and staff incentives that encourage learning from a wide range of external sources including research and researchers;
- international policies and processes (e.g. of donors) that increase the demand for evaluation of programmes;
- approaches to doing research such as rapid appraisal, designed to match the pace of policy decision making.

Improving the relationship between research and policy

Since the mid-1990s in the health field, there has been an explosion of interest in using the insights from the different models of the research–policy relationship discussed above, especially the idea of the 'two communities', to try to reduce the barriers to the use of research in policy making and health system management in line with the goal of 'evidence-based' or 'evidence-informed' policy. In the early stages of this movement, the emphasis was simply on improving the flow of information to policy makers through better *dissemination* of research findings (e.g. researchers were encouraged to produce user-friendly summaries of their research findings and to try to draw out the policy and practical implications of their work). This emphasis was consistent with improving the functioning of the engineering model of research and policy. The focus then shifted to more active strategies of '*knowledge transfer*' (Denis and Lomas 2003) which began to focus attention on how the relationships between researchers and policy makers affect the extent to which the contribution of research is taken into account in the policy process and how these relationships can be modified.

Practical steps inspired by the 'two communities' perspective to reduce the 'gap' between research and policy

Table 9.3 summarizes the practical steps which researchers and, importantly, policy makers, have been encouraged to take in order to improve dissemination and diffusion of research into policy and practice. In some cases, researchers and policy makers have a similar responsibility, such as in improving the quality of media reporting of research. In other cases, the onus lies on one group or the other.

It is increasingly the norm that funders of research require researchers to demonstrate how they plan to ensure that their findings are disseminated widely to appropriate audiences. Sometimes funders, especially of larger programmes, go further and require researchers to demonstrate how they will try to ensure that their research has actual impact on policy or practice (e.g. the UK Department for International Development consortia).

Table 9.3 Practical steps advocated to reduce the 'gap' between research and policy

Steps to be taken by researchers	Steps to be taken by policy makers
Provide a range of different types of research reports including newsletters, executive summaries, short policy papers, etc. all written in an accessible, jargon-free style and easily available	Set up formal communication channels and advisory mechanisms involving researchers and policy makers working jointly to identify researchable questions, develop research designs, and plan dissemination and use of findings
Stage conferences, seminars, briefings and practical workshops to disseminate research findings and educate policy makers about research	Ensure that officials are able critically to appraise evidence, are familiar with the evidence in their area and are encouraged to use evidence in developing their policy advice. More strongly, require that major policy proposals demonstrate a basis in evidence

(Continued overleaf)

Table 9.3 Continued.

Steps to be taken by researchers	Steps to be taken by policy makers
Produce interim reports to ensure that findings are timely	Be willing to fund researchers not just to produce research but also to take part in 'knowledge transfer' activities
Include specific policy implications in research reports	Ensure that all major policies and programmes have evaluations built into their budgets and implementation plans
Identify opinion leaders and innovators, and ensure that they understand the implications of research findings	Identify opinion leaders and innovators, and ensure that they understand the implications of research findings
Undertake systematic reviews of research findings on policy-relevant questions to enable policy makers to access information more easily	Publish the findings of all public programme evaluations and view evaluation as an opportunity for policy learning rather than a threat
Keep in close contact with potential policy makers throughout the research process	Commission research and evaluation and consider having additional in-house research capacity
Design studies to maximize their policy relevance and utility (e.g. ensure that trials are of interventions feasible in a wide range of settings)	Establish 'clearing houses' to help summarize, package and disseminate evidence or agencies designed to increase the demand for, and use of, evidence. (e.g. the National Institute for Health and Clinical Excellence in England and Wales systematically synthesizes the available evidence on 'best practice' and determines its clinical and management implications. It then advises patients, health professionals and the NHS on which treatments, drugs and other interventions should be provided)
Use a range of research methods, including 'action-research' (i.e. participative, practically-oriented, non-exploitative research which directly involves the subjects of research at all stages with a view to producing new knowledge that empowers people to improve their situation) and other innovative methods	Provide more opportunities for the public and civil society organizations to learn about research and to participate more actively in research and policy processes
Research topics that are important and relevant for future policy development and give career recognition to researchers whose work is focused on practical application	Encourage the mass media to improve the quality of reporting and interpretation of research findings and their policy implications through devoting more time and effort to media briefing

'Linkage and exchange' model of health research transfer

The steps outlined in Table 9.3 tend to emphasize better communication and translation of research findings, but offer little by way of a response to the political and ideological barriers discussed earlier. Perhaps the most sophisticated practical approach to
improving research utilization is the 'linkage and exchange' approach developed by

Lomas (2000b) through the Canadian Health Services Research Foundation (CHSRF). This approach recognizes the interactive nature of policy development. It focuses on mutual exchange and the joint creation of knowledge between policy makers and researchers. Using a variety of 'cross-boundary' techniques, researchers and policy makers are encouraged to work together to plan and develop research projects. They remain in direct contact throughout the life of projects. The objectives are to grow the research literacy of decision makers, enhance the relevance and utility of the research undertaken, increase the policy and managerial awareness and experience of researchers, and increase the likelihood that the knowledge from research will be successfully transferred and translated into appropriate action. The CHSRF sees a crucial new role for various forms of 'knowledge broker' whose activities span the boundaries of different organizations in the worlds of research, and policy and management.

An extension of the 'linkage and exchange' approach to the problem of knowledge transfer and evidence-based policy making, advocates the 'co-production' of research knowledge. In this researchers and official policy makers work together to undertake research and develop policy, not just to plan studies, thereby transcending the distinction between the 'two communities'. A number of techniques have been devised to support 'co-production' such as locating researchers in policy agencies, and using exchange and secondment arrangements in which staff spend time in each other's environments working together, thereby, it is hoped, increasing mutual understanding and the ability to collaborate in future.

Activity 9.6

What are the pros and cons of 'co-production' of research knowledge for policy?

Feedback

On the positive side, 'co-production' should increase the relevance, comprehensibility and likelihood of use of a piece of research. It should bring new approaches into the policy process from outside government. On the negative side, there is a risk that challenging research questions are not asked and researchers become increasingly 'captured' by policy makers, thereby losing their independence. There is a risk that the researchers not only lose credibility with other researchers and interests, but they gradually lose value for policy makers because they cease to offer distinctive insights from their vantage point outside the machinery of government.

Much will depend on the power relations between, say, a ministry of health and a university or think tank, and the nature of any agreement reached between the two to support 'co-production' of knowledge for policy application. The ideal is probably a continuously adjusted balance between closeness to decision making and independence of view on the part of the researchers (Bennett et al. 2011).

Although a large part of the CHSRF approach is informed directly by the 'two communities' idea, it does recognize that policy makers are *not* homogeneous. The approach encourages researchers to identify the different target groups among decision makers for their work and to use appropriate strategies for each. The 'linkage and exchange' approach has been tested in a series of experiments with some encouraging results (Denis and Lomas 2003).

There have been many similar attempts to develop models of the knowledge transfer process. A systematic review (Ward et al. 2009) identified five common components of these models:

1   *problem identification and communication* – e.g. problems are identified through a system of communication and interaction between decision makers and researchers;
2   *knowledge/research development and selection* – the process of producing the knowledge and the characteristics of the knowledge itself (e.g. its compatibility with previous beliefs, complexity and relative advantage it bestows);
3   *analysis of context* – e.g. organizational, individual, environmental or structural factors which determine the context of transferring knowledge into action including the political context;
4   *knowledge transfer activities or interventions* – typically two main types of activities or interventions: distribution-type interventions which involve targeted dissemination, marketing and the use of local 'champions' or advocates; and linkage-type interventions which involve interaction, dialogue and the use of intermediaries (e.g. 'policy entrepreneurs');
5   *knowledge/research utilization* – different types of use such as conceptual use, direct use, political use or procedural use, or the various actions associated with knowledge utilization.

From this, Ward et al. developed a conceptual framework of the main elements and processes in the knowledge transfer process (see Figure 9.1).

There is no indication in the framework of the relative importance of the five components or their applicability to specific cases. The authors argue that knowledge transfer is not a linear process, but rather an interactive and multi-directional one.

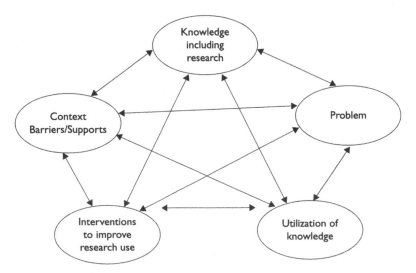

Figure 9.1 Conceptual model of the knowledge transfer process

Source: Ward et al. (2009)

However, as Gibson (2003) points out, the 'knowledge transfer' approach still tends to see the problem of knowledge transfer and evidence-based policy making as relating to the *separation* between the two worlds of research and policy making, hence the interest in notions of brokerage and knowledge transfer as ways of making links. This fails adequately to take into account the degree of conflict *among* both researchers and policy makers, and the *alliances* between sub-groups of both researchers and policy makers that can arise on specific issues in particular political contexts. For example, most academic disciplines are notable for controversies and disputes between rival groups of researchers and theorists. This is even more so in fields of enquiry occupied by different disciplines, each of which brings a range of perspectives to bear on each substantive topic. To the contrary, the 'knowledge transfer' approach still shies away from explicitly recognizing the inherently political nature of the policy process that has been demonstrated in the preceding chapters of this book.

Beyond the 'two communities': are policy communities, issue networks and advocacy coalitions a better representation of reality?

Rather than seeing resistance to research as lying in the relationship (or lack of it) between the research world and the policy world, perspectives on the policy process from a political science perspective locate the barriers and facilitators to the uptake of research for policy as lying in the relationships, conflicts and bargaining that take place in particular political contexts between groups which involve both researchers and others more closely involved with the policy process.

Policy networks and policy communities

Conceiving of the policy process more in terms of *issue networks* and *policy communities* (see Chapter 6), focuses attention on the pattern of formal and informal relationships that shape policy agenda setting, formulation, decisions, implementation and evaluation in an area of policy. Research and researchers can be involved in each of these activities. Marsh and Rhodes (1992) identify a continuum between fields of policy which are characterized by policy communities which have stable and restricted memberships and those which feature issue networks that are much looser, less stable and less exclusive sets of interests. Where a particular policy area sits on the continuum between tight and loose groups shapes the way in which policy is made in that area and the way in which research evidence is considered. The looser the relationships within the group, the more divergent are the views represented and the wider the range of different types of research that are likely to be used by those advocating different policy directions (Nutley and Webb 2000). Tighter, more consensual groupings are better placed to take advantage of 'policy windows' to get research-based responses to problems onto the government's agenda (see above). The key point is that the differences of view between groups are not based on the distinction between whether people are researchers or policy makers. This insight is taken further in the Advocacy Coalition Framework.

The Advocacy Coalition Framework

As you learnt in Chapter 7, the *Advocacy Coalition Framework* sees each area of public policy as occupied by a number of reasonably distinct networked groups of actors interacting with varying degrees of intensity over time (Sabatier and Jenkins-Smith 1993). Rather than seeing researchers pitted against bureaucrats or politicians, *advocacy coalitions* are seen as comprising a diverse range of actors including politicians, civil servants, pressure groups, journalists, academics, think tanks and others united by their beliefs and ideas for change. Each advocacy coalition thus interprets and uses research to advance its policy goals in different ways.

Implications of these theories for ways of enhancing the impact of research on policy

Gibson (2003) concludes that theories of the policy process that abandon the 'two communities' perspective are perhaps a more accurate picture of reality, particularly in controversial areas of policy and have a number of implications for those who wish to increase the impact of research on policy:

1 Researchers who wish to influence policy must analyse the policy area politically to identify the advocacy coalitions and their core values and beliefs about the nature of the policy problem, its causes and potential solutions.
2 Researchers must be engaged directly with advocacy coalitions if they wish to have influence rather than focusing exclusively on managing the boundary between research and policy activities.
3 Research evidence owes its influence in the policy process to its ability to be turned into arguments and advocacy rather than its ability to reveal an uncontested 'truth'.
4 A strategy to enhance the role of research in policy is as much about influencing values and beliefs, and producing good arguments, as it is about improving the knowledge base and its transmission.

Summary

You have learnt how researchers and research are only one among a wide variety of influences on policy processes. Yet, there is no doubt that the policy making process is influenced by research and other sources of evidence: research can help define a phe-nomenon as a policy problem potentially worthy of attention and research provides 'enlightenment', with many ideas from research affecting policy makers indirectly and over long periods of time. This is facilitated by the links between policy makers and researchers, the role of the media, timing and how the research is communicated. There are also many impediments to research being acted upon, including political and ideo-logical factors, policy uncertainty, uncertainty about scientific findings, the perceived utility of research and how easy it is to communicate. There is considerable enthusiasm at present for using a variety of brokerage and knowledge exchange mechanisms to improve the productivity of the relationship between researchers and policy makers.

The idea that researchers and policy makers comprise two culturally distinct 'com-munities' is potentially misleading though it can be useful for identifying some practical actions to improve communication and interaction. Neither group is homogeneous, politically. Sub-sets of researchers and policy makers can be found together participat-ing in competing 'advocacy coalitions' or looser groupings around issues. This perspec-tive suggests that research enters policy as much through influencing political argument as through the transmission of knowledge. This indicates that recent efforts to use techniques of 'linkage' and 'exchange' to bridge the supposed 'gap' between research (and wider evidence) and policy are unlikely to succeed as much as their proponents would like. Such efforts have to accommodate the fact that policy making, even at its best, is the messy product of 'the interplay between institutions, interests and ideas' (John 1998).

References

Bennett S, Corluka A, Doherty J, Tangcharoensathien V, Patcharanarumol W, Jesani A, Kyabaggu J, Namaganda G, Hussain AMZ and de-Graft Aikins A (2011) Influencing policy change: the experience of health think tanks in low- and middle-income countries. *Health Policy and Planning*, advance access published 10 May 2011 doi: 10.1093/heapol/czr035.

Black N (2001) Evidence based policy: proceed with care. *BMJ* 323: 275–8.

Court J, Hovland I and Young J (2005) *Bridging Research and Policy in Development*. London: ODI.

Daniels K, Lewin S and the Practice Policy Group (2008) Translating research into maternal health care policy: a qualitative case study of the use of evidence in policies for the treatment of eclampsia and pre-eclampsia in South Africa. *Health Research Policy and Systems* 6: 12 doi:10.1186/1478-4505-6-12. Available at: http://www.health-policy systems.com/content/6/1/12.

Davies PT (1999) What is evidence-based education? *British Journal of Educational Studies* 47: 108–21.

Denis JL and Lomas J (eds) (2003) Researcher: decision-maker partnerships. *Journal of Health Services Research & Policy* 8 (suppl 2).

Gibson B (2003) Beyond 'two communities'. In Lin V and Gibson B (eds) *Evidence-Based Health Policy: Problems and Possibilities*. Melbourne: Oxford University Press, pp. 18–32.

Global Forum for Health Research (2004a) *Monitoring Financial Flows for Health Research*. Geneva: Global Forum for Health Research. Available at: www.globalforumhealth.org/ accessed 08/11/2004.

Global Forum for Health Research (2004b) *The 10/90 Report on Health Research 2003–2004*. Geneva: Global Forum for Health Research. Available at: www.globalforumhealth.org/ accessed 08/11/2004.

Harrison S (2001) Implementing the results of research and development in clinical and managerial practice. In Baker MR and Kirk S (eds) *Research and Development for the NHS: Evidence, Evaluation and Effectiveness*. Abingdon: Radcliffe Medical Press.

Hyder AA, Corluka A, Winch PJ, El-Shinnawy, Ghassany H, Malekafzali H, Lim M-K, Mfutso-Bengo J, Segura E and Ghaffar A (2011) National policy-makers speak out: are researchers giving them what they need? *Health Policy and Planning* 26: 73–82.

Innvaer S, Vist G, Trommald M and Oxman A (2002) Health policy makers' perceptions of their use of evidence: a systematic review. *Journal of Health Services Research & Policy* 7: 239–44.

John P (1998) *Analysing Public Policy*. London: Cassell.

Lavis J, Davies H, Oxman A, Denis J-L, Golden-Biddle K and Ferlie E (2005) Towards systematic reviews that inform health care management and policy-making. *Journal of Health Services Research & Policy* 10: 35–48.

Lomas J (2000a) Connecting research and policy. *Isuma: Canadian Journal of Policy Research* 1: 140–4.

Lomas J (2000b) Using linkage and exchange to move research into policy at a Canadian Foundation. *Health Affairs* 19: 236–40.

Marsh D and Rhodes RAW (1992) Policy communities and issue networks: beyond typology. In Marsh D and Rhodes RAW (eds) *Policy Networks in British Government*. Oxford: Oxford University Press.

Nutley S and Webb J (2000) Evidence and the policy process. In Davies HTO, Nutley SM and Smith PC (eds) *What Works? Evidence-Based Policy and Practice in Public Services*. Bristol: The Policy Press, pp. 13–41.

Parkhurst J (2002) The Ugandan success story? Evidence and claims of HIV-1 prevention. *Lancet* 360: 78–80.

Petersen M (2002) Madison Ave. plays growing role in drug research. *New York Times* Online www.nyt.com.

Rampton S and Stauber J (2001) *Trust Us, We're Experts: How Industry Manipulates Science and Gambles with Your Future*. New York: Putnam.

Roberts L, Lafta R, Garfield R, Khudhairi J and Burnham G (2004) Mortality before and after the 2003 invasion of Iraq: cluster sample survey. *Lancet*. Published online October 29, 2004. Available at: http://image.thelancet.com/extras/04art10342web.pdf.

Rossi P and Wright S (1979) Evaluation research: an assessment of theory, practice and politics. In Pollitt C, Lewis L, Negro J and Pattern J (eds) *Public Policy in Theory and Practice*. London: Hodder and Stoughton.

Sabatier PA and Jenkins-Smith HC (eds) (1993) *Policy Change and Learning: An Advocacy Coalition Approach*. Boulder, CO: Westview Press.

Schneider H (2002) On the fault line: the politics of AIDS policy in contemporary South Africa. *African Studies* 61: 145–67.

Short S (1997) Elective affinities: research and health policy development. In Gardner H (ed.) *Health Policy in Australia*. Melbourne: Oxford University Press.

Trostle J, Bronfman M and Langer A (1999) How do researchers influence decision makers? Case studies of Mexican policies. *Health Policy and Planning* 14(2): 103–14.

Ward V, House H and Hamer S (2009) Knowledge brokering: the missing link in the evidence to action chain? *Evidence & Policy* 5(3): 267–79.

Weiss CH (1979) The many meanings of research utilization. *Public Administration Review* 39: 426–31.

Weiss CH (1991) Policy research: data, ideas or arguments? In Wagner P, Hirschon Weiss C, Wittrock B and Wollman H (eds) *Social Sciences and Modern States*. Cambridge: Cambridge University Press.

Doing policy analysis 10

Overview

In this chapter you will be introduced to a political science-based approach to policy analysis and a range of tools for gathering, organizing and analysing health policy data. The chapter aims to assist you to analyse policy processes and to develop better political strategies to bring about health policy change in your professional life.

Learning objectives

After working through this chapter you will be better able to:

- gather and present data for policy analysis
- undertake retrospective and prospective policy analysis
- identify policy actors, and assess their political resources and current positions on a given policy
- develop successful political strategies to manage policy change.

Key terms

Analysis. Separation of a problem into its constituent parts so as to better understand it as a whole.

Crowdsourcing. Canvassing suggestions from the general public via Twitter or other social media to help decide a course of action.

Social media. Web-based and mobile technologies which enable virtual dialogue through the creation and exchange of user-generated rather than professional content.

Social network analysis. Methods used for mapping, measuring and analysing the social relationships between people, groups and organizations.

Stakeholder. An individual or group with a substantive interest in an issue, including those with some role in making a decision or its execution. Used synonymously with actor and interest group.

Stakeholder analysis. Process through which those making policy or affected by it are identified and their likely position and levels of interest and influence are assessed.

Introduction

By now you will appreciate that policy change is political, dynamic and highly complex. Policy change in the health sector is challenging because health systems are technically complex, and changing one part of the system invariably affects other parts and many different actors. Experience with health sector reform suggests that the costs of reform often fall on powerful and well-organized groups (e.g. doctors and drug companies) while the benefits are often intended for widely dispersed and disadvantaged populations with little political clout (e.g., pregnant women). Achieving successful policy reform is, therefore, often difficult.

After reiterating the way that policy analysis can be used, this chapter introduces you to tools that are employed in policy analysis, primarily to improve the prospects of successful policy change. These tools permit you to gather, use and apply knowledge in systematic ways. You will be introduced first to stakeholder analysis. Identifying actors is at the centre of the 'policy triangle' and therefore considerable emphasis is placed on this method. The chapter then presents an approach to developing political strategies and guidance for gathering evidence for analysis, as well as some suggestions for using the 'policy triangle' to present the results of the analysis. The chapter concludes with some thoughts on the ethics of policy analysis. The chapter does not deal with rational-comprehensive approaches to policy analysis, such as applied economic techniques (e.g. cost-benefit analysis), because they do not incorporate any analysis of the politics of decision making. These are well covered elsewhere (Weimer and Vining 2010).

Retrospective and prospective policy analysis

In Chapter 1 you learned that there are two types of policy analysis; these were characterized as analysis *of* policy and analysis *for* policy. Analysis of policy tends to be retrospective, descriptive and explanatory. Analysis of policy looks back at why or how a policy made its way onto the agenda, its content, and whether or not and why it achieved its goals (e.g. a summative evaluation). For example, disappointing results with health sector reform in some countries have prompted the World Bank to undertake analysis of past reform processes to diagnose the political dimensions of the problem. Analysis *of* policy comprises the bulk of this book.

Analysis *for* policy tends to be prospective. It is usually carried out to inform the formulation of a policy (e.g. a formative evaluation) or anticipate how a policy might fare if introduced (e.g. how other actors might respond to the proposed changes). Typically, analysis for policy will be undertaken, or sponsored, by interested parties to assess the prospects and manage the politics of policy change in a way that meets their goals. At times, such analysis will result in the decision to abandon a particular course of action due to its poor political feasibility.

It is likely that you will want to use what you have learned from this book to undertake analysis for policy – to increase the chances that evidence from your research is used to influence policy or more generally that your advocacy plans are brought to fruition. Having read the preceding chapters, you will appreciate that an astute policy reformer will engage in prospective analysis at all stages of the policy cycle – from problem identification, through agenda setting, formulation, implementation and evaluation – as each of these stages are subject to the flow of political events. Hence, successful policy change depends on continuous and systematic political analysis (Roberts et al. 2004).

Analysis in the early stages of policy making, particularly in problem definition and agenda setting, is particularly important. It was argued in Chapter 4 that epidemiological or economic facts do not simply speak for themselves in setting priorities, but will be used or not depending on political processes. The role of the media in agenda setting was highlighted as critical to raising and framing problems in public debates and in policy circles. Similarly, policy 'entrepreneurs' actively promote particular problems and solutions and look out for 'windows of opportunity' to get issues onto the agenda and ensure the formulation of a policy response that suits their interests or ideas (Kingdon 1995).

If you want to successfully influence policy outcomes, you will need to:

- engage in framing problems;
- understand how agendas are set;
- learn to recognize political windows of opportunity;
- understand how to manipulate political processes to encourage wider acceptance of your definition of a problem and proposed solution;
- understand the positions, interests and power of other interested parties (including the media) based on the potential distribution of costs and benefits of the proposed policy;
- adapt your solutions to make them more politically feasible.

Undertaking these tasks constitutes analysis *for* policy, and will provide the basis for developing politically informed strategies to influence or even manage policy change. While such analyses may enhance your success in influencing policy outcomes, they cannot guarantee such outcomes – for success depends on many factors beyond your control – including serendipity.

Stakeholder analysis

Irrespective of whether or not analysis is retrospective or prospective, it will be based on an analysis of relevant stakeholders. Stakeholders include those individuals and groups with an interest in an issue or policy, those who might be affected by a policy and those who may play a role in relation to making or implementing the policy – in other words, actors in the policy process. Although a variety of approaches to *stakeholder analysis* have been described (Varvasovszky and Brugha 2000), three distinct activities recur (Roberts et al. 2004). These are: (1) identifying the policy actors; (2) assessing their political resources; and (3) understanding their position and interests with respect to the issue.

Identifying stakeholders

A number of chapters in this book have focused on the range of stakeholders in health policy – from those inside government to the spectrum of interest groups in civil society and the private sector. Stakeholders will be specific to the particular policy and the context within which it is being discussed. Identifying stakeholders who are, or might become, involved in a particular policy process, requires judgement. For example, it may be necessary to identify groups within organizations which may have different interests (e.g. the ministry of health would rarely be treated as one actor as there are likely to be different groups and programmes within any ministry pursuing differing interests). The idea is to discover independent actors who wield considerable influence while keeping the number sufficiently small to make the analysis manageable (for a greater number of actors, a social network analysis approach is more useful – see below). Identifying an initial set of stakeholders can be conducted through a brainstorming session with knowledgeable informants.

To compile a list of stakeholders, you will need to think about the likely implications of the content of the proposed policy – in particular how it will affect different actors or groups. Relevant actors will include those who are likely to be affected by the policy either positively or negatively and those who might take action or could be mobilized to do so. Particular importance needs to be devoted to individuals or organizations which can either block policy adoption (often leaders of political parties, heads of agencies, etc.) or implementation (often bureaucrats, service providers and users, but other groups as well depending on the policy).

Activity 10.1

Choose a health policy with which you are familiar. Using the above guidelines identify 15–20 individuals or groups who have an interest in the issue or a role to play in adopting or implementing the policy.

Feedback

Health sector reform often involves the following types of groups, some of which you may have identified as having a stake in the issue you are analysing (Reich 1996): consumer organizations (e.g. patient groups); producer groups (e.g. nurses, doctors, pharmaceutical companies); economic groups (e.g. workers who may be affected, industries, companies with health insurance schemes); and ideological groups (e.g. single issue campaign organizations, political parties, researchers).

Assessing power

The second step in a stakeholder analysis consists of assessing the power of each actor. You learned in Chapters 2 and 6 that political resources take many forms but can be divided into tangible (e.g. votes, finance, infrastructure, members) and intangible assets (expertise and legitimacy in relation to the policy issue, access to the mass media, networks and political decision makers). Access to these resources increases stakeholders' influence in the policy process. For example, groups with a developed organization and infrastructure will often have more power than groups which have yet to organize themselves. Doctors, for example, often have health policy-relevant expertise and are, therefore, often viewed as legitimate; they are often organized into long-standing professional organizations, and, because they usually have high social status, frequently have access to financial resources and relationships with decision makers. As a result of these political resources, doctors are usually characterized as a group with considerable political power on most health policy issues. Pharmaceutical companies have great expertise and considerable finance, but often limited legitimacy – at least in so far as civil society and activist groups are concerned. The type of strategy any group will employ in wielding its power will depend on the nature of the political resources at its disposal. The context will often determine the precise value of any particular resource. To take an extreme example, where corruption is rife, finance becomes a very useful political resource to influence or buy policy decisions.

Activity 10.2

Select ten of the stakeholders you identified in Activity 10.1. For each, make an inventory of the major resources at their disposal. Differentiate between tangible and intangible resources. Given these political assets, characterize each of your stakeholders as having high, medium or low power in relation to the health policy under consideration.

Feedback

Clearly your inventory will depend on the stakeholders you select. The example of a patient group serves to illustrate one potential stakeholder with medium power:

- tangible resources, e.g. large number of members and electoral votes;
- intangible resources, e.g. passion, first-hand experience, access to media, public sympathy and support, highly legitimate interest.

Assessing interests, position and commitment

Each actor's interests, position and level of commitment to a particular policy issue will determine how they will deploy their political resources. Assessing these attributes constitutes the third and final stage in a stakeholder analysis.

You learned about interest groups in Chapter 6 – here we are concerned not just with so-called cause and sectional interest groups, but the 'interests' of any relevant actor in a particular policy issue. Interests are those things which benefit an individual or group (as distinct from their wants or preferences). Often it is the expected economic effect of a policy on an actor's interests which plays an overriding role in determining his/her position on a policy. Determining what these interests are can be complex. At times, actors may conceal their real interests for tactical purposes, perhaps because they are illegal (e.g. illicit payment for referrals). At other times, interests may be difficult to discern because the policy content may be fuzzy or there may be a number of variants of the policy under discussion. For example, a minister of health may be committed to a policy of contracting out publicly funded service delivery to non-state organizations. Doctors employed in the public sector who practise privately may not be sure whether or not to support such a policy unless they have assurances that they will be eligible to compete for contracts with NGOs or private practitioners and/or have assurances that their employment in the public sector will not be compromised by the new policy. These may be details that the minister may not wish to elaborate upon until s/he undertakes a stakeholder analysis.

Activity 10.3

Select any five of the stakeholders you have identified in Activity 10.2 and list their interests in relation to your chosen policy. Seek to reveal what they would stand to gain or lose from the policy change you are considering.

Feedback

Often the financial or material impacts of policy change constitute central interests to individuals and groups. In the example of a policy to contract out publicly financed services, public sector doctors might perceive their interests at risk if they think that the policy's aim is to reduce their number (i.e. they could lose their jobs) or if they fear that one outcome of such a policy would be to increase the competition that they face in their private practices (i.e. limiting the amount they can earn by practising illegally). Yet other interests might also be perceived to be under threat. For example, the potential loss of a public sector position may not be compensated for by improved employment prospects in the private sector due to the credibility, prestige and symbolic value of a public sector post in many countries – as well as other perks which might include housing, invitations to conferences, further education, etc.

The impact of an issue on stakeholders' interests will determine their position with respect to the proposed policy – whether they are supportive, neutral or opposed. As with identifying interests, positions may not be easily determined as they may be concealed or because publicly aired positions may be different from privately held ones (the latter often determining what a group may actually do). For example, a minister may publicly support a policy so as to win favour with voters or specific interest groups but may be quietly working against the policy within government on the grounds that it is unaffordable. At times, actors may not be certain of their position if they are still not sure how a policy might affect their interests. This may happen if the policy content is vague or if there are a number of policy options being discussed, each with different repercussions on the actor's interests.

Activity 10.4

Identify the likely publicly aired and privately held positions of the five stakeholders you analysed in Activity 10.3.

An example will illustrate the difference in public and private positions a stakeholder might hold. Doctors in a publicly-funded system might complain publicly about a lack of resources and patients having to wait for treatment. However, in private they might resist any attempt by policy makers to appoint extra doctors as this would jeopardize the size of their private practice and income.

In addition to assessing interests and positions, it is necessary to assess the importance of the issue to each stakeholder in terms of other priorities they hold. What you want to find out is the intensity of actors' commitments to the policy and how much of their political resources they are likely to devote to pursuing their interests through the policy. While a powerful actor may be opposed to a particular policy, the issue may be of marginal importance and the stakeholder may do little to block policy adoption or implementation. One can gauge the level of commitment of an actor by asking them, or from assessing how critical the issue is likely to be to the pursuit of the organization's mandate, or from the time that senior organizational figures devote to it, and so on.

It is important to attempt to determine each stakeholder's real interests, position and level of commitment to a proposed policy. This knowledge will play a central part in understanding the likely success of the proposed policy and in designing politically oriented strategies and tactics to bring about policy change.

Activity 10.5

For each of the stakeholders analysed in Activity 10.4, list the interests they hold (what they gain or lose from policy change), their position (opposed, supportive, neutral), and their level of commitment to the policy issue (high, medium, low). Construct a table with the data including position and power (from Activity 10.1) for each of the actors – this is commonly referred to as a position map. As for Activity 10.4, you may need to undertake some research.

Feedback

Each position map will look different depending on the policy content, actors and context. A position map of players in relation to health sector reform in the Dominican Republic in the mid-1990s is presented in Figure 10.1. Although there is bound to be a degree of uncertainty in relation to each of the variables, the position map provides a good starting point for thinking about who might form a coalition in favour of reform and which groups might try to undermine a reform.

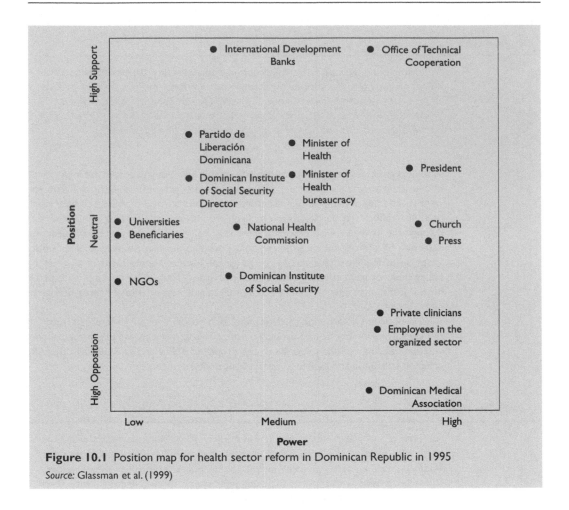

Figure 10.1 Position map for health sector reform in Dominican Republic in 1995

Source: Glassman et al. (1999)

The next step in a more sophisticated stakeholder analysis would aim to model how each actor's commitment and position would shift with a modification to the content of the policy. This issue will be returned to in the section on designing strategies for political reform.

Given the centrality of networks and advocacy coalitions in influencing policy, stakeholder analysis can be extended with a social network analysis. Such analysis maps, measures and analyses quantitatively and visually the social relationships between people, groups and organizations – typically to determine the position of actors within networks as this conditions their access to information and power. In particular, analysts use computer software to analyse network features including 'between-ness', centrality, density, distance and 'reachability' to characterize participants and their relationships in a network. Using a social network analysis approach, Blanchet and James (2011) examined the evolving network engaged in eye care policy implementation in Ghana between 2008 and 2010. They observed a shift in relations and power balance between managers, nurses and doctors and international organizations. Examining distance between actors and the centrality and reachability of actors through social network analysis can help to assess the cohesion of a network as well as the key individuals – the brokers and opinion leaders – and organizations at the centre of networks who can influence change.

Before we move on to thinking about how to use the results of stakeholder analysis to bring about policy change, it is useful to consider some of the limitations inherent in stakeholder analysis. On the one hand, it is obvious that any analysis is only as good as the analyst's attention, creativity, tenacity and access to information on the interests, positions, influence and commitment in relation to a particular policy. On the other hand, stakeholder analysis only provides data on actors and reveals little about the context and process of policy making which, you will appreciate, play equally important roles in policy change.

Developing political strategies for policy change

Roberts et al. (2004) suggest that the political feasibility of policy change is determined by 'position, power, players and perception'. The viability of a proposed policy change can be improved by developing strategies to manage the position of relevant actors, the power or political resources at the disposal of key stakeholders, the number of players actively involved in the policy arena and the perceptions held by stakeholders of the problem and solution. Based on their experience with health sector reform in numerous countries, Roberts and his colleagues provide useful guidance in terms of managing these variables.

Activity 10.6

While reading through the following summary of Roberts et al.'s work, make notes on which strategies you have used in your past efforts to effect policy change and/ or others which you think might be useful in the policy context where you operate.

Case Study 10: position, power, players and perception

Position strategies
Roberts et al. (2004) begin by presenting four types of bargains that can be used to shift the position of actors with respect to a particular policy. Deals can be made with actors who are opposed or neutral so as to make them more supportive or less opposed by altering a particular component of the policy. For example, provider managers may drop their opposition to a proposal to introduce user fees if they are allowed to retain a percentage of the revenue to improve quality or provide perks for their staff. Second, deals can be struck through which support is sought for one issue in return for concessions on another. For example, a medical association may drop its opposition to a ministry of health proposal to train paramedical staff to assume additional medical functions, if the ministry agrees to drop its proposal to curb spending on teaching institutions – which is in the interests of the association's members. Third, promises can be made. If the medical association drops its opposition to the paramedic upgrading programme, the ministry can promise to consider the need to increase the number of specialists in particular areas. In contrast, threats

can also be used to change the positions of actors. In Bangladesh, development agencies threatened to suspend aid if the ministry did not proceed with agreed reforms while ministry staff threatened to strike if the reforms went ahead. A variety of deals can be made and compromises reached to change the position of actors without altering the balance of power in a given arena. These can involve changing the content of policy so that it is more closely aligned to the interests of some of the players.

Power strategies

A range of strategies can be used to affect the distribution of political assets of the players involved to strengthen supportive groups and undermine opposition groups. These involve providing supportive actors with:

• funds, personnel and facilities;
• information to increase expertise;
• access to decision makers and the media;
• links to supportive networks;
• public relations material which highlights supportive actors' expertise, legitimacy, victim status or heroic nature.

Roberts et al. suggest that actions can also be taken to limit the political resources of opponents, for example, by:

• challenging their legitimacy, expertise, integrity or motives, for example, by characterizing them as self-interested and self-serving;
• reducing their access to decision makers;
• refusing to cooperate or share information with them – or withholding information. For example, some governments practise internet bandwidth throttling to disable the use of social networking sites by the opposition during moments of perceived crisis.

Player strategies

Player strategies attempt to impact on the number of actors involved in a policy arena, in particular to mobilize those that are neutral and to demobilize those groups who are opposed. Recruiting unmobilized actors can be achieved at times by simply informing a group that an item is on the agenda and what their stake in the issue is likely to be. For example, an association of private providers may not be aware that a particular policy is being discussed which may have consequences for its members. Player strategies can, however, be difficult to execute if new organizations need to be formed or if they involve demobilizing a group which has already publicly taken a position on an issue. It may be possible to persuade the group that its stake or impact is different to that which it had previously calculated – but then efforts at face-saving will also have to be made. Alternatively, it may be possible to undermine opponents by dividing them. For example, it may be possible to identify a sub-group within the larger group which might benefit from your proposal and whom you might win to your side. Roberts et al. suggest that another player strategy involves changing the venue of decision making. This was a tactic employed by the donors in Bangladesh when confronted with opposition to reform in the ministry of health – they sought allies in the ministry of finance and the parliament who might support their cause. Player strategies aim to alter the balance of mobilized players by introducing sympathetic ones and sidelining opposing ones.

Perception strategies

Throughout this book the force of ideas and the role that the perceptions of a problem and its solution have on the position and power of important stakeholders have been highlighted. A variety of techniques are used to alter perceptions. Data and arguments can, for example, be questioned as can the relative importance of a problem or the practicality of a policy solution. The appropriateness of public or private action can be attacked using economic theory or philosophy to shift players' perceptions on an issue. Associations can also be altered to give an issue a greater chance of political and social acceptability. For example, those seeking to eliminate congenital syphilis (i.e. syphilis transmitted from mother to infant) may highlight that this is a condition 'inflicted' upon 'innocent' infants, and may not stress the fact that the infection in the mother is sexually transmitted since sexually transmitted infections historically are both low on policy agendas and attract moral opprobrium. Appealing to prevailing values can also work. Advocates for congenital syphilis, for example, stress the principles of fairness and equity – arguing that the elimination of congenital syphilis deserves the same attention as the elimination of mother-to-child transmission of HIV – an issue that has received much public and policy concern. Invoking symbols can also change perceptions of issues. Thus, reforms can be linked to nationalist sentiments, imperatives or celebrities. Employing celebrities to endorse new reforms and initiatives is becoming common as is the branding of public health interventions. The latter places great emphasis on simple messages and the feasibility of a particular course of action so as to appeal to policy makers and the public. Carla Bruni, France's First Lady, for example, launched the 'Born HIV-Free' campaign in 2010 to close the implementation gap between women receiving or not receiving anti-retrovirals (ARVs) during labour (so that their babies would be born HIV-free). Within days, a petition with over 700,000 signatures had been presented to UN Secretary-General Ban Ki-moon urging him to take action.

Feedback

You have now reviewed the range of tools which Roberts et al. have identified as useful in influencing the position, power, players and perceptions associated with policy change. Some strategies are open to most players, for example, sharing or refusing to share information, changing the perception of an issue, or mobilizing groups. Some strategies may, however, only be available to certain groups. For example, the tactics to increase the political resources of supportive actors require that you have access to resources to distribute to them. Similarly, many strategies which aim to change the position of actors require access to decision making over other issues that can be traded. Even changing the perception of an issue requires communication skill as well as access to the media. Some degree of power is usually necessary to deliver credible threats.

Software programmes are now available (free of charge) to support both stakeholder analysis and policy influencing strategies, such as Policy Maker (http://polimap.books. officelive.com/politour.aspx).

Data for policy analysis

It will come as no surprise to you that the quality of your policy analysis will depend on the accuracy, comprehensiveness and relevance of the information that you are able to collect. These, in turn, depend on the time and resources available to you, your official mandate, as well as your contacts in the relevant policy domain. The steps describing a stakeholder analysis, above, can be conducted through brainstorming sessions to elicit differing perspectives – but it is also useful for analysts to work independently as well before comparing their responses. Evidence for policy analysis usually emanates from documents and people – and increasingly from resources available through the Internet, though these need to be interpreted with care.

Policy documents

Policy-relevant documents are those which provide clues as to the likely stakeholders in any policy process as well as their interests, positions and commitment to the policy in question. Much can be learned about policy actors, process, context and content from academic books and journals (such as the *Journal of Health Politics, Policy and Law, Social Science and Medicine, Health Affairs, Health Policy, Journal of Health Services Research and Policy, Health Policy and Planning, Journal of Public Health Policy, Bulletin of the World Health Organization, Global Public Health, Global Health Governance*). Reports and evaluations produced by interest groups or independent evaluators, think tanks and consultants, government and inter-governmental organizations (e.g. the WHO), can also be useful. Press releases and editorials in the mass media provide additional material.

A literature search would likely start with a topic search on your health problem or policy using a combination of bibliographic services such as the *Social Science Citation Index*, the US National Library of Medicine's MEDLINE (www.nlm.nih.gov) or Google Scholar. There is likely to be a wealth of information about most policies and many policy contexts available on the Internet which may be searched with web-based search engines. Yet in contrast to journals, the information on the Internet is neither necessarily subject to peer review nor is it always obvious which group or individual has published the material (which may have a bearing on its credibility).

Unpublished reports, email messages, minutes of meetings, memoranda and other 'internal' documents can be particularly useful in revealing the true interests and positions of actors – but are generally difficult to access, though some countries have freedom of information legislation allowing citizens to request documents produced by public bodies that can be used by researchers. Internal tobacco industry documents, made public as a result of litigation against companies in the US in 1998, provided a rare and rich account of the industry's aims, interests and activities related to a number of health policies and organizations (e.g. undermining the Framework Convention on Tobacco Control and exerting influence over WHO). Figure 10.2 is a copy of one such internal document which reveals the mechanisms through which Philip Morris sought to influence the policy decisions of legislators in the US.

Depending on the issue, you may also wish to consult statistical data sources, for example, to verify the magnitude of a problem so as to assist in framing a problem or undermining an opponent's argument. International organizations, such as the WHO and the World Bank, provide policy relevant data as do most governments and sub-national agencies of government (much of which is available on their websites).

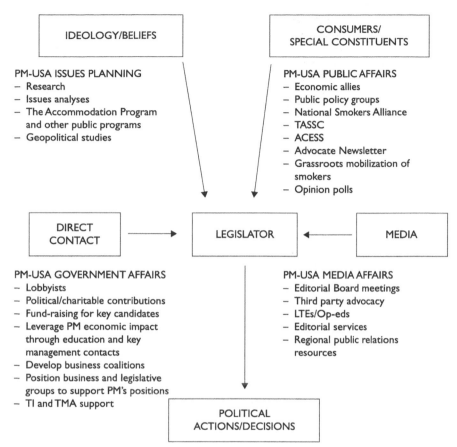

Figure 10.2 Tools to affect legislative decisions

Note: Since this is an internal industry document, not all the acronyms are explained. The following seem likely: PM, Philip Morris; TMA, Tobacco Manufacturing Association; LTE, letter to editor; TASSC, the Advancement of Sound Science Coalition; TI, Tobacco Industry; ACESS, unknown.

Source: Philip Morris (PM) (no date)

The purpose of documentary analysis is to provide evidence that explains or predicts policy change. Therefore, you are looking for evidence on relevant contextual variables (situational, structural, cultural and exogenous), actors (their power, interests, positions and commitment), content (policy aims and means), and process. Although there are a number of approaches to extracting data from documentary sources, most policy analysts will rely on content analysis, of which there are two types. First, quantitative content analysis is a systematic approach that seeks to quantify the content within documents according to predetermined categories. A policy analyst might, for example, search through a sample of national newspapers to record the number of column inches devoted to different health policy issues, such as AIDS, over a particular time span so as to gauge media and public interest in a policy issue. Here the predetermined category is AIDS. Alternatively, an analyst may go through a broader range of document types to reveal specific stakeholders' positions with respect to a particular policy over a period of time – in which case the policy, the actors and their positions would be the predetermined categories.

In contrast, qualitative content analysis aims to uncover underlying themes and structures of argument used in documentary material. The policy analyst searching through newspapers for coverage of AIDS, for example, may examine the editorials to understand whether there is support for the government's policy on AIDS or to determine whether the press is spreading scientifically inaccurate messages in relation to the disease. Alternatively, an analyst might search documents for evidence of the philosophical arguments used to support or frame a particular policy stance. The themes extracted using qualitative content analysis are often depicted using illustrative quotations from the document.

The utility of documentary analysis rests upon the quality and quantity (i.e. completeness) of the documents used. Bryman (2008) suggests that a number of questions should be posed to assess documentary sources critically, including:

• Who wrote and published the document?
• Why was the document produced?
• Was the author in a position to be authoritative about the subject?
• Is the material authentic?
• What interests did the author have (and did the author declare them)?
• Is the document representative or atypical – and, if so, in what way?
• Is the meaning of the material clear?
• Can the contents be corroborated through other sources?
• Are competing interpretations of the document possible?

Another factor to take into account is whether the document has been edited for public release (known as redaction).

Gathering data from people

Talking to actors and undertaking surveys of key stakeholders can provide rich information for policy analysis. These methods may be the only way to gather valid information on the political interests and resources of relevant actors or to gather historical and contextual information. Large-scale surveys represent a quantitative method for collection of information predominantly by questionnaire or structured interview. Surveys, which can be administered in person or by post, email or the Internet for self-completion, are used by policy analysts to generate basic information in relation to stakeholders' views of a problem or their position in relation to a policy if this information cannot be obtained from documentary sources.

Semi-structured interviews are generally more useful than questionnaire surveys in eliciting information of a more sensitive nature. The goal of the semi-structured interview is to obtain useful and valid data on stakeholders' perceptions of a given policy issue and how it might affect them. Typically, what is called a topic or interview guide will be used to prompt the analyst to cover a given set of issues with each respondent, as opposed to using a predetermined set of questions. The idea is to allow flexibility and fluidity in the interview so that it resembles a conversation in which the respondent feels sufficiently comfortable to provide a detailed account and to tell their story. Hence, questions should be open (i.e. those which do not invite a 'yes' or 'no' response) and should be sequenced in such a way as to deal with more factual and less contentious issues before tackling more difficult areas and at deeper levels of under-standing.

Health policy interviews tend to be undertaken with senior decision makers and representatives of powerful interest groups and are, therefore, of a special nature. These are sometimes called elite interviews. Elite interviews pose particular challenges. First, it is often difficult to recruit respondents into the study as they may be wary of how the results might be used, particularly if they are concerned that the analysis may undermine their own policy aims. Second, elites may not have sufficient time for an interview. Third, policy elites may simply provide official positions which may be more efficiently obtained through policy documents. Often it is more productive to inter-view such officials outside the office (or office hours) which may encourage them to provide 'off the record' comments which are more informative. Fourth, interviewees may be reluctant to be interviewed on the grounds that it will be difficult to maintain their anonymity since, by definition, senior representatives and leaders of organizations are few in number.

Relevant individuals to interview can be initially identified through the literature and document review which should reveal organizations and actors with an interest in the policy issue. These individuals will likely be able to identify further informants who may in turn identify others (called 'snowball' sampling). Interviewing retired staff from inter-ested organizations can yield more forthright and analytical perspectives as these indi-viduals will have had time to reflect and may not fear reprisals – and may also have more time available to allow them to participate in an interview. The most informed informants are likely to be drawn from a sub-group of the stakeholders identified in the stakeholder analysis. It has been suggested that it is best to approach first those indi-viduals with rich sources of information and power, and who are supportive of the proposed policy, while those who may be hostile or may block access to other inter-viewees should be interviewed later in the process.

Thought needs to be given to introducing the purpose of the interview in such a way that is honest and ethical, and yet yields good data. Similarly, it will be necessary to inform the respondent how you will use the information and whether s/he wishes to keep his/her responses anonymous and out of the public domain. The pros and cons of using a tape recorder need to be weighed up but whatever decision is taken, the importance of transcribing the results or writing up notes taken during the interview immediately afterwards cannot be overemphasized. Even if an interview has been taped, it is helpful for the interviewer to write a few notes covering their impressions of the main findings from the interview and its implications for further data collection (e.g. questions that did not seem to elicit revealing responses and which might be cut).

The central limitation of interview data is that they concern what people say and how they say it, as opposed to what people actually do or think. This problem can be overcome by 'triangulating' the responses with responses from other informants, or with data gathered through other means, including observations of meetings or docu-mentary sources. It is harder to negotiate access to meetings and other events than to obtain interviews, unless the meetings are held in public.

Social media as a source for policy analysis

Social media provide a potentially rich source of material for policy analysis. This type of media is evolving very rapidly and takes many different forms, including weblogs, forums, microblogging, wikis, podcasts, etc. Kaplan and Haenlein (2010) have identified six different types of social media: collaborative projects (e.g. Wikipedia and Wikileaks); blogs and microblogs (e.g. Twitter); content communities (e.g. YouTube); social networking sites (e.g. Facebook); virtual game worlds; and virtual social worlds. The technologies employed vary, but the point is that valuable information about stakeholders' positions, interests and commitment may be readily discernible from material they post (e.g., Tweets) or the virtual social networks in which they participate. Indeed online interaction may help identify relevant stakeholders in a policy process and provide clues as to the nature of the networks surrounding a policy issue. The Internet is also useful for testing policy proposals. For example it was central to the development of Iceland's Constitution in 2011. The responsible council posted draft clauses on its website for public comment and invited citizens to join discussion on the council's Facebook page, as well as posting Tweets. This is the first use of social media to canvass public opinion and generate language to develop a national constitution but it is by no means the first use of 'crowdsourcing' to develop policy.

In summary, documents and people are equally important sources of evidence for policy analysis, and both quantitative and qualitative approaches will be required to gather data. Multiple sources and methods can increase understanding and the validity of the results. Once you engage in a real policy analysis, you will likely have additional questions on gathering data and would be well advised to consult a social research methods guide, such as that by Bryman (2008).

Data analysis: applying the 'policy triangle'

Although the 'policy analysis triangle' (Figure 1.1) provides an extremely useful structure to make your exploration of health policy issues and collection of data more systematic, it is more difficult to apply when you come to analysing and presenting your data because the different aspects, such as actors and processes, are so integrally intertwined and the goal of the analysis is generally to draw out their inter-relationships.

A few scholars have presented a policy analysis by talking separately about content, actors, processes and context. Trostle et al. (1999) analysed policies on AIDS, cholera, family planning and immunization in Mexico to understand the extent to which researchers influence decision makers. They found a number of common factors enabling or impeding interactions between these two sets of actors and analysed their data by looking at:

• the content of each policy and the factors that promoted (e.g. good quality research) or constrained (e.g. academic jargon, unrealistic recommendations) the relationship;
• the actors involved in each policy and the factors that enabled (e.g. networks that agreed on priority issues) or impeded (e.g. lack of technical background among decision makers) the relationship;
• processes, which included communication channels and events that intervened to promote or impede the use of research;
• contextual factors that enabled (e.g. the stability of the state) or constrained the ability of research to influence policy (e.g. centralization of power and information).

Another way of presenting your policy analysis is by applying a different, more explanatory framework, for example, the one by Shiffman and Smith (2007) (see Chapter 4).

While similar to the 'policy triangle', it offers more explicit guidance as to what you might include.

There are different ways to organize your material. On the whole, it is usually easier to approach your analysis like a narrative if it is a retrospective policy analysis: a story with a beginning, middle and end. For example, if you arrange your data and analysis chronologically, using the 'stages heuristic' (see Chapter 1), you will start with problem identification and issue recognition (agenda setting), go on to policy formulation and implementation, and end with an evaluation of what happened in this particular policy 'story'. This last part could be an overall discussion of how to understand what happened in this particular issue.

In gathering your data, you may well have produced a time-line: writing down the dates over a period of time of a series of events such as meetings or conferences, results from research studies, media stories, a change in government or the availability of funding, and decisions which will have informed your analysis of how the issue got on to the policy agenda and was handled. You may start your narrative by describing the background to the issue you are looking at, referring to some or all of Leichter's four contextual factors – situational, structural, cultural or external – that you learned about in Chapter 1. Having done that, you will move on to the problem identification phase, saying how the issue got on to the agenda, whether there was a single focusing event or several, where ideas came from and how they were framed, what role particular actors played in getting attention for the issue, whether the media were involved, and so on.

Having established how and why the issue reached the policy agenda, you can go on to describe who was involved in formulating the policy: was it largely prepared within a government department, how far did it involve others, such as the finance or social welfare ministries or interest groups? You may refer to the extent to which researchers, non-government organizations or the private sector were consulted or involved directly, or not; or how far they tried to influence the formulation of the policy and go on to describe its content (e.g. the policy mechanism, who was covered by it, or the cost implications).

The third stage is that of implementation. What happened once the policy was formulated? How was it executed? Was there good communication between policy makers and those putting it into practice or was this a top-down instruction, which implementers were expected to carry out without discussion?

A good example of this sort of analytical narrative is that by David Pelletier and colleagues (2011). They explored the policy process in five low and middle income countries to understand why under-nutrition – a major contributor to the global burden of disease – was neglected in these countries. The research was undertaken in Bangladesh, Bolivia, Guatemala, Peru and Vietnam, and sought to identify the challenges in the policy process and ways to overcome them. The authors looked specifically at the commitment of governments to under-nutrition policies, and then at the processes of agenda setting, policy formulation and implementation. Among their findings, they suggested that high level political attention to nutrition could be generated in a number of ways, but required sustained efforts from policy entrepreneurs and champions. Further, they observed that there were many hurdles in the process of policy formulation, and that mid-level actors from ministries and external partners had difficulty in translating windows of opportunity for nutrition into concrete operational plans. This was often due to capacity constraints, differing professional views of under-nutrition and disagreements over interventions, ownership, roles and responsibilities. Finally, when it came to implementation, the pace and quality of execution were often constrained by weaknesses in human and organizational capacities from national to front-line levels.

In taking such an approach to your narrative, you will be looking very closely at both processes and actors – and having analysed your data from interviews and documents – you will be making a judgement about who exercised their power or influence at each stage of the process. Remember you need to demonstrate that you are presenting your analysis based on your data and not just making a judgement according to your own beliefs. You need to support your analysis by giving the sources of your analysis such as: 'Fourteen (out of sixteen) interviewees suggested that the Prime Minister and her commitment to this policy was the single most important factor in getting it on to the policy agenda.'

Politics and ethics of policy analysis

In this book you have learned that policy change is political and in this chapter that analysis for policy typically serves political ends. Making policy alternatives and their consequences more explicit and improving the political feasibility of policy are neither value-neutral nor immune to politics. Policy analysis, therefore, will not invariably lead to better policy (e.g. policy which improves efficiency, equity or addresses problems of public health importance), or to better policy processes (e.g. fairer decision making processes in which all stakeholders are provided opportunities to air their views and influence decisions). The substance and process of policy analysis are influenced by who finances, executes, uses and interprets the analysis.

As you will appreciate from this chapter, ongoing, systematic analysis of a policy can be a resource-intensive endeavour. Not all policy actors are equally endowed with resources. Everything else being equal, policy analysis may serve to reinforce the prevailing distribution of political power and economic resources: those with political resources are more likely to be those who can finance analysis, and influence who will use the analysis and how it will be used. Those groups with more political resources are in a better position to develop politically informed strategies to manage the positions, players, power and perceptions surrounding a policy issue. In this way, policy analysis may reinforce the status quo.

Policy analysis is influenced not just by interests and power but also by interpretation. These issues raise questions about the role of the analyst, or of the organization for which the analyst works, in the analysis. If the analysis is for policy, it is almost inevitable that the analyst will have a preferred policy outcome. The policy goal may be at odds with some definitions of 'good policy' as discussed above (e.g. many well-intentioned health professionals champion services with poor cost-effectiveness). As no-one is value-neutral, it is difficult to produce policy analysis which is entirely unbiased. While there are ways to minimize bias, for example, by triangulating methods and sources of information and testing results with peers, it is probably necessary to accept the fact that the results of policy analysis, especially prospective analysis, will reflect to some degree the perspective of the analyst (e.g. the weight she/he gives to equity versus efficiency in analysing the likely impact of a policy). It is the responsibility of the analyst to make clear the values that have shaped her/his approach to the analysis.

Analysis for policy raises other kinds of ethical issues. For example, is it ethical to allow any group to participate in the policy process so as to develop a more powerful coalition? Is it ethical to undermine the legitimacy of opponents or to withhold information from public discourse for tactical purposes? How far should one compromise on evidence-informed policy content so as to accommodate and win over a policy opponent? Your values will dictate how you answer these questions. In thinking about your response, it may be useful to assume that other actors use these and other techniques to manipulate the substance and process of policy to their advantage. This may lead you to decide to join in the process of strategically managing the policy process to achieve your aims. Alternatively, you may decide to undertake prospective policy analysis to monitor and describe a policy process and leave it to other actors in the policy arena to use the knowledge in the process of policy debate. You may, however, feel uncomfortable with some of the strategies and decide that the ends do not justify the means. While these means may relate to values and ethics, they may also relate to the time, resources and emotional costs of pursuing, and at times failing to achieve, a particular policy change. There is nothing inherently wrong with abandoning or adopting a political strategy – particularly as it will now be based on a solid grasp of the fact that successful policy change requires a political approach.

Summary

In this chapter you have reviewed the retrospective and prospective uses of policy analysis. A stakeholder approach to policy analysis was presented. You used this approach to identify policy actors, assess their power, interests and position with respect to a policy issue of your choice, and developed a position map on the basis of this analysis. A range of strategies to manage the position, power, players and perceptions associated with policy change were reviewed as were sources of information for policy analysis. With these tools in hand, you are now better equipped to pursue policy change as well as to analyse what happened in the past. While the tools call for both creativity and evidence – the art and science of policy analysis – they also demand judgement, and will be infused with values and ethical questions. While analysis may more often serve to reinforce the status quo, without the use of policy analysis tools groups without power will remain at a perpetual disadvantage.

References

Blanchet K and James P (2012) The role of social networks in the governance of health systems: the case of eye care systems in Ghana. *Health Policy and Planning* 1–14. doi:10.1093/heapol/czs031. Advance Access published 12 March 2012.

Bryman A (2008) *Social Research Methods*, 3rd edn. Oxford: Oxford University Press.

Glassman A, Reich MR, Laserson K and Rojas F (1999) Political analysis of health reform in the Dominican Republic. *Health Policy and Planning* 14: 115–26.

Kaplan AM and Haenlein M (2010) Users of the world, unite! The challenges and opportunities of Social Media. *Business Horizons* 50(1): 59–68.

Kingdon JW (1995) *Agendas, Alternatives, and Public Policies*, 2nd edn. New York: HarperCollins.

Pelletier D, Frongillo EA, Suzanne Gervais S et al. (2011) Nutrition agenda setting, policy formulation and implementation: lessons from the Mainstreaming Nutrition Initiative. *Health Policy and Planning* 1–13. doi:10.1093/heapol/czr011.

Philip Morris (no date) PM tools to affect legislative decisions. October 2003. Bates No. 204770711. Available at: http://legacy.library.ucsf.edu/tid/.

Reich MR (1996) Applied political analysis for health policy reform. *Current Issues in Public Health* 2: 186–91.

Roberts MJ, Hsiao W, Berman P and Reich MR (2004) *Getting Health Reform Right: A Guide to Improving Performance and Equity*. Oxford: Oxford University Press.

Shiffman J and Smith S (2007) Generation of political priority for global health initiatives: a framework and case study of maternal mortality. *Lancet* 370: 1370–9.

Trostle J, Bronfman M and Langer A (1999) How do researchers influence decision makers? Case studies of Mexican policies. *Health Policy and Planning* 14: 103–14.

Varvasovszky Z and Brugha R (2000) How to do a stakeholder analysis. *Health Policy and Planning* 15(3): 338–45.

Weimer DL and Vining AR (2010) *Policy Analysis: Concepts and Practices*, 5th edn. Englewood Cliffs, NJ: Prentice Hall.

Glossary

Actor Shorthand term used to denote any participant in the policy process that affects policy, including individuals, organizations, groups and even the state or government.

Advocacy coalition Group within a policy sub-system distinguished by a shared set of norms, beliefs and resources. Can include politicians, civil servants, members of interest groups, journalists and academics who share ideas about policy goals and to a lesser extent about solutions.

Agenda setting Process by which certain issues come onto the policy agenda from the much larger number of issues potentially worthy of attention by policy makers.

Analysis Separating a problem into its constituent parts so as to better understand its whole.

Audit Examination of the extent to which an activity corresponds with predetermined standards or criteria.

Authority Where power concerns the ability to influence others, authority concerns the right to do so.

Bicameral/unicameral legislature In a unicameral legislature, there is only one 'house' or chamber, whereas in a bicameral legislature, there is a second or upper chamber, the role of which is to critique and check the quality of draft legislation promulgated by the lower house. Normally, only the lower house can determine whether draft legislation becomes law.

Bottom-up approach to understanding implementation Approach to analysing and explaining policy implementation that focuses on how local level actors and contextual factors influence policy implementation. Recognizes the strong likelihood that implementing actors at subordinate levels have discretion and play an active part in the process of implementation producing policy results, which may be different from those envisaged.

Bounded rationality Policy makers intend to be rational but make decisions that are satisfactory as opposed to optimum due to imperfect knowledge.

Bureaucracy Comprises the public officials, often known as civil servants, whose job it is to advise ministers (the executive) on how best to take forward their policy goals and then to manage the process of policy implementation.

Cause group Interest or pressure group whose main goal is to promote a particular cause.

Civil society That part of society between the private sphere of the family or household and the sphere of government and operating outside the market economy.

Civil society group A group or organization which is outside government and beyond the family/household. It may or may not be involved in public policy (e.g. sports clubs are civil society organizations, but not primarily pressure groups). Private sector groups involved in the market (e.g. industry groups) are sometimes included in civil society, but are generally treated separately.

Company Generic term for a business which may be run as a sole proprietorship, partnership or corporation.

Content Substance of a particular policy which details its constituent parts (e.g. its specific objectives and methods of implementation).

Context Systemic factors – political, economic, social or cultural, both national and international – which may have an effect on health policy.

Corporation An association of stockholders (shareholders) which is regarded as a 'person' under most national laws. Ownership is marked by ease of transferability and the limited liability of stockholders.

Crowdsourcing Canvassing suggestions from the general public via Twitter or other social media to help decide a course of action.

Decentralization The transfer of power and responsibilities from central government to local organizations.

Dissemination Process by which research findings are made known to key audiences, including policy makers.

Elitism The theory that power is concentrated in a minority group in society.

Epistemic community Policy community marked by shared political values, and a shared understanding of a problem, its definition and its causes. These are sometimes referred to as 'discourse communities'.

Evaluation Research designed specifically to assess the operation and/or impact of a programme or policy in order to determine whether the programme or policy is worth pursuing further.

Evidence Any form of knowledge, including, but not confined to research, of sufficient quality to be used to inform decisions.

Evidence-based medicine Movement within medicine and related professions to base clinical practice on the most rigorous scientific basis, principally informed by the results of randomized controlled trials of effectiveness of interventions.

Evidence-based (or evidence-informed) policy Movement within public policy to give evidence greater weight in shaping policy decisions, better described as 'evidence-informed' policy than 'evidence-based' since it is more obvious in public policy that evidence is only one factor influencing decision making.

Executive Leadership of a country (i.e. the president and/or prime minister and other ministers). The prime minister/president and senior ministers are often referred to as the cabinet.

Feasibility A characteristic of issues for which there is a practical solution.

Federal systems The sub-national or provincial level of government is not subordinate to the national government but has substantial powers of its own which the national government cannot take away.

Formative evaluation Evaluation designed to assess how a programme or policy is being implemented with a view to modifying or developing the programme or policy in order to improve its implementation.

Global civil society Civil society groups which are global in their aims, communication or organization.

Global public goods Goods which are undersupplied by markets, inefficiently produced by individual states, and which have benefits which are strongly universal.

Globalization Complex set of processes which increase interconnectedness and interdependencies between countries and people.

Governance Often contrasted with hierarchical, directive 'government' which is argued to have been superseded. Governance refers to the increasing requirement for governments to manage through policy networks, and is often characterized as a shift from 'command and control' to 'steering, influencing and negotiation' as prevalent processes of decision making. A similar shift is observed in the running of organizations of all types, not just government.

Government The institutions and procedures for making and enforcing rules and other collective decisions. This is a narrower concept than the state since the state also includes the judiciary, military and other public bodies.

Ideas The values, evidence, anecdote and argument that shape policy, including the way a policy problem or policy solution is presented.

Implementation Process of turning a policy into practice or action.

Implementation gap Difference between what the policy architect intended and the end-result of a policy.

Incrementalism The theory that decisions are not made through a rational process but by small adjustments to the status quo in the light of political realities.

Industry Groups of firms that are closely related and in competition in a particular sector of the economy due to use of similar technology of production or producing similar products.

Insider group Interest groups which pursue a strategy designed to win themselves the status of legitimate participants in the policy process, closely involved with governments.

Interest What an actor or group stands to gain or lose from a policy change.

Interest (pressure) group Any group outside the state including market and civil society groups that attempts to influence the policy process to achieve specific goals.

Interest network Policy community based on some common material interest.

Institutions The 'rules of the game' determining how government and the wider state operate. Institutions can be formal structures and procedures, but also informal norms of behaviour that may not be written down.

Iron triangle Small, stable and exclusive policy community usually involving executive agencies, legislative committees and interest groups (e.g. around defence procurement).

Issue network Loose network comprising a large number of quite diverse members who usually come together to try to draw attention to an issue, address a specific problem or promote a particular solution.

Judiciary Comprises judges and courts which are responsible for ensuring that the government of the day (the executive) acts according to the laws passed by the legislature.

Knowledge transfer Strategy usually incorporating a variety of 'linkage' and 'exchange' activities designed to reduce the social, cultural and technical 'gap' between researchers and policy makers.

Legislature Body that enacts the laws that govern a country and oversees the executive. Normally democratically elected in order to represent the people of the country and commonly referred to as the parliament or assembly. Often there will be two chambers or 'houses' of parliament.

Legitimacy A characteristic of issues that policy makers see as appropriate for government to act on.

Majoritarian An electoral system based on the 'winner takes all' principle, unlike proportional representation electoral systems in which the number of parliamentary seats is allocated in proportion to the votes gained by each party.

Monitoring Routine collection of data on an activity usually against a plan or contract.

Multinational corporation Business which controls operations in more than one country, even if it does not own them but controls through a franchise.

New public management An approach to government involving the application of private sector management techniques.

Non-governmental organization (NGO) Originally, any not for-profit organization outside government, but, increasingly, used to refer to structured organizations providing services. Sometimes referred to as Third Sector organizations.

Outsider group Interest groups which have either failed to attain insider status or have deliberately chosen a path of confrontation with government.

Parliamentary system The executive are also members of the legislature and are chosen on the basis that the majority of members of the legislature support them.

Path dependency The process by which decisions taken in one period shape and limit the range of policy choices available to interest groups and operating systems later.

Peak (apex) association Interest group composed of, and usually representative, of other interest groups (e.g. the Confederation of British Industry).

Pluralism The theory that power is widely distributed in society.

Policy Broad statement of goals, objectives and means that create the framework for activity. Often takes the form of explicit written documents but may also be implicit or unwritten.

Policy agenda List of issues to which an organization is giving serious attention at any one time with a view to taking some sort of action.

Policy community (and sub-system) Relatively stable network of organizations and individuals involved in a recognizable field of wider public policy such as health policy. Within each of these fields, there will be identifiable sub-systems, such as for mental health policy, with their own policy communities.

Policy instrument One of the range of options at the disposal of policy makers in order to give effect to a policy goal (e.g., privatization, regulation, subsidy, etc.).

Policy elites Specific group of policy makers who have high positions in an organization or policy system, and often have privileged access to other top members of the same and other organizations.

Policy makers Those who make policies in organizations such as central or local government, multinational companies or local businesses, schools, clinics, or hospitals.

Policy network Generic term for interdependent organizations involved in an area of policy that exchange resources and bargain to varying degrees to attain their specific goals.

Policy process The way in which policies are initiated, formulated, developed, negotiated, communicated, implemented and evaluated.

Policy stream The set of possible policy solutions or alternatives developed by experts, politicians, bureaucrats and interest groups, together with the activities of those interested in these options (e.g. debates between researchers).

Policy windows Points in time when the opportunity arises for an issue to come onto the policy agenda and be taken seriously with a view to action.

Political system The processes through which governments transform 'inputs' from citizens into 'outputs' in the form of policies.

Politics stream Political events such as shifts in the national mood or public opinion, elections and changes in government, social uprisings, demonstrations and campaigns by interest groups.

Power The ability to influence people, and in particular to control resources to achieve a desired outcome.

Presidential system The president or head of state is directly elected in a separate process from the election of members of the legislature.

Principal–agent theory Theory of organizational and government behaviour that focuses on the relationship between principals (e.g. purchasers) and their agents (e.g. providers), together with the contracts or agreements that enable the purchaser to specify what is to be provided and check that this has been accomplished.

Private sector That part of the economy which is not under direct government control.

Privatization Sale of publicly owned property to the private sector.

Problem stream Indicators of the scale and significance of an issue which give it visibility.

Proportional representation Voting system which is designed to ensure as far as possible that the proportion of votes received by each political party equates to their share of the seats in the legislature.

Punctuated equilibrium A decision-making theory which explains why long periods of policy stability are upset by abrupt adjustment, and policy reversals and reforms in response to external 'shocks' to the system.

Rationalism The theory that decisions are (and should be) made through a rational process by considering all the options and their consequences and then choosing the best.

Regulation Government intervention enforcing rules and standards (e.g. in the private sector).

Research Systematic activity designed to generate rigorous new knowledge and relate it to existing knowledge in order to improve understanding of the physical or social world.

Sectional group Interest group whose main goal is to protect and enhance the interests of its members and/or the section of society it represents (sometimes referred to as a 'vested interest').

Social media Web-based and mobile technologies which enable virtual dialogue through the creation and exchange of user-generated rather than professional content.

Social movement Loose grouping of individuals sharing certain views and attempting to influence others but without a formal organizational structure.

Social network analysis Methods used for mapping, measuring and analysing the social relationships between people, groups and organizations.

Sovereignty Entails rule or control over a geographical area that is supreme, comprehensive, unqualified and exclusive.

Stakeholder An individual or group with a substantive interest in an issue (i.e., interest group), including those with some role in making a decision or its execution. Used synonymously with actor and interest group.

Stakeholder analysis Process through which those making policy or affected by it are identified and their likely position and levels of interest and influence are assessed.

State A set of institutions that enjoy legal sovereignty over a fixed territorial area. The state includes a wider set of institutions than the government and includes the parliament, judiciary, military as well as other public bodies.

Stewardship The role of governments in directing and overseeing the health system, improving its performance and ensuring that it is maintained in good order for future generations (e.g. by ensuring a future supply of trained health workers).

Street level bureaucrats Front-line staff involved in delivering public services to members of the public who have some discretion in how they apply the objectives and principles of policies handed down to them.

Summative evaluation Evaluation designed to produce an overall verdict on a policy or programme in terms of the balance of costs and benefits.

Support A characteristic of issues that the public and other key political interests want to see responded to.

Top-down approach to understanding implementation Approach to analysing and explaining policy implementation structured according to a largely linear, rational perspective on the policy process which follows policy initiated at higher levels of the policy system (e.g. national government) through its subsequent execution at subordinate levels. This perspective recognizes a relatively clear division between policy formulation and implementation and focuses on how aspects of policy design at higher levels affect local implementation.

Transaction cost economics Branch of economic theory based on the insight that efficient production of goods and services depends on lowering the costs of transactions between buyers and sellers by removing as much uncertainty as possible on both sides, and by maximizing the ability of the buyer to monitor and control transactions.

Transnational corporation Business which owns branch companies in more than one country.

Unitary system The lower levels of government are constitutionally subordinate to the national government. Lower levels of government receive their authority from central government.

Vested/sectional group Interest group whose main goal is to protect and enhance the interests of its members and/or the section of society it represents (sometimes referred to as a 'vested interest').

Acronyms

ABC	Abstinence, Be faithful, and Condom use
ABPI	Association of British Pharmaceutical Industry
ACF	Advocacy Coalition Framework
ACMD	Advisory Committee on the Misuse of Drugs
ACTUP	AIDS Coalition to Unleash Power
AIDS	Acquired Immune Deficiency Syndrome
ARISE	Associates for Research into the Science of Enjoyment
ART	Antiretroviral Therapy
ARV	Antiretroviral drugs
ASH	Action on Smoking and Health
AZT	Azidothymidene
BIO	Biotechnology industry organization
BRICS	Brazil, Russia, India, China and South Africa
BUGAUP	Billboard Utilizing Graffitists Against Unhealthy Promotions
CD4	Cluster of 4 Differentiation
CHSRF	Canadian Health Services Research Foundation
CSO	Civil Society Organization
DfID	Department for International Development, UK
DHB	District Health Board, New Zealand
DOTS	Directly Observed Therapy, Short-course
ECOSOC	Economic and Social Council (UN)
EU	European Union
FAO	Food and Agriculture Organization (UN)
FCTC	Framework Convention on Tobacco Control
G8	Group of Eight
G20	Group of Twenty Finance Ministers and Central Bank Governors
GAVI	Global Alliance for Vaccines and Immunization (also known as the GAVI Alliance)
GHP	Global Health Partnership
GIPA	Greater Involvement of People living with AIDS
GK	Gonoshasthaya Kendra
GNP	Gross National Product
GP	General Practitioner
HIA	Health Impact Assessment
HIV	Human Immunodeficiency Virus
ICC	International Chamber of Commerce
IDB	Inter-American Development Bank
IHR	International Health Regulations
ILSI	International Life Sciences Institute
IMF	International Monetary Fund
IPC	Intellectual Property Committee
IPR	Intellectual Property Rights

IT	Information Technology
MDG	Millennium Development Goal
MEDLINE	US National Library of Medicine
MMR	Mumps, Measles and Rubella
MNC	Multinational Corporation
MoH	Ministry of Health
MSF	Médecins Sans Frontières
NGO	Non-Governmental Organization
NHS	National Health Service
NPM	New Public Management
OECD	Organisation for Economic Cooperation and Development
PEPFAR	President's Emergency Plan for AIDS Relief
PFI	Private Finance Initiative
PhRMA	American Pharmaceutical Manufacturers Association
PLWA	People Living with AIDS
RJR	R.J. Reynolds Tobacco Company
SARS	Severe Acute Respiratory Syndrome
SIDA	Swedish International Development Agency
SMS	Short Message Service
STI	Sexually Transmitted Infection
SWAP	Sector-Wide Approach
TAC	Treatment Action Campaign
TAG	Treatment Action Group
TB	Tuberculosis
TNC	Transnational Corporation
TRIPS	Agreement on Trade-Related Intellectual Property Rights
UIA	Union of International Associations
UN	United Nations
UNAIDS	Joint United Nations Programme on HIV/AIDS
UNDP	United Nations Development Programme
UNFPA	United Nations Population Fund
UNICEF	United Nations Children's Fund
UNODC	United Nations Office on Drugs and Crime
UK	United Kingdom
US	United States of America
USAID	United States Agency for International Development
WFP	World Food Programme
WHA	World Health Assembly
WHO	World Health Organization
WTO	World Trade Organization

Index

Page numbers in *italics* refer to figures and tables.

actors
 agenda setting 75–80
 definition 4
 industry 56
 policy process 9–11
 see also stakeholders
Advisory Council on the Misuse of
 Drugs (ACMD), UK 177
advocacy coalition framework (ACF)
 128, 142–5, 187–8
agenda, definition 65–6
agenda setting
 activities and feedback 65–6, 68,
 71–3, 74, 75, 82
 actors 75–80
 definition 64
 and issues 66–74
 Baumgartner and Jones model
 42–3
 crisis model 73–4
 Hall et al. model 67–9, 72
 Kingdon model 69–71, 73
 key terms 64–5
 non-decision making 74–5
 priorities 80–2
AIDS *see* HIV or AIDS
air pollution, US (case study) 26–7
Alford R 120
authoritarian-inegalitarian regimes
 37–8
authority
 definition 20
 forms of 23–4
Avaaz 77, 160–1

Bachrach P and Baratz MS 23, 35
Baumgartner FR and Jones BD 42–3
bicameral/unicameral legislature 84,
 91–2
bilateral cooperation, UN system
 155–6
Bill and Melinda Gates Foundation
 75–6, 158–9
'black box' decision making 35–6, 38

Black N 173
Blair, T/Blair government 40, 74
'bottom-up' approaches to policy
 implementation 128, 133–6,
 141–5
'bounded rationality' 20, 41
Bryman A 204, 206
bureaucracy
 civil service 28–9, 85, 94–6
 'street-level bureaucrats' 129, 133
Buse K
 et al. 18
 and Tanaka S 165
business interests 119–20

Canadian Health Services Research
 Foundation (CHSRF) 184–6
Cattaui MS 162
cause groups 106, 113
chief executive, role of 94
civil service/bureaucracy 28–9, 85,
 94–6
civil society 106
 global 148, 157–61
 and interest groups 108–10
'co-production' of research knowledge
 185
co-regulation 61–2
Collin J et al. 159–60
commercial interests *see* business
 interests; industry
communication and reputation in
 research 181
communities *see* policy communities
community health advocates 120
content of policy 4, 7
contextual factors 4, 11–13
cooperation *see* global health policy
corporate rationalizers 120
Council on Foreign Relations 110
Cox T 56
Crenson M 26–7
crowdsourcing 191, 206
cultural factors 11–12

Dahl R 22–3, 27, 28
data sources and analysis 202–8
Davies PT 171
decentralization 47, 53
decision making
 models 38–44
 non-decision making 22–3, 74–5
 power as 22
DeLeon P 129
Department of Health 61–2
documentary analysis 202–4
drug policy, Bangladesh (case study)
 71–3
drug users
 HIV or AIDS 143–4
 UK Advisory Council on the Misuse
 of Drugs (ACMD) 177
Dye T 6

Easton D 34, 35–6
egalitarian-authoritarian regimes 37
elective affinity model 174
elite interviews 205
elitism 20, 29–33
'entrepreneurs' 69, 96, 180, 193
equal health advocates 120
ethics of policy analysis 208–9
Etzioni A 42, 43
evaluation 170, 171
 see also research
evidence-based medicine 170, 171
evidence-based policy 170
 and knowledge transfer 185–7
evidence-informed policy 170
executive
 definition 85
 influence 93–4
 legislature and judiciary systems,
 relationship between 88–9

feasibility 64, 68
federal *vs* unitary government systems
 85, 86–7, 90–1
feminist perspective 31–2

food industry 25, 162
foreign policy instrument, health as 156
formative and summative evaluation
    170, 171
Framework Convention on Tobacco
    Control (case study) 159–60
Fukuyama F 38

Gates Foundation 75–6, 158–9
gendered policy implementation, India
    (case study) 31–2
Gibson B 187, 188
Giddens A 109
Global Forum on Health Research 177,
    178
global health policy 148–9
    activities and feedback 150, 151–2,
        156–7, 159–60, 161, 162–4, 165,
        167
    key terms 148
    mixed-scanning decision making 44
    modern cooperation 157–66
    process 166–8
    traditional cooperation 152–7
global public-private health
    partnerships (GHPs) 164–6
globalization 148, 149–50
    and health 150–2
governance 106, 118
government/state
    activities and feedback 88–90, 92–3,
        95, 98, 99, 100–3
    agenda setting 76–7
    definitions 20, 21
    and interest groups, relationship
        between 114–16, 117–19
    key terms 84–5
    legislature, executive and judiciary
        systems, relationship between
        88–9
    and private sector 48–9
        activities and feedback 50, 51,
            54–5, 57, 59–60
        key terms 47–8
    role in health systems 49–51
        critique of 51–2
        reinvention and reform 52–5,
            138–41
    systems 86–91
    see also ministries of health; entries
        beginning public

Hall P et al. 67–9, 72
harm reduction approach 143–4
Harrison S 172

health care lobbyists, US (case study)
    30
health insurance 53–4
health policy
    activity and feedback 8
    analysis 7–8, 18
    definition 5–7
    importance of 5
    key terms 4–5
'health policy triangle' 8–9, 18, 206–7
high politics 29, 66, 83, 96, 103, 107, 143
HIV or AIDS
    activities and feedback 10–11, 12–13,
        119, 123–4, 144, 176–7
    conceptions of 67
    decision making 41–2
    documentary analysis 203–4
    drug users 143–4
    interest/civil society groups 115, 119,
        159, 161
        case study 121–4
    research 174
    UNAIDS 154
Hogwood B and Gunn L 76, 132
Howlett M et al. 14, 15, 137–8

ideological barriers to research 176–8
implementation see policy
    implementation
implementation gap 129–30
incremental decision making 20, 41–3
industry 47, 56
    food 25, 162
    pharmaceutical 54, 57–8, 60, 115,
        164, 177–8
    tobacco 23, 159–60
    transnational corporations (TNCs)
        48, 161–4
infectious diseases 150–1
'insider' and 'outsider' groups 106,
    114–16
institutions 86
    definition 5, 85
    'stickiness' 42
intellectual property rights (IPRs)
    162–4
interest groups 107–8
    activities and feedback 107–8, 112,
        114, 115–16, 117, 119, 124–5
    advantages and disadvantages 124–5
    and civil society groups 108–10
    definition 106
    functions 116–17
    and government, relationship
        between 114–16, 117–19

    impact 121–4
    influential 119–21
    key terms 106–7
    NGOs 18, 107, 109–10, 117, 143
    strategies 114–16
    types 110–14
interests
    definition 4
    position and commitment of
        stakeholders 195–9
International Chamber of Commerce
    (ICC) 162
international factors 12
    see also global health policy;
        globalization
international health financing reform
    (case study) 32–3
International Health Regulations (IHR)
    152
interviews 204–5
iron triangle 106, 118
issue networks 106, 118–19, 187
issues see agenda setting, and issues

John P 14, 15, 189

Kaplan AM and Haenlein M 205–6
Keck ME and Sikkind KI 160
Kingdon J 65, 69–71, 73, 193
knowledge transfer 170, 185–7

Lakoff G 24
Lasswell HD 34
Lee K and Goodman H 32–3
legislature
    bicameral/unicameral 84, 91–2
    executive and judiciary systems,
        relationship between 88–9
    role of 91–4
legitimacy 64, 67–8
Leichter H 11–12
Levine P 12
liberal democratic regimes 37
Lindblom CE 14, 41
    and Woodhouse EJ 42
Linder SH and Peters BG 141
'linkage and exchange' model of
    research transfer 184–6
Lipsky M 133
Lomas J 172, 184–6
low politics 29, 66, 83, 96, 107
Lukes S 24, 25

McDonalds 25
McKee M et al. 18

majoritarian *vs* proportional electoral systems 87
markets *see* new public management
Marsh D and Rhodes RAW 118–19, 187
mass media
    agenda setting 77–80
    risk conceptions 179
Maucher HO 162
Millennium Development Goals (MDGs) 82, 130, 167
Mills AJ and Ranson MK 49–50
ministries of health
    low and middle income countries 166
    and other ministries, relationship between 98–100
    position of 96–8
    professional vs other sources of advice 100
mixed-scanning approach to decision making 43–4

National Health Service (NHS), UK 54, 55, 62, 74, 94, 112–13, 139, 140
networks
    maps 32–3
    policy 106, 118, 187
    social network analysis 191, 198–9
new public management (NPM) 47, 53, 138–41
non-decision making 22–3, 74–5
non-government organizations (NGOs) 18, 106, 107, 109–10, 117, 143
Nutt D 177
Nye J 23, 25

Odgen J et al. 15–17
Olson M 28
Organization for Economic Cooperation and Development (OECD) 99, 167
organogram/organizational chart 101–3
'outsider' and 'insider' groups 106, 114–16

path dependency 21, 42
Pelletier D et al. 207–8
performance-based funding 139–40
Peterson MA 116, 117, 177
pharmaceutical industry 54, 57–8, 60, 115, 164, 177–8
pluralism 21, 28

policy analysis 192
    activities and feedback 194, 195, 196–8, 199–201
    data analysis 206–8
    data sources 202–6
    key terms 191
    political strategies for policy change 199–201
    politics and ethics of 208–9
    retrospective and prospective 192–3
    see also stakeholder analysis
'policy brokers' 142
policy communities 106, 118–19, 187
    and research community 174–5, 183–4
    and sub-systems 118, 142–5
policy documents 202–4
policy 'entrepreneurs' 69, 96, 180, 193
policy implementation 129–30
    activities and feedback 130, 131–2, 134–5, 137–8, 140–1, 144–5
    approaches
        early 131–6
        other 136–41
        synthesis 141–5
    key terms 128–9
    and policy makers 145
    strategies 146
policy networks 106, 118–19, 187
policy process 9–11, 13–17
    definition 5
    global 166–8
    'streams' 65, 69–71
policy sub-systems 118, 142–5
policy windows 65, 69, 70, 73, 82, 180
political barriers to research 176–9
political parties 91
political strategies for policy change 199–201
political systems 21, 34–6
    classification 37–8
politics and ethics of policy analysis 208–9
'politics-as-usual' agenda setting 66–7
populist regimes 37
position
    interests and commitment of stakeholders 195–9
    maps 197, 198
    power, players and perception strategies (case study) 199–201
power 21–2
    activities and feedback 23, 25, 26–7, 31–2, 34, 36, 44
    definition and types 22–7

key terms 20–1
of private sector 57–8
theories 27–34
see also political systems
Pressman JL and Wildavsky A 129, 131
pressure groups *see* interest groups
principal-agent theory 129, 136–8
private sector 52–3
    definition 48, 55–7
    involvement of 58–62
    policies 6
    power of 57–8
    see also government/state, and private sector
professional monopolists 120–1
professional vs other sources of advice 100
proportional representation
    definition 85
    vs majoritarian electoral systems 87
prospective policy analysis 192-3
public choice 28–9
public expenditure 53
public policy 85–6
    definition 6
    and private sector 61
public-private health partnerships
    global (GHPs) 164–6
    PFI 54
punctuated equilibrium 21, 42–3

rational decision making 21, 38–41
regulation of private sector 48, 58–62
Reich M 71–3
research 170–1
    activities and feedback 173, 174–5, 181–2, 185
    barriers to use 176–82
    and evaluation 170, 171
    key terms 170
    and policy
        improving relationship between 183–8
        influence 172–5
    risk conceptions 179
Roberts MJ et al. 52, 180, 192–3, 199–201
Rossi P and Wright S 171
Rushing W 67

Sabatier PA
    and Jenkins-Smith HC 13, 142, 187–8
    and Mazmanian DA 131
Safe Motherhood Initiative 80–2
Schlosser E 25

scientific uncertainty 178–9
sectional groups 21, 107, 111–13
'sector-wide approaches' (SWAPs)
    166–7
self-regulation 58–61
Sell S 163
Sen A 79
Sethi PS 59–60
sex-selective abortions, India (case
    study) 31–2
Shiffman J 80
    et al. 12, 43
    and Smith S 14–15, 80–2, 206
Simon HA 38, 40–1
situational factors 11
social media 191, 205–6
social network analysis 191, 198–9
'soft power' 23, 25
stakeholder analysis 191, 193–9
stakeholders
    assessment of power 194–5
    definition 191
    identifying 193–4
    interests, position and commitment
        195–9
    interviews 205
    policy implementation 145
state see government/state
strategic model 173–4
'streams' in policy process 65, 69–71
'street-level bureaucrats' 129, 133
structural factors 11
structural interests 120–1
sub-systems 118, 142–5

summative and formative evaluation
    170, 171
support 65, 68–9

thought control, power as 24–6
timing of research 180
tobacco industry 23, 159–60
'top-down' approaches to policy
    implementation 129, 131–2,
    134–5, 141–5
traditional-inegalitarian regimes 37
transnational corporations (TNCs) 48,
    161–4
Treatment Action Campaign (TAC) 11,
    115, 160
Trostle J et al. 206
tuberculosis (TB), DOTS policy (case
    study) 15–17
two communities of research and
    policy 174–5, 183–4

unitary vs federal government systems
    85, 86–7, 90–1
United Nations (UN) 152–5
    Framework Convention on Climate
        Change 113
    Global Compact 162
    and International Chamber of
        Commerce (ICC) 162
    Millennium Development Goals
        (MDGs) 82, 130, 167
    UNAIDS 154
    UNDP 107
    UNICEF 154

    WHO 153-4
    utility of research 179–80

voluntary codes 59–60

Walker L and Gilson L 133
Walt G 7, 29, 145, 146
    and Gilson L 9
Ward V et al. 186
Waxman HA 162
Weber M 23–4
Weiss CH 172–3, 179–80
windows of opportunity see policy
    windows
World Bank 9, 16, 32–3, 40, 51, 53, 58,
    154–5
World Health Assembly (WHA) 153
World Health Organization (WHO)
    153–4
    annual budget 57–8
    and commercial interests 23, 159–60,
        162
    health care workers 151
    Framework Convention on Tobacco
        Control 159-60
    International Health Regulations
        (IHR) 152
    non-communicable diseases 44
    TB programme 16
World Trade Organization (WTO) 155,
    157, 162, 163

Zeltner T et al. 23
Zuniga J 121

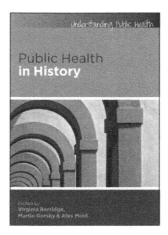

PUBLIC HEALTH IN HISTORY

Virginia Berridge, Martin Gorsky
and Alex Mold

9780335242641 (Paperback)
2011

eBook also available

This fascinating book offers a wide ranging exploration of the history of public health and the development of health services over the past two centuries. The book surveys the rise and redefinition of public health since the sanitary revolution of the mid-nineteenth century, assessing the reforms in the post World War II years and the coming of welfare states.

Written by experts from the London School of Hygiene and Tropical Medicine, this is the definitive history of public health.

Key features:

- Case studies on malaria, sexual health, alcohol and substance abuse
- A comparative examination of why healthcare has taken such different trajectories in different countries
- Exercises enabling readers to easily interact with and critically assess historical source material

www.openup.co.uk

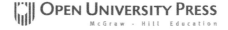

OPEN UNIVERSITY PRESS
McGraw - Hill Education

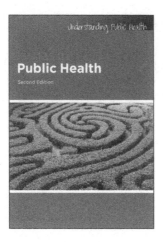

ISSUES IN PUBLIC HEALTH
Second Edition

Fiona Sim and Martin McKee

9780335244225 (Paperback)
September 2011

eBook also available

What is public health and why is it important? By looking at the foundations of public health, its historical evolution, the themes that underpin public health and the increasing importance of globalization, this book provides thorough answers to these two important questions.

Written by experts in the field, the book discusses the core issues of modern public health, such as tackling vested interests head on, empowering people so they can make healthy decisions, and recognising the political nature of the issues. The new edition has been updated to identify good modern public health practice, evolving from evidence

Key features:

- New chapters on the expanding role of public health, covering the issues of sustainability and climate change, human rights, genetics and armed conflict
- Examination of the impact of globalization on higher and lower income countries
- Expanded UK and International examples

www.openup.co.uk

OPEN UNIVERSITY PRESS
McGraw · Hill Education

WHERE HEAVEN AND EARTH TOUCH

תא אחוי לך היכא דנשקא ארעא ורקיעא אהדדי

(Baba Batra 74a)

An Anthology of Midrash and Halachah

by

DANNY SIEGEL

THE TOWN HOUSE PRESS
Spring Valley, New York

ACKNOWLEDGEMENTS

To my handful of private students over the years — Arthur Kurz-weil, Beth Huppin, Miriam Laufer, Nechama Katz, Polly Okunieff, Ruth Mendelsohn, Sally Mendelsohn, and Amy Eilberg — my gratitude. With them I have begun to explore many of the texts in this volume. They are all rare individuals, gentle teachers.

Second printing, 1984

Cover illustration by Fran Schultzberg.

For Ordering:
The Town House Press
28 Midway Rd.
Spring Valley NY 10977
914-425-2232

DEDICATION

To Nahum N. Glatzer—*Yasher Koach* and *Biz Hundert Und Tzvantzig*—great strength to him, till age one hundred and twenty in his lifelong work of inspiring students! While I was not graced with the opportunity to study with him, partaking of his auraed enthusiasm, generations of students at Brandeis and other universities were granted such magic Torah-moments. The one time I did hear him speak, I was deeply moved—for his words, and for the ever-so-obvious fact that he embodied the Torah he was teaching. This volume is dedicated to him.

I also dedicate this work to Dr. David HaLivni, *my* teacher. There seems to be no end to his knowledge, his sweep of the worlds of Torah material. At once profound and humble, he is always a Mensch, *Edel* to the highest degree, patient with slow-to-understand students such as myself, caring for the individual, sensitive to the most delicate nuances of the soul. He personifies the principle of "Torah and Greatness in one person." I am blessed, grateful.

TABLE OF CONTENTS

Introduction 1

Torah 3
Human Qualities 11
Sensitivity 14
Money 16
The Angel 20
Heaven and Hell 23
Praying 24
Torah and Life 25
Aphorisms and Other Brief Insights 26
A Miscellany 28
Children 34
Old Age 35
Marriage and Divorce 36
Our Souls 38
The Creator 39
Shabbat 41
The Troubles of the Jews 42
The Exodus 43
Revolt 46
Death and Mourning 48

INTRODUCTION

"Passionate, Gutsy Torah" would have been an appropriate additional subtitle for this pamphlet, or "Torah and Life-Values." These passages taken from the Talmud, Midrash, Law Codes, and other traditional volumes—including many off-the-beaten-track texts—have been anthologized for one purpose: exploring the relationship between Torah and the search for Menschlichkeit, human being, decency, caring, a benevolent reaching out. My hope is that people will be intellectually stimulated, but even more so, to be moved, touched, given pause to consider what Judaism has to say about how we live our lives as Jews. Insight and lyric are the topics more than plain acquisition of facts.

Wisdom is the subject. Menschlichkeit, a goal always only partially attainable, is the essence of Torah-study as I see it, an immense struggle, worthwhile despite the immensity. Surrounded as we are by paganism, cynicism, arrogance, and a culture that breeds egocentricity, this is a modest attempt to redirect our vision. Ignorance destroys—that is a truism. But there is also a kind of destructive knowledge, and I would wish by the easy availability of the pamphlet to bring to light a different view of knowledge, one that points to actions that allow us to rise above ourselves and the insufficient values swirling around us every day.

This is a pamphlet for adults, though it may be used as a text in Hebrew highschools, too. The Talmud, Maimonides, and Shulchan Aruch all incontrovertibly rule that adult education is more important than education of the children. Selection #1 says exactly that. I believe it is a source of great detriment to the welfare of our communities that we have not taken this insight to heart. Rarely do adult education courses center on the topics of Menschlichkeit, Edelkeit—Jewish nobility of soul, Ehrlichkeit—honesty and uprightness, Ziesskeit—human sweetness, and Shaynkeit—the inner beauty of the individual soul. It is hoped that this pamphlet will be used for courses and minicourses, in synagogues and Chavurot and small home study groups, in one-on-one *chavruta*-exchanges, and by individuals. We are in great need of the "Redignification of Adult Jewish Study," and this is perhaps a small first step.

The pamphlet is also intended as a leaf-through book. Allowing the eye and mind to fall randomly on some selection, to consider a change of vision, an adjustment of our actions—this, too, would be worthwhile—as well as more formalized study settings.

I am not a scholar, but rather a student of Torah and a poet. Nearly twenty years ago I purchased a copy of Professor Nahum N. Glatzer's *Hammer On The Rock, A Midrash Reader.* . . . texts without commentary. My copy is well-worn from re-reading and teaching and re-teaching the material. As I read or leafed through the slender book, modest doors and brilliantly shining gates both opened to me, views of worlds I did not suspect existed in Jewish life. I would allow my mind to roll and bend and turn and wander, and wonder at the profundities and suggestibilities of the texts presented to me. Over the years, the texts changed meanings, re-arranged themselves into different priorities and possibilities, moving me in different ways. I would hope that this volume, too, will do the same for others to some degree, though I do not pretend to have at my disposal the vast storehouse of Torah knowledge and wisdom that Professor Glatzer has.

As a student of Torah, I have remained essentially faithful to the text, translating as carefully as my abilities allowed, but also freeing myself from literalistic tendencies when I felt the lyricism of the words demanded a more intuitive, singing rendition. I began my writing career as a poet, and see now that with certain passages I needed to be free, grasping for the spirit of the words as well as the exact sense. I have also knowingly taken many selections out of context. While scholars may view this with an element of disfavor, I believe, nevertheless, that the pedagogical goal justifies this approach.

The selections are varied and out of balance—too much here, too little there. *Where Heaven and Earth Touch* is a rather personal selection, though, intended to whet the appetite, to offer the student and casual peruser an opportunity to go beyond this selection—to the *Encyclopaedia Judaica*, *Hammer on the Rock*, Klagsbrun's excellent *Voices of Wisdom*, Montefiore and Loewe's *A Rabbinic Anthology*, Ginzberg's work of genius *The Legends of the Jews*, other anthologies, and, of course, the sources in the original. While it is hoped that all Jews will enjoy the unique pleasure of opening the giant volumes of Talmud, Midrash, and Law Codes in the Hebrew and Aramaic, for now, English translations will have to serve as an intermediate step. No one should be robbed of the privilege of passionate Torah study.

As I have been allowed into the world of Torah values and the glorious struggle to interact with those values, so, too, may you, with the moderate assistance of this volume, enjoy the wonders of Torah.

Danny Siegel
March 7, 1983

TORAH

1. If a parent wished to study Torah, and he has a child who must also learn—the parent takes precedence. However, if the child is more insightful or quicker to grasp what there is to be learned, the child takes precedence. Even though the child gains priority thereby, the parent must not ignore his own study, for just as it is a Mitzvah to educate the child, so, too, is the parent commanded to teach himself.

Maimonides, Mishna Torah,
Laws of Torah Study 1:4

2. Rav Ya'acov the son of Rav Acha bar Ya'acov was sent by his father to study with Abayye.

When his father came to observe, he saw that his son was not learning well.

He said, "I can do better than you. Return home, and I will take your place."

Kiddushin 29b

3. Who is truly wise?

One who learns from all people.

Pirke Avot 4:1

One who foresees the consequences of his acts.

Tamid 32a

One who lives out what he has learned.

Sifray, Deuteronomy 1, Piska 13

4. Rabbah the son of Rav Huna said:

Whoever possesses Torah-knowledge but has no fear of sin is like a treasurer who has been given the keys to the inner doors, but not to the outer doors. How could he possibly get in to reach the treasure?

Shabbat 31a–b

3

5. When a teacher is teaching, and the students do not understand, he should not be angry at them or become upset, but rather he should go over the material again and again—even many times—until they understand the depth of the law. Similarly, a student should not say, "I understand," if he has not understood. He should ask again—many times, if necessary. And if the teacher becomes angry and disturbed, the student should say, "My teacher, this is Torah, and I must learn it, but my capacities are limited."

Maimonides Mishna Torah,
Laws of Torah Study 4:4

6. A student should not be embarrassed if a fellow student has understood something on the first or second time and he has not grasped it even after a number of attempts. If he is embarrassed because of this, it will turn out that he will have spent his time in the house of study without learning anything at all.

Shulchan Aruch,
Yoreh De'ah 246:11

7. People should not go to study with a teacher who does not walk in the good way—even though he might be a great sage and might be needed by the people. They must not study with him until he reforms his ways.

Shulchan Aruch
Yoreh De'ah 246:8

8. People should first learn Torah-texts under the supervision of a teacher. Only afterwards should they begin to apply their own powers of reason, logic, and analogy.

Avoda Zara 19a
(with Rashi)

9. Rava said:

If there are two teachers available for hire—one who has studied extensively but is not meticulous about mistakes, and another who is meticulous about mistakes but has not studied as much, we hire the one who has studied extensively but is not as meticulous because mistakes have a way of working themselves out.

Rav Dimi of Neharde'a said:

We hire the one who is meticulous about mistakes, because once a mistake enters the students' minds, it stays there.

Bava Batra 21a

10. A person who reviews his subject matter one hundred times does not achieve the same understanding as a person who reviews it one hundred and one times.

Chagiga 9b

11. Rabbi Preda had a certain student to whom he had to teach everything four hundred times. One day, Rabbi Preda was going to be needed for a Mitzvah related to Tzedakah. He taught the student, but the student could not grasp the material.

He asked, "What is the matter?"

The student answered, "From the moment they said to you there is a Mitzvah to be done, I could not concentrate because I thought, 'Now he will have to go. Now he will have to go.'"

Rabbi Preda said to him, "Pay attention, and I will teach you again." He then reviewed the material another four hundred times.

A Voice from Heaven was heard to say to Rabbi Preda, "Would you prefer to have four hundred years added to your life, or that you and your entire generation be assured life in the World to Come?"

He answered, "May my generation and I be privileged to enter the World to Come."

The Holy One, blessed be He, said, "Give him both rewards."

Eruvin 54b

12. Rabbi Abbahu said:

The entire forty days that Moses was On High, he would study the Torah and then forget it.

He said, "Master of the world, I have been here forty days, and I know nothing."

What did the Holy One, blessed be He, do?

At the end of the forty days He gave Moses the Torah as a gift.

Exodus Rabba, Ki Tissa 41:6

13. Our rabbis have taught:

A person's Rebbi [Quintessential Teacher] is defined as one who teaches him wisdom, and not one who taught him the Written and the Oral Torah. This is Rabbi Meir's opinion.

Rabbi Yehudah says:

Whoever has taught him most of his wisdom.

Rabbi Yossi says:

Even if he did no more than make his eyes light up from an explanation of a single selection from the Oral Torah—he is still considered to be his Rebbi.

Bava Metzia 33a

14. Rabbi Akiva said:

I once followed my teacher, Rabbi Yehoshua, into the bathroom and learned three things about personal care from him. . . .

Ben Azzai said to Rabbi Akiva:

How could you dare to do such a thing with your teacher?

He said to him:

This, too, is Torah, and I needed to learn.

Berachot 62a

15. "And acquire a friend for yourself." (*Pirke Avot 1:6*)

How may this be accomplished?

A person should find another who will eat with him, drink with him, study the Written and Oral Torah with him, sleep with him, and reveal all his secrets to him—both the secrets of the Torah and the secrets of the ways of the world.

Avot DeRabbi Natan A:8

16. Whenever Rabbi Yoshiah and Rabbi Mattiah ben Cheresh would study Torah together, they studied with great passion. And when they parted, they treated each other like childhood friends.

Avot DeRabbi Natan A:1

17. One who reports a statement of Torah he has heard from someone else should imagine that person standing in front of him as he speaks.

Y. Shabbat 1:2

18. Solomon did not only survey the words of Torah, but rather, "everything that was done under the heavens." (*Ecclesiastes 1:13*) He even investigated how to sweeten mustard and lupine-plants.

Song of Songs Rabba 1:1, Section 7

19. It was said that Rabban Yochanan ben Zakkai's studies included the following:

Bible, Mishna, Gemara [explication of the Mishna], legal and homiletical material, the intricacies of the Written and Oral Torah, various rules of Torah-logic, astronomy, arithmetic, washer's proverbs, fox fables, the languages of demons, palm trees, and angels, and great and small matters. "Great matters" refers to the study of God's divine chariot, and "small matters" refers to the intricate legal discussions between Rava and Abayye.

Bava Batra 134a

20. People can learn Torah well only if the material at hand is of particular interest to them.

Avoda Zara 19a

21. From what age should a parent begin to teach his child?

From the moment he begins to speak.

He begins by teaching him, "Moses instructed us in Torah, the heritage of the congregation of Jacob," (Deuteronomy 33:4) and the first verse of the Shema.

Afterwards he teaches him little by little until he is six or seven, and then takes him to a school for elementary Torah studies.

Shulchan Aruch,
Yoreh De'ah 245:5

22. When a child knows how to speak, his parent should teach him the Shema, Torah, and Hebrew, and if he does not do so, it were better that the child were not even born.

Tosefta Chagiga 1:1

23. "In his sickness, You have overturned his bed." (Psalm 41:4)

Rav Yosef said, "This means that he forgets his studies."

Rav Yosef himself became ill and forgot his Torah-knowledge, but Abayye re-taught it to him.

This is the meaning of the frequently mentioned statement that Rav Yosef made time and again, "I have not heard this law,"—and Abayye would remind him, "But you yourself taught it to us, deriving it from such-and-such a source."

Nedarim 41a

24. The question was raised:

Does a person who feeds another have to wash his hands or not?

Shmuel's father once found Shmuel crying.

He asked him, "Why are you crying?"

"Because my teacher hit me."

"Why did he do that?"

"Because he said to me, 'You were feeding my son and did not wash your hands before doing so.'"

Shmuel's father asked, "And why did you not wash?"

Shmuel replied, "It was he who was eating, so why should I wash?"

His father said, "It is not enough that the teacher does not know the law, but he also hit you!"

Chulin 107b

25. It is taught:

Every day an angel goes forth from the presence of the Blessed One, setting out to destroy the world—to return it to its primeval chaos.

However, when the Blessed One sees young children studying with their teachers, and the students of the wise sitting in their houses of study, his anger immediately changes to mercy.

Kallah Rabbati 2

26. Rabbi Shimon bar Yochai said:

Moses would show respect to Aaron by saying, "Teach me," and Aaron would show similar respect to Moses by saying, "Teach me." As a result, God's words came from between them, and it was as if both of them were speaking.

Mechilta,
Massechta d'Pischa 3
Lauterbach I:23

27. It was said of Yonatan ben Uzziel that, whenever he would sit to study Torah, any bird that flew overhead would be instantly incinerated.

Sukkah 28a

28. "Surrounded by lilies" (*Song of Songs 7:3*):

This refers to the words of Torah.
They are as delicate as lilies.

Song of Songs Rabba 7

29. Rabbi Mana said:

"It (Torah) is not an empty thing for you. It is your life."
(Deuteronomy 32:47)

If it is empty, it is because of you.

Why is that so? Because you do not work at it.

"It is your life. . . ." When is it your life? When you work hard at it.

Y. Ketubot 8:11

30. Rabbi Shefatyah said in the name of Rabbi Yochanan:

The verse—"I gave them laws which were not good" (Ezekiel 20:25)— refers to someone who studies the Written Torah without the appropriate melody, and studies the Oral Torah without a tune.

Megillah 32a

HUMAN QUALITIES

31. In life, you discover that people are called by three names:

One is the name the person is called by his father and mother; one is the name people call him, and one is the name he acquires for himself.

The best one is the one he acquires for himself.

Tanchuma, Vayakhel, 1

32. Rabbi Ila'i said:

A person may be known by three things—
by his cup,
by his pocket,
and by his anger.
And some say:
Also by his laughter.

Eruvin 65b

33. When Rabbi Meir died, the last great fable-teller died.
When Ben Azzai died, the last ultra-diligent student died.
When Ben Zoma died, the last great sermonizer died.
When Rabbi Yehoshua died, goodness left the world.
When Rabban Shimon ben Gamliel died, locusts came and troubles
    increased.
When Rabbi Elazar ben Azaryah died, great wealth ceased among the
    sages.
When Rabbi Akiva died, the glory of the Torah ceased.
When Rabbi Chanina ben Dosa died, great wonder-workers were no
    more.
When Rabbi Yossi Ketanta died, true piety ceased. . . . for he embodied
    the essence of the pious.
When Rabban Yochanan ben Zakkai died, the radiance of wisdom
    ceased.
When Rabban Gamliel the Elder died, the glory of the Torah ceased
    and purity and abstinence passed away.
When Rabbi Yishmael ben Pavi died, the radiance of the priesthood
    ceased.
When Rabbi Yehuda the Prince died, humility and the fear of sin
    ceased.

Mishna Sota 9, End

11

34. Rabbah the son of Rava (and some say: Rabbi Hillel the son of Rabbi Vallas said):

From the days of Moses until Rabbi Yehudah the Prince we have not found Torah and greatness in one place.

Sanhedrin 36a

35. Take note:

Even though the House of Shammai and the House of Hillel often disagreed on important matters, this did not prevent them from marrying members of each other's circle.

Yevamot 14b

36. Rabbah the son of Rav Huna said:

It is permitted to call an arrogant person "evil."

Rav Nachman the son of Yitzchak said:

It is permitted to hate him.

Ta'anit 7b

37. Rav Yehuda said in Rav's name:

Whoever is arrogant—
if he is a sage, he will lose his wisdom;
if he is a prophet, he will lose his power of prophecy.

Pesachim 66b

38. The townspeople of Simoniah came to Rabbi Yehuda HaNassi and said, "We would like to hire someone who can interpret Torah for us, judge us, supervise our synagogue affairs, teach us elementary and advanced Torah, and oversee whatever might be our needs."

He gave them Levi Bar Sisi.

The Simonians made him a large Bima, sat him upon it, and approached him with a question of Halacha.

He gave no answer.

They asked him another such question, and, again, he did not reply. They said, "Perhaps he is not an expert in Halacha. Let us ask him to explain a verse from the Book of Daniel."

They did so, but, still, he had no answer for them.

They went back to Rabbi Yehuda HaNassi and said, "Is this the way you satisfy our request?"

He replied, "I swear I have given you someone as good as myself. Bring him here."

Rabbi Yehuda asked him the same three questions, and he immediately gave substantial, appropriate answers.

So Rabbi Yehuda asked, "Why did you not answer them when they asked?"

He replied, "They made me this huge Bima and sat me upon it, and I became so enthralled by my own self-importance, I could not function properly.

Y. Yevamot 12:6

SENSITIVITY

39. We are taught:

If the eye only had the power to see, no one could survive because of the Evil Spirits.

Berachot 6a

40. Rabbi Yossi says,

"Woe to God's creatures who see and do not know what they see!"

Chagiga 12b

41. Our rabbis have taught:

Seven things are hidden from human beings—the day of death, the day of comfort, the extent of judgment; one human being does not know what is in another's heart, nor does he know from what he will earn a living, nor when the Kingdom of David will return, nor when the Evil Kingdom will end.

Pesachim 54b

42. Three kinds of people live lives that are not really living:
Oversensitive people,
irascible people,
and physically delicate people.

Pesachim 113b

43. Rabbi Yannai says:

"All the days of the poor are bad" (*Proverbs 15:15*)—
This refers to a person who is physically delicate.
"But one with a good heart has an eternal feast" (*Proverbs 15:15*)—
This refers to a person who has a hardy constitution.

Rabbi Yochanan says:

"All the days of the poor are bad" (*Proverbs 15:15*)—
This refers to a person who is compassionate.
"But one with a good heart has an eternal feast (*Proverbs 15:15*)—
This refers to a person who is cruel.

Bava Batra 145b

MONEY

44. We are taught:

Who is to be considered truly wealthy?

He who derives peace of mind from his wealth. This is the opinion of Rabbi Meir.

Rabbi Tarfon says: He who has a hundred vineyards, a hundred fields, and a hundred workers working in them.

Rabbi Akiva says: He who has a spouse who does exquisite deeds.

Rabbi Yossi says: He who has a bathroom near his diningroom table.

Shabbat 25b

45. The One Who has created the day has also created the means for a living.

Rabbi Elazar used to say:

Whoever has enough to eat for today and says, "What will I eat tomorrow?" is a person of little faith.

Mechilta,
Massechta DeVayissa 3
Lauterbach II: 103

46. Rabbi Yishmael said:

One who wishes to acquire wisdom should study the way money works, for there is no greater area of Torah-study than this. It is like an ever-flowing stream. And one who wishes to study money matters should apprentice himself to Rabbi Shimon ben Nannas.

Bava Batra 175b

47. Rabbi Yochanan was once robbed by a gang of thieves. When he went into the Study House, Resh Lakish asked him a question, but he did not respond. He asked him another, but, again, he did not answer.

Resh Lakish asked him, "What's wrong?"

Rabbi Yochanan answered, "All the parts of the body depend on the heart, and the heart depends on the pocket."

"What happened?"

"I was robbed by thieves."

"Which way did they go?"

He showed Resh Lakish which way they had gone, and when Resh Lakish saw them from a distance, he screamed at them.

The thieves said, "If it is Rabbi Yochanan's money, we will return half of it."

Resh Lakish said, "If you value your lives, I will take it all back." He then took it all back from them.

Jerusalem Talmud,
Terumot 8:4

48. Alexander the Great once stood at the door of the Garden of Eden and shouted, "Open the gate for me."

They replied, "This is the gate of the Lord, only the righteous are entitled to enter." (*Psalm 118:20*)

He said, "I am a king. I am someone of great importance. Give me something."

They gave him an eyeball.

He weighed all his silver and gold against it, but they did not weigh as much.

He said to the rabbis, "What is the meaning of all this?"

They replied, "This is a human eyeball, which is never satisfied."

He asked, "How do you know this is true?"

They took a little dust and covered it. It was immediately weighed down.

Tamid 32b

49. Rabbi Akiva said to his wife, "If I only had the means, I would buy you a Jerusalem of gold."

Nedarim 50a

50. Rabbi Yudan has said in the name of Rabbi Aibo:

People never leave this world with half their cravings satisfied.

If they have a hundred, they want two hundred, and if they have two hundred, they want four hundred.

Ecclesiastes Rabba 3:12

51. Rabbi Natan bar Abba said in the name of Rav, "The wealthy of Babylonia deserve to go to Hell!

"See, for example, when Shabbetai bar Maraynus came to Babylonia—he looked for help in setting up a business, but they did not help. And even when he asked for help for food, they did not give him any."

Betzah 32b

52. Rabbi Yehuda used to say:

Ten strong things were created in the world—
A mountain is strong, but iron cuts through it.
Iron is strong, but fire causes it to bubble.
Fire is strong, but water extinguishes it.
Water is strong, but clouds contain it.
Clouds are strong, but the wind (ruach) scatters them.
Breath (ruach) is strong, but the body holds it in.
The body is strong, but fear breaks it.
Fear is strong, but wine dissipates its effects.
Wine is strong, but sleep overcomes its power.
Death is harder than all of them.
But Tzedakah saves from death, as it is written,
"And Tzedakah saves from death." (*Proverbs 10:2*)

Bava Batra 10a

53. It was taught in the name of Rabbi Yehoshua:

The poor person [standing at the door] does more for the householder than the householder does for the poor person.

Leviticus Rabba 34:8

54. Rabbi Abba bar Acha said:

It is impossible to understand the nature of this people—
when they are asked to contribute to the Golden Calf,
they give,
and when they are asked to contribute to the building of
the Tabernacle,
they give.

Shekalim 1:1

THE ANGEL

55. While the fetus is still in the womb, it is taught the entire Torah. As it emerges into the air of this world, an angel comes and slaps it on the mouth, making it forget all the Torah it had learned. It does not leave the womb until it is made to take an oath. And what is this oath?

"Be righteous and do not be wicked.

And even if the whole world calls you righteous, do not consider yourself to be what they say.

Know that the Holy One, blessed be He, is pure, and His servants are pure, and the soul which He has given to you is pure. If you preserve its purity—fine. If not, it will be taken away from you."

Then the Holy One, blessed be He, summons the angel who is in charge of souls and says, "Bring me So-and-So's soul." The soul immediately comes before the Holy One, blessed be He, and bows before Him.

The Holy One, blessed be he, says to it, "Enter this drop." The soul then says, "Master of the World, since I was created, this world has been good to me. If it is all right with You, please do not put me into this stinking drop, because I am holy and pure."

The Holy One, blessed be He, says to the soul, "The world which you will enter is better than this world, and, besides, when I created you, I only created you for this drop."

The Holy One, blessed be He, then forces the soul into the drop, and the angel returns the drop, with the soul, into the mother's womb. He also stations two angels there to prevent miscarriages.

A candle sits on its head, and by its light the developing fetus sees from one end of the world to the other.

In the morning, the angel takes it on a tour of the Garden of Eden, showing it the Righteous sitting in great majesty.

The angel says, "Do you know whose soul that one is?"

"No," he replies.

The angel says, "The one you see there treated with such honor and majesty was created just like you in the mother's womb. And this one, and that one, too. And they kept God's way carefully. If you do as they did, then, after your death, as after theirs, you will be privileged to enjoy

20

all this grandeur and this honor—just as you see it now. But if you do not act that way, you will find yourself in another place. . . . which I will show you.

In the evening, he takes it to Gehinnom and shows it wicked people being beaten with fiery clubs by angels of destruction. They are screaming, "Oy V'avoi!" No mercy is shown to them.

The angel says, "My child, do you know who these people are who are being burned?"

And he answers, "No, I do not."

The angel responds, "Know that these, too, were created from a stinking drop in the mother's womb. They entered the world, but did not keep the ways of the Holy One, blessed be He. That is why they have been reduced to such degradation."

The angel takes him around to every place where he will ever be, and to his future home, and to where he will be buried, and then takes him back to the womb.

Then the Holy One, blessed be He, sets up double doors and a cross-bar to the womb and says, "For now, you may go only this far—no farther."

When it is time for the fetus to be born, the same angel comes and says, "Go! Your time to be born has arrived."

But the fetus says, "But have I not already told the Holy One, blessed be He, "I am satisfied in the world where I am'?"

The angel replies, "The world I am taking you into is beautiful. Furthermore, whether you wanted it or not, you were created, and, against your will, you will be born."

At the moment of birth, the infant weeps.

Why does he weep?

He weeps for that world he is leaving.

And he weeps because, at that moment, they show him seven worlds: In the first world, he is like a king—everyone looks after him and runs to see him, and hugs and kisses him. . . . until he is a year old.

In the second world, he is like a pig—always in the garbage, and a mess to clean. . . . until he is two.

In the third world, he is like a baby goat dancing in the meadow—always dancing everywhere. . . . until he is five.

In the fourth world, he is like a horse, proudly prancing down the road—this is what a child is like, full of pride and sure of the powers of youth. . . . until he is eighteen.

In the fifth world, he is like a mule with a saddle on his back—with a wife and sons and daughters, running around looking for a livelihood to support the members of his household.

In the sixth world, he is like a dog, still grabbing for a livelihood wherever he can, sometimes being pushy, taking and stealing from one and then others without shame.

In the seventh world, he does not resemble anything, having become different from all other things—even his family curses him and wishes he were dead, and even infants make fun of him.

Finally, when his time comes to die, the angel comes to him and says, "Do you recognize me?"

And he answers, "Yes. but why have you come to me today?"

The angel answers, "To take you away from this world."

He weeps deeply—a weeping that can be heard around the world, though no human being can hear it—and he says to the angel, "Have you not already taken me from two worlds and put me in this one?"

And the angel replies, "But have I not already told you, 'Against your will you were created, and were born, and will die, and will—against your will—give an accounting to the King of Kings of Kings, the Holy One Blessed be He'?"

Niddah 30b,
Seder Yetzirat HaVelad,
Bet Hamidrash I:153–155

HEAVEN AND HELL

56. The sun is red at sunrise because it passes by the roses of the Garden of Eden, and at sunset because it passes by the gate of Hell.

Bava Batra 84a

57. In Elijah's academy it was taught:

Hell is above the sky. Some say it is behind the Mountains of Darkness.

Tamid 32b

58. Rabbi Yirmiah ben Elazar said:

There are three doors to Hell—one in the desert, one in the sea, and one in Jerusalem.

Eruvin 19a

59. A certain caravan merchant once said to Rabbah bar bar Channah, "Come, I will show you the place where heaven and earth touch so closely it appears that they are kissing."

Bava Batra 74a

PRAYING

60. The Holy One, blessed be He, said to the Jews:

I have said to you—
When you pray, pray in the synagogue in your city.
If you cannot pray in the synagogue, pray in your field.
If you cannot pray in your field, pray in your house.
And if you cannot pray in your house, pray on your bed.
And if you cannot pray on your bed, reflect in your heart.

Midrash on Psalms 4:9

61. Rabbi Chiyya bar Abba said in the name of Rabbi Yochanan:

One should only pray in a house where there are windows.

Berachot 34b

62. One who is praying should keep his eyes turned down and his heart turned up.

Yevamot 105b

TORAH AND LIFE

63. What is an example of a foolish religious person?

When a woman is drowning in the river, and he says, "It is not proper for me to look at her . . . so I cannot save her."

Sotah 21b

64. What is an example of a foolish religious person?

One who sees a child bobbing up and down in the river and says, "Once I get my Tfillin off, I will save him. . . ."—by the time he removes his Tfillin, the child will have drowned.

Jersualem Talmud,
Sotah 3:4

65. Rabbi Tarfon said,

"Akiva, whoever separates himself from you—it is as though he disconnects himself from Life itself."

Kiddushin 66b

66. Rabbi Tarfon said,

"Akiva, whoever separates himself from you—it is as though he disconnects himself from his own life."

Zevachim 13a

67. Rabbi Yehuda said:

One who would wish to become a saintly person should live the words of Nezikin [The Talmudic material on damages and interpersonal relations.]

Rava said:

The words of Avot [the Talmudic selection called, "Sayings of the Fathers."]

And some say [he said]:

The words of Brachot [the Talmudic material concerning blessings.]

Bava Kamma 30a

APHORISMS
and other Brief Insights

68. In Rabbi Shayla's academy it was taught:

Whoever avoids evil is considered by others to be a fool.

Sanhedrin 97a

69. The greater the person, the greater the inclination to do wrong.

Sukkah 52a

70. Honor your doctor before you need him.

Jerusalem Talmud,
Ta'anit 3:6

71. Only a portion of another's praise may be offered in his presence, though all of it may be stated in his absence.

Eruvin 18b

72. At times, adding on detracts.

Sanhedrin 29a

73. A person should use his face, hands, and feet only to honor his Creator.

Tosefta Brachot 4:1

74. Eat quickly, drink quickly, for the world we leave is like a wedding feast.

Eruvin 54a

75. Our Rabbis have taught:

It is forbidden to enjoy anything in this world without a Bracha.

Berachot 35a

76. Tongs are made with other tongs. Who, then, made the first tongs?

Pesachim 54a

77. Rabbah bar Bar Channah said in Rabbi Yochanan's name in the name of Rabbi Yehuda bar Ila'i:

Eat onions and live in your own house, and do not eat geese and fowl so that your heart pursues you. Eat less, but spend more on your home.

Pesachim 114a

78. If you spit into the air, it will fall on your face.

Ecclesiastes Rabba 7:21

79. Sixty runners may run after you, but they will not catch up with you if you have eaten an early breakfast.

Though a duck walks low to the ground, its eyes sweep great distances.

A person's tooth feels sixty toothaches when he hears another eating but he himself does not eat.

Don't throw clods of dirt into a well from which you have drunk.

Bava Kamma 92b

80. There are many old camels bearing the hides of young camels on their backs.

Sanhedrin 52a

81. Even among thorns a willow is still called a willow.

Sanhedrin 44a

82. When our love was strong, we could have slept on the blade of a sword. Now that our love is no longer strong, a bed sixty cubits wide is not large enough for us.

Sanhedrin 7a

83. A folk saying goes:

She whores for apples, then gives them to the sick.

Leviticus Rabba 3:1

A MISCELLANY

84. Rabbi Abbahu was sitting and teaching in one of the synagogues in Caesarea. He noticed a man carrying a stick who was about to hit someone. Behind that man he saw a demon carrying an iron club. Rabbi Abbahu immediately got up and appealed to the man, saying, "Do you want to kill this man?"

The man replied, "With a stick like this, can anyone kill anyone else?"

Rabbi Abbahu answered, "There is a demon standing behind you with an iron club in his hands. If you hit the man with your stick, he will hit him from the other side with his club, and the man will die."

Lamentations Rabba 1:30

85. Rabbi Yehoshua said:

Always consider others as if they were thieves, but honor them as if they were as great as Rabban Gamliel.

Derech Eretz Rabba 5

86. Rava bar Mechasia said in the name of Chama bar Goria who said in the name of Rav:

One should never show favoritism among one's children, for because of two coins' worth of fine wool that Jacob gave to Joseph beyond what he gave to the other sons—the brothers became jealous, and one thing led to another until our ancestors became slaves in Egypt.

Shabbat 10b

87. Rabbi Yossi bar Chanina said:

During the second plague, the croaking was worse than the frogs themselves.

Pesikta deRav Kahana 7:11

88. "And when the Lord has brought you into the land of the Canaanites, as He swore to you and your fathers, and has given it to you. . . ." (*Exodus 13:11*)

The Land should not be thought of as an inheritance from your ancestors, but rather as if it were given to *you* this very day.

Mechilta, Massechta d'Pischa 18
Lauterbach I:159

89. Do not be troubled with tomorrow's woes because you do not know what the day will bring forth. It may be that tomorrow will come, and you will be no more and you will have troubled yourself about a world which is not yours. (Ben Sira)

Yevamot 63b

90. Rav Chizkiya or Rav Cohen said in the name of Rav:

In the Future, everyone will have to give an accounting for everything his eyes saw, but of which he did not eat. Rabbi Le'azar paid particular attention to this statement, setting aside money so that he could eat every kind of food at least once a year.

Jerusalem Talmud,
Kiddushin 4, end

91. Rabbah said:

When the Rabbis in Pumpeditha would take leave of each other, they would recite the following—

"May He Who gives life to the living give you a long, good, and stable life."

Yoma 71a

92. A person should not be awake among those who are asleep,
nor asleep among those who are awake,
nor weeping among those who are laughing,
nor laughing among those who are weeping,
nor sitting among those who are standing,
nor standing among those who are sitting,
nor reading the Written Torah among those studying the Oral Torah,
nor reading the Oral Torah among those studying the Written Torah.

Derech Eretz Zuta 5

93. Rabbi Ila'i said in the name of Rabbi Elazar the son of Rabbi Shimon:

Just as it is a Mitzvah to say something which will be listened to, so, too,
is it a Mitzvah not to say something which will not be listened to.

Yevamot 65b

94. Rabbi Chiyya bar Abba became ill.
Rabbi Yochanan went to visit him.
He said, "Do you appreciate your suffering?"
He replied, "Neither the suffering nor any reward I might receive
for the suffering."
Rabbi Yochanan said, "Give me your hand."
He gave him his hand and Rabbi Yochanan raised him from his sickbed.

Berachot 5b

95. One who would wish to sense the delicate beauty of Rabbi Yochanan
should take a silver goblet—just at the moment the silversmith has
finished polishing it—fill it with the seeds of a red pomegranate, circle
its brim with a crown of red roses, and set it between the sunlight and
the shade. That radiance resembles the beauty of Rabbi Yochanan.

Bava Metzia 84a

96. Rabbi Shimon bar Yochai said:

Had I stood at Mount Sinai at the moment the Torah was being given, I would have asked the Merciful God to create two mouths for people—one for Torah and the other for day-to-day needs.

Later on he said:

I see now that the world struggles so much to survive when people have only one mouth—because of their outrageous slander. How much worse it would be if they had two mouths!

Jerusalem Talmud,
Shabbat 1:2

97. Rav Chanan bar Rav said:

Everyone knows why a bride enters the Chuppah, but, nevertheless, anyone who speaks obscenely of the event—even if he were entitled by Heaven to seventy good years—all that good will be turned into misfortune.

Ketubot 8b

98. Rabbi Pinchas said:

It once happened that two prostitutes from Ashkelon were arguing with each other. In the course of the argument one of them said to the other, "You should not go out on the streets because you have a Jewish face!"

A few days later, after they had settled their differences, the second prostitute said, "I forgive you for everything you said except for your snide remark that I have a Jewish face." This is the meaning of the verse, "See, O God, how despicable I have become." (Lamentations 1:11)

Lamentations Rabba 1:41

99. We are taught:

[The High Priest] would recite a brief prayer in the outer enclosure of the Temple.

What would he say?

Rabin bar Ada and Rava bar Ada said in the name of Rav Yehuda, "May it be Your will, O Lord, our God, that if this year will be a hot one, let it also be rainy and filled with dew, and do not listen to the prayers of travellers."

Ta'anit 24b

100. Whoever sees a rainbow in the clouds should fall on his face in awe, as the verse says, "The appearance of the brilliance was like the appearance of a rainbow in the clouds on a rainy day—that was the likeness of God's Glory that I saw, and I fell on my face [and heard a voice speaking.]" (Ezekiel 1:28)

Berachot 59a

101. When Rav Yosef would hear the footsteps of his mother, he would say, "I shall arise before God's approaching Presence."

Kiddushin 31b

102. Rabbi Yochanan said in the name of Rabbi Shimon ben Yehotzadak:

A community leader may not be appointed unless he has a basket of unclean reptiles hanging over his back, so that if he becomes arrogant, he can be told, "Just turn around!"

Yoma 22b

103. When a person goes to the bathroom, he says [to the two angels that are always with him],

"Guard me, guard me. Help me, help me. Be reliable, be reliable. Wait for me, wait for me, until I go in and come out—for this is what human beings have to do."

Berachot 60

104. Rabbi Nathan said:

Jonah went down to the sea in order to drown himself.

Mechilta, Massechta d'Pischa
Lauterbach I:10

105. A wise person [Talmid Chacham] is not permitted to live in a city that does not have the following ten things:

1. A court empowered to and capable of punishing the guilty
2. A communal Tzedakah fund, monies for which are collected by two people and distributed by three
3. A synagogue
4. A bath house
5. Sufficient bathroom facilities
6. A doctor
7. A blood-letter
8. A scribe
9. A butcher
10. A Torah teacher for children

It was stated in Rabbi Akiva's name:

Also, a variety of fruits, because a variety of fruits brightens the eyes.

Sanhedrin 17b

CHILDREN

106. Rabbi Abbahu said, "Though a baby emerges from its mother's womb covered with mucus and blood, everyone hugs and kisses it."

Leviticus Rabba 14:4

107. We are taught:

After a child would be born on Shabbat, the wealthy would store the placenta in oil, and the poor would store it in straw and sand. After Shabbat, both would bury it in the earth, as a guarantee to the earth.

Jerusalem Talmud,
Shabbat 18:3

108. Rabbi Yochanan said:

Since the time of the destruction of the Temple, prophecy has been taken away from the prophets and given over to fools and infants.

Bava Batra 12b

109. Rabbi Yochanan said in the name of Rabbi Yossi ben Katzarta:

There are six kinds of tears—
    three are beneficial, and three are harmful.
Tears caused by smoke, weeping from grief, and straining in the
    bathroom are harmful.
Tears caused by certain chemicals, laughter, and certain plants [such as
    onions and mustard] are beneficial.
Tears from laughter are the best of all;
    tears from the death of a child are the worst of all.

Shabbat 151b–152a
Lamentations Rabba 2:19

OLD AGE

110. Rabbi Yossi ben Kisma says:

    Two are better than three.
    Woe for the one that leaves us and does not return.
    What is that?

    Rav Chisda said: our youth.
    When Rav Dimi came from Israel, he said:
    Youth is a crown of roses.
    Old age is a crown of thorns.

    Shabbat 152a

111. When we were young, we were told to act like adults.
    Now that we are old, we are treated like infants.

    Bava Kamma 92b

112. It was said of Rabbi Chanina that at the age of eighty he could still stand on one foot and remove and replace the shoe on his other foot.

    Rabbi Chanina said, "The warm baths and oil with which my mother rubbed me have served me well in my old age."

    Chullin 24b

113. One who is delivering a divorce document for someone who is old—even 100 years old—still delivers it with the assumption that the man is alive. . . . since, if he has lived so long, he is bound to continue living longer.

    Gittin 28a

114. "A man went from the land of the Hittites and built a city. He called it Luz, and that is its name to this very day." (Judges 1:26) We are taught. . . . :

    The Angel of Death does not have permission to go there. When the old no longer wish to go on living, they go outside the city walls and die.

    Sotah 46b

MARRIAGE AND DIVORCE

115. Rabbi Yossi HaGlili's wife caused him great anguish.

Rabbi Elazar ben Azariah went to visit him and said, "Divorce her, because she does not treat you with dignity."

He said to him, "But I cannot afford to pay the settlement."

He said, "I will pay it for you. Just divorce her."

Rabbi Elazar ben Azariah paid the settlement for him, and he divorced his wife.

She eventually married one of the town guards who later became poor and blind. She would lead him around town begging for money.

Once, she took him through the entire town without finding any money.

He said to her, "Are there any other neighborhoods where we have not been?"

She said, "There is one neighborhood left, but I do not have the strength to go there."

He began to beat her, just as Rabbi Yossi HaGlili was passing by.

He heard her shouts and saw the way she was being humiliated.

Because of this, he took them in and gave them accomodations in one of his houses and provided for them for the rest of their lives.

Jerusalem Talmud,
Ketubot 11:3

116. Rabbi Iddi said:

Once upon a time a certain woman in Tzidon was married to a certain man, but they had no children. They came to Rabbi Shimon bar Yochai and requested a divorce.

He said, "By your lives, just as you were married in the midst of a great feast, so, too, shall you begin your separation with a great feast."

They followed his instructions and made a feast. During the meal the woman gave the man too much to drink. As he began to get sober he said, "My beloved, survey all the precious things in this house, take that which is most dear to you, and return to your father's house."

What did she do?

After he fell asleep, she told her servants, "Carry him on his bed to my father's house."

In the middle of the night, he awoke, and, as he became more sober, he asked, "My beloved, where am I?"

She said, "In my father's house."

He asked, "What am I doing in your father's house?"

She said, "Did you not say to me this evening, 'Choose whatever is most precious to you and take it with you to your father's house'? There is nothing more precious to me in the entire world than you."

They then went back to Rabbi Shimon bar Yochai, who prayed for them, and they had children.

Song of Songs Rabba 1:4

OUR SOULS

117. Rabbi Alexandri said:

When you leave new things in a human being's possession for safe-keeping, though they might have been new when they were delivered, they are often returned used and worn out.

The Holy One, blessed be He, though, works differently:

Though we leave things in His hand all worn out and tattered,
He returns them to us new.

This is obvious to us—

a worker will work all day and come home exhausted;
when he is asleep, though, he is at peace, since his soul is in the hands of the Holy One, blessed be He.

Indeed, at dawn, the soul returns, a new creation to the worker's body, as the verse indicates, "[Souls] are new every morning; great is Your reliability." (Lamentations 3:23)

Midrash on Psalms 25:2

118. "To You, O Lord, I lift my soul." (Psalm 25:1)

This verse may be understood by referring to the words, "Into Your hand I entrust my spirit." (Psalm 31:6)

This is the way of the world:

If one leaves some items for another to watch, sometimes the latter mixes them up with someone else's possessions for some objects are not easily distinguishable from others. But the Holy One, blessed be He, does not work that way, but, rather, "God is a God of truth." (Psalm 31:6)

Has anyone ever awakened in the morning and looked for his soul and not found it? Or has anyone ever found his soul in another's possession or another's in his possession? "You redeem me, O Lord, reliable God." (Psalm 31:6)

Midrash on Psalms 25:2

THE CREATOR

119. "There is no rock (*Tzur*) like our God." (I Samuel 2:2)

There is no artist (*Tzayyar*) like our God:

A human being can cut a form on a wall but cannot make breath, a soul, organs or intestines for it. But the Holy One, blessed be He, fashions forms within forms and gives them breath, a soul, and all the organs needed for life.

Megillah 14a

120. "There is no rock (*Tzur*) like our God." (I Samuel 2:2)

There is no artist (*Tzayyar*) like our God.

This is the way of human beings:

A person goes to a sculptor and says, "Make a statue of my father for me."

The sculptor says, "Let your father come to pose for me, or bring me some image of him."

But the One Who spoke and brought the world into being is different:

He gives a person a child formed from a drop of fluid, and it resembles the parent.

Mechilta Shirata 8
Lauterbach II:65

121. God and human beings do not act the same:

The creations of human beings outlive them, but the Holy One, blessed be He, outlives His creations.

Megillah 14a

122. "Awesome in splendor, working wonders!" (Exodus 15:11)
Human beings function in the following manner:

A worker works for his landowner, plowing, sowing, weeding, and hoeing for him, and his employer gives him money, and he goes his way.

It is different, however, with the One Who spoke and created the world thereby:

If a person desires children, He can give them to him; if he desires wisdom, He can give it to him; possessions, He can give them to him.

Mechilta, Shirata 8
Lauterbach II:63–64

123. You have confused the creation with its creator.

Deuteronomy Rabba 1:3

SHABBAT

124. Rabbi Shimon ben Lakish said:

Before Shabbat begins, the Holy One, blessed be He, gives every person an additional soul, and when Shabbat is over, it is taken back from him.

Betzah 16a

125. Your Shabbat clothes should not be the same as your weekday clothes.

Shabbat 113a

126. We are permitted to comfort mourners on Shabbat. So, too, are we allowed to visit the sick on Shabbat.

Shulchan Aruch,
Orach Chaim 287:1

127. We are permitted to weep on Shabbat if weeping is a pleasure because it releases pain in the heart.

Isserles, Shulchan Aruch,
Orach Chaim 288:2

128. The Jews have been assured that Elijah will not come on the eve of Shabbat nor on the eve of holidays.

Eruvin 43b

THE TROUBLES OF THE JEWS

129. Our teachers have said:

Once, while Moses, our Teacher, was tending Yitro's sheep, one of the sheep ran away. Moses ran after it until it reached a small, shaded place. There the lamb came across a pool of water and began to drink. As Moses approached the lamb, he said, "I did not know you ran away because you were thirsty. You are so exhausted!" He then put the lamb on his shoulders and carried him back.

The Holy One, blessed be He, said, "Since you tend the sheep of human beings with such overwhelming love—by your life, I swear you shall be the shepherd of My sheep, Israel."

Exodus Rabba 2:2

130. [*While Moses was tending the flocks of his father-in-law, Yitro, in Midian, God took note of Moses's concern for the anguish of the Children of Israel in Egypt.*]

The Holy One, blessed be He, said, "Since Moses is disheartened and troubled by the woes of Israel in Egypt, he is worthy to be their shepherd."

Exodus Rabba 2:11

131. When the Jews are in trouble, a person should not say, "I will go to my home, eat, drink, and be at peace with myself."

Ta'anit 11a

132. When the Jews are in trouble, and one individual distances himself from them, the two angels who always accompany everybody come and put their hands on that person's head and say, "This person who separated himself from the people shall not be entitled to witness the consolation of the people."

Ta'anit 11a

THE EXODUS

133. Only one out of five of the Children of Israel left Egypt.
Some say one out of fifty.
And some say only one out of five hundred.

Rabbi Nehorai says:
Not even one out of five hundred.

Mechilta, Massechta dePischa 12
Lauterback I:95

134. When the Israelites fled from Egypt, they were outnumbered three to one.
Some say thirty to one.
And some say three hundred to one.

Mechilta, Beshallach 2
Lauterback I:202

135. "They shall take some of the blood and put it on the two doorposts and on the lintel." (Exodus 12:7)

On the inside, as it says, "And I shall see the blood" (12:13). . . . the blood that I [the Lord] will see, and not the blood others will see.

These are the words of Rabbi Yishmael.

Rabbi Yonatan says:

On the inside, as it says, "And the blood shall be a sign for you."

Rabbi Yitzchak says:

It certainly means on the outside, so that the Egyptians would see it and be terrified.

Mechilta, Massechta dePischa 6
Lauterback I:44

136. Once the Angel of Destruction is allowed to begin his work, he does not differentiate between the Righteous and the Wicked.

Mechilta, Massechta dePischa 11
Lauterbach I:85

137. At the Red Sea the Israelites divided into four factions:
One group said, "Let us throw ourselves into the sea."
Another said, "Let us go back to Egypt."
Another said, "Let us fight them."
And the fourth said, "Let us make a lot of noise [to scare them.]"

Mechilta, BeShallach 3
Lauterbach I:214

138. At the Red Sea the Egyptians divided into three factions:

One said, "Let us take their money and take back our money, but let us not kill them."

Another said, "Let us kill them but not take their money."

And the third said, "Let us kill them and take their money."

Mechilta Shirata 7
Lauterbach II:57

139. The Israelites saw the Egyptians dying on the seashore, but they did not see them dead.

Mechilta BeShallach 7
Lauterbach I:250

140. "The Lord said to Moses, 'Why do you cry out to me?'" (Exodus 14:15)

Rabbi Eliezer says:

The Holy One, blessed be He, said to Moses,

"Moses, my children are in mortal danger—the sea is on one side and the enemy is pursuing from the other—and you stand here and take time to say lengthy prayers? Why do you cry out to me?"

As Rabbi Eliezer used to say:

There are appropriate times for short prayers and appropriate times for long prayers.

Mechilta BeShallach 4
Lauterbach I:216

141. When the tribes stood at the shore of the Red Sea, they began to argue, each saying, "I will go in first!"

While they were arguing, the tribe of Benjamin jumped in first.

The leaders of the tribe of Judah then began to throw stones at them.

Mechilta BeShallach 6
Lauterbach I:232

142. Rabbi Yehuda ben Betayra says:

"But they would not listen to Moses, their spirits crushed." (Exodus 6:9)

Is it possible that someone would hear good news and not be overjoyed?—

"A son has been born to you. . . ."—and he should not be overjoyed?

"Your master is setting you free. . . ."—and he should not be overjoyed?

So why, then, should the Torah say, "They would not listen to Moses"? Because it was difficult for them to tear themselves away from their idols.

Mechilta, Massechta dePischa 5
Lauterbach I:38

143. Why did God speak to Moses outside of the city?

Because the city was filled with abominations and idols.

Mechilta, Massechta dePischa 1
Lauterbach I:4

REVOLT

144. During the three and a half years that Hadrian besieged Bethar during the Bar Kochba revolt, Rabbi Elazar of Modi'in dressed in sackcloth and sat in ashes, praying every day, "Master of all worlds, do not sit in judgment today! Do not sit in judgment today!"

Jerusalem Talmud,
Ta'anit 4:4

145. Rabbi Tzadok fasted for forty years so that Jerusalem might not be destroyed.

Gittin 56a

146. Rabbi Yehuda and Rabbi Yossi and Rabbi Shimon were sitting together, along with Rabbi Yehuda ben Gerim.

Rabbi Yehuda began the conversation, "What exquisite things Rome accomplishes! They have set up marketplaces, bridges, and bath houses!"

Rabbi Yossi remained silent.

Rabbi Shimon Bar Yochai replied,
"Whatever they do is only for selfish reasons.

They set up markets only to make a place for their whores.
They build bath houses only to pamper themselves.
They set up bridges only to collect tolls."

Shabbat 33b

147. When Rabbi Akiva would see Bar Kochba, he would say, "This is the King Messiah."

Rabbi Yochanan ben Torata said to him,

"Akiva—grass will grow from your cheeks before the Son of David will come."

Jerusalem Talmud,
Ta'anit 4:4

148. The Romans continued to slaughter the Jews until their horses sank to their snouts in blood. The blood gushed to such a degree that huge boulders rolled in the flow, and the blood washed all the way to the sea forty Roman miles away.

It was said that they found the brains of three hundred children splattered on one rock.

Jerusalem Talmud,
Ta'anit 4:4

149. For seven years after the Bar Kochba revolt, the Romans did not need fertilizer for their vineyards—because of all the Jewish blood that was spilled.

Gittin 57a

150. The Emperor Hadrian had a vineyard eighteen Roman miles square that he encircled with bodies from Bethar.

He would not allow them to be buried, until a new emperor rose to power and allowed them to be buried.

Lamentations Rabba 2:5

DEATH AND MOURNING

151. We are not permitted to leave a person who is near death, so that he should not have to die alone. And it is a Mitzvah to stand by a person at the moment of death.

Shulchan Aruch,
Yoreh De'ah 339:4

152. If we are in the presence of someone who is dying, we are required to tear our garment at the moment of death.

What is this like?

It is like a Sefer Torah that has been burned, an occasion for which we are also required to tear our garment.

Mo'ed Katan 25a

153. We may desecrate the Sabbath for a day-old infant, if he is still alive, but if he has already died, we may not do so even for someone as great as David, King of Israel.

Shabbat 151b

154. Rava said to Rav Nachman, "Show yourself to me [in a dream after you die]."

He showed himself to Rava.

Rava asked him, "Was death painful?"

Rav Nachman replied, "It was as painless as lifting a hair from a cup of milk. But were the Holy One, blessed be He, to say to me, 'You may return to that world where you were before,' I would not wish to do it. The fear of death is too great."

Mo'ed Katan 28a

155. Rav Sheshet noticed the Angel of Death in the marketplace. He said, "Do you want to take me here in the marketplace like an animal? Come home with me!"

Mo'ed Katan 28a

156. Rabbi Levi said:

"And David the King" is mentioned nearly fifty-two times. However, when he was dying, what is recorded is only this—"When David's life was drawing to a close. . . ."—indicating that no one wields power on the day of death.

I Kings 2:1
Ecclesiastes Rabba 8:11

157. Two good things are near to you and far from you, far from you and near to you:

Repentance is near to you and far from you, far from you and near to you.

Death is near to you and far from you, far from you and near to you.

Ecclesiastes Rabba 8:17

158. The rabbis said to Rav Hamnuna Zuti at the wedding of Mar the son of Ravina, "Please sing for us!"

He said, "Woe for us that we are to die! Woe for us that we are to die!"

They said to him, "What is our chorus?"

He said, "Where is the Torah and the Mitzvah that will protect us?"

Berachot 31a

159. Our rabbis have taught:

God decided to create three things, and even had He not decided to do so, it would have been only right for Him to consider them—

That corpses should decompose,
That the dead should be forgotten from the heart,
And that produce should rot with the passage of time.

Pesachim 54b

160. It is improper for someone to walk in a cemetery with his Tfillin on or carrying a Sefer Torah and reading from it. If he does so, he violates the negative Mitzvah of, "One who disparages the unfortunate, blasphemes his Creator." (Proverbs 17:5)

Berachot 18a

161. At the resurrection of the dead, the handicapped will arise still handicapped, and then they will be cured.

Sanhedrin 91b

162. A certain non-Jew once asked Rabbi Yehoshua ben Korcha, "Do you not claim that the Holy One, blessed be He, sees into the future?"

"Yes, certainly," the rabbi replied.

The man said, "But it is written, 'And the Lord regretted that He had made people on earth, and His heart was saddened'"? (Genesis 6:6)

The rabbi asked, "Have you ever had a son?"

He replied, "Yes."

"And what did you do when he was born?"

He answered, "I was overjoyed and made everyone else joyous."

The rabbi asked, "And did you not know that some day the child would die?"

He answered, "At the time when one should be joyous—be joyous. And when it is time to mourn—mourn."

The rabbi said, "So, too, with the Holy One, blessed be He."

Genesis Rabba 27:7

163. Rabbi Yochanan said:

A person's feet are responsible for him. They will lead him to the place where he is wanted.

Sukkah 53a

164. Concerning the Future it is said,
"He will destroy death forever.
My Lord God will wipe away the tears from all faces." (Isaiah 25:8)

Mishna Mo'ed Katan 3:9

165. Our rabbis have taught:

A funeral procession must make way for a wedding procession.

Ketubot 17a

166. At first, burying the dead was more difficult for the relatives than the death itself—because of the enormous expense. Relatives even abandoned the bodies and ran away. Finally, Rabban Gamliel adopted a simple style, and the people carried him to his grave in linen garments. Subsequently everyone followed his example and carried out the dead in similar fashion—even in rough cloth worth only a Zuz.

Ketubot 8b

167. Rabbi Yannai said to his children:

My children, do not bury me either in white or black garments—white, because I may not be privileged, and I would be like a bridegroom among mourners,

and black, because I may be privileged, and I would be like a mourner among bridegrooms.

Rather bury me in the red garments that are imported from the sea provinces.

Shabbat 114a

168. It has been the custom in some places for a number of people to be buried in coffins which were made from the tables upon which they studied, or upon which they fed the poor, or upon which they worked faithfully at their trade.

Kav HaYashar, Chapter 46
(Kol Bo Al Avaylut, p. 182)

169. We need not make monuments for the righteous—their words serve as their memorial.

Shekalim 2:5

170. Comforters in a Shiva-house should not begin speaking until the mourner begins the conversation. The mourner sits in a central place, and once the mourner shakes his head to indicate that the comforters should leave, the comforters are no longer permitted to sit with him. (Neither a mourner nor a sick person is required to stand, even in the presence of the Nasi [the leader of the Jewish community].)

Shulchan Aruch,
Yoreh De'ah 376:1

171. Do not attempt to comfort a person whose dead relative still lies before him.

Pirke Avot 4:23

172. If someone who is not well sustains a loss, he should not be informed of it, to prevent him from becoming frantic.

Mo'ed Katan 26b

173. Simcha is forbidden to a mourner. Therefore, he should not pick up an infant, so that he will not begin to laugh.

Mo'ed Katan 26b

174. A person should not mourn too much for the deceased, and anyone who mourns too much, weeps [or: will weep] for someone else.

Rather, there should be three days for tears, seven days for lamenting, and thirty days to refrain from cutting the hair and wearing pressed clothes.

Shulchan Aruch,
Yoreh De'ah 394:1

175. Anyone who weeps and mourns for a worthy person shall have his sins forgiven because of the honor he has shown for that person.

Mo'ed Katan 25a

Danny Siegel is a free-lance author, poet, and lecturer living in Rockville, Maryland. He is the author of five books of poetry: *Nine Entered Paradise Alive, Between Dust and Dance, And God Braided Eve's hair, Soulstoned,* and an anthology of selected writings: *Unlocked Doors,* two books of essays: *Gym Shoes and Irises: Personalized Tzedakah,* and *Angels,* and this anthology of Midrash and Talmud, *Where Heaven and Earth Touch.* He is also co-author with Allan Gould of Toronto of a book of humor, *The Unorthodox Book of Jewish Records and Lists.*

Siegel is a popular lecturer at synagogues, Jewish community centers, conventions, and retreats, where he teaches Tzedakah and Jewish values and recites from his works. His books and talks have received considerable acclaim throughout the entire North American Jewish community.